Complementary

for

ent

Commissioning Editor: Claire Wilson
Project Development Manager: Kerry McGechie
Project Manager: Jess Thompson
Design Direction: George Ajayi
Illustration Manager: Merlyn Harvey
Illustrator: David Gardner

Complementary Therapies for Pain Management

An Evidence-Based Approach

Editors

Edzard Ernst MD PhD FRCP FRCPEd
Professor of Complementary Medicine, Peninsula Medical School, Universities of Exeter and Plymouth, Exeter, UK

Max H Pittler MD PhD
Senior Research Fellow in Complementary Medicine, Peninsula Medical School, Universities of Exeter and Plymouth, Exeter, UK

Barbara Wider MA
Research Fellow in Complementary Medicine, Peninsula Medical School, Universities of Exeter and Plymouth, Exeter, UK

Assistant Editor

Kate Boddy MA
Academic Assistant in Complementary Medicine, Peninsula Medical School, Universities of Exeter and Plymouth, Exeter, UK

Foreword by

Andrew Moore
Pain Research Unit, The Churchill, Oxford, UK

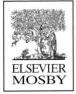

ELSEVIER
MOSBY

EDINBURGH LONDON NEW YORK OXFORD PHILADELPHIA ST LOUIS SYDNEY TORONTO 2007

ELSEVIER
MOSBY

An imprint of Elsevier Limited

First published 2007
Reprinted 2007

ISBN-13: 978-0-7234-3400-9

British Library Cataloguing in Publication Data
A catalogue record for this book is available from the British Library

Library of Congress Cataloging in Publication Data
A catalog record for this book is available from the Library of Congress

Knowledge and best practice in this field are constantly changing. As new research and experience broaden our knowledge, changes in practice, treatment and drug therapy may become necessary or appropriate. Readers are advised to check the most current information provided (i) on procedures featured or (ii) by the manufacturer of each product to be administered, to verify the recommended dose or formula, the method and duration of administration, and contraindications. It is the responsibility of the practitioner, relying on their own experience and knowledge of the patient, to make diagnoses, to determine dosages and the best treatment for each individual patient, and to take all appropriate safety precautions. To the fullest extent of the law, neither the Publisher nor the Editors assume any liability for any injury and/or damage to persons or property arising out of or related to any use of the material contained in this book.

The Publisher

Working together to grow
libraries in developing countries

www.elsevier.com | www.bookaid.org | www.sabre.org

 ELSEVIER   BOOK AID International   Sabre Foundation

your source for books,
journals and multimedia
in the health sciences
www.elsevierhealth.com

The
Publisher's
policy is to use
**paper manufactured
from sustainable forests**

Printed in China

Contents

Contributors

Daniel J Benor MD, ABHM
American wholistic psychiatric psychothera-pist, Editor of *The International Journal of Healing and Caring* – online, Coordinator of the Council for Healing and Founder of the Doctor-Healer Network – UK and North America, USA

Martien Brands MD, PhD, MFHom
Senior Clinical Lecturer in Homeopathy, Division of Primary Care, School of Population, Community & Behavioural Sciences, University of Liverpool, UK

Luis F Buenaver PhD
Postdoctoral Fellow at the Department of Psychiatry & Behavioral Sciences, Johns Hopkins University School of Medicine, Baltimore, MD, USA

Peter H Canter PhD
Research Fellow, Complementary Medicine, Peninsula Medical School, Universities of Exeter and Plymouth, UK (Chapter Meditation)

Robert R Edwards PhD
Assistant Professor at the Department of Psychiatry & Behavioral Sciences, Johns Hopkins University School of Medicine, Baltimore, MD, USA

Peter Heusser MD, MME
Medical doctor, Master of Medical Education and Professor of Anthroposophic Medicine at the Institute of Complementary Medicine KIKOM at the University of Berne, Switzerland, Head of the Lukas Klinik, an oncological hospital specialising in anthropo-sophic medicine in Arlesheim, Switzerland

Anita Holdcroft MB, ChB, MD, FRCA
Reader in Anaesthesia and Honorary Consultant Anaesthetist, Imperial College London, and Chelsea and Westminster Hospital, London, UK

Edward K Hui MD
Clinical Instructor, Division of General Internal Medicine and Health Services Research and Center for East–West Medicine, Department of Medicine, David Geffen School of Medicine, University of California at Los Angeles, USA

Ka-Kit Hui MD, FACP
Wallis Annenberg Chair in Integrative East–West Medicine, Professor of Clinical Medicine and Director, Center for East–West Medicine, Department of Medicine, David Geffen School of Medicine, University of California at Los Angeles, USA

CM Janine Leach DO, ND, PhD
Osteopath and naturopath, Senior Research Fellow in Osteopathy at the University of Brighton, Associate Editor of the *International Journal of Osteopathic Medicine*, Member of the National Council for Osteopathic Research, and President of the British Naturopathic Association

Stephen Morley BSc, MPhil, PhD, FBPsS, CPsychol
Professor of Clinical Psychology, Institute of Health Sciences, University of Leeds, UK

Ram Harsh Singh MD(Hons), PhD, DLitt, FNAIM
Visiting Professor, Wonkwang Digital University, Iksan, Republic of Korea; Professor-Head and Dean, Faculty of Ayurveda, Banaras Hindu University, Varanasi, India

Bernhard Uehleke MD, PhD, Dipl Phys, Dipl Kfm, FFPM
Research coordinator of the Department of Naturopathy, Charité Berlin, Campus Benjamin Franklin, Berlin, Germany

Acknowledgements

We would like to thank all authors who contributed chapters to section 2, *General topics and Alternative concepts of pain*. All other chapters in sections 1, 2, 3, 4, and 5 were jointly written by Edzard Ernst, Max H Pittler and Barbara Wider. Kate Boddy performed the literature searches and compiled section 6.

Foreword

The thing about pain is that there is a lot of it about. Most people (lay and professional) think immediately about cancer pain or acute pain, but the stark fact is that these two areas are dwarfed in scope by the amount of chronic non-malignant pain that occurs in the community. A recent, large, European survey[1] found that almost one in five adults had pain of at least moderate intensity, occurring almost every day, and lasting for 6 months or longer. Of course, chronic pain is a bigger problem for older people, with about half of people of retirement age having some chronic pain problem, most often musculoskeletal.[2]

Moreover, this chronic pain in the community is not well treated. In one community survey,[2] at least half of the patients had either high-intensity pain or were limited in their activities of daily living, and British general practitioners (GPs) when asked about treating chronic pain in the community come up with a similar estimate.[3] A survey of over 3000 patients with osteoarthritis showed that the majority suffered interference in the activities of daily living,[4] which makes it understandable why chronic pain conditions have the most negative impact on quality of life of chronic conditions in the community, including cancer and heart disease.[5]

Clinical trials of analgesic interventions for chronic pain often show limited improvement over placebo. For instance, a recent systematic review of interventions in knee osteoarthritis showed that, on average, interventions produced just over 10 mm more pain relief on a 100-mm visual analogue scale than did placebo,[6] while analysis of recent non-steroidal anti-inflammatory drugs (NSAIDs) versus placebo trials in osteoarthritis showed that only 11% more patients had pain relief greater than 10 mm with NSAIDs.[7]

In these circumstances, it is not surprising that many patients seek additional help for their pain outside formal health-care provision. In the European survey, for instance, 40% of patients used over-the-counter analgesics as well as their usual prescribed medicines.[1] In addition, 60% also used some other form of treatment, namely, in descending order, massage, physical therapy, acupuncture, topical analgesics, heat and exercise. A number of other less conventional therapies were used in small numbers of patients.

One obvious retort is to question how well those additional therapies work, because the patients are spending significant amounts of money for this additional care and should be getting value for their money. In the UK, about 20% of the population uses these therapies, spending over £500 million a year. In the USA 40% of the population regularly use some form of complementary therapy, spending £15–20 billion a year between them. There are now more complementary practitioners than GPs in the UK, and some treatments are even delivered on the National Health Service.

Pain is the major driver for all this, and a book that delivers concise evidence-based information is clearly going to be helpful but there are always going to be difficulties, however good authors are. It is worth thinking briefly about a few of the issues.

- To be trustworthy, trials and reviews need to fulfil criteria of quality (to avoid bias), size (to avoid the random play of chance) and validity (we need sensible answers to sensible questions, not just whatever is available). The biggest problem with complementary therapies is that most trials, and most reviews, are deficient in some or all of these areas, and consequently the potential to mislead is large.

- For many therapy/condition combinations, therefore, it is inevitable that the conclusion will be that we do not know with any certainty whether they work. There is an absence of robust evidence from clinical trials, though clearly many practitioners, and some patients, will testify anecdotally to a therapy's success in particular cases.
- Absence of evidence is a major problem, not just for efficacy but especially for harm. Absence of good data relating to harm, from clinical trials or observational studies, means that there are real dangers from rare but serious adverse events. Here, not only is anecdote unhelpful, it is positively misleading, laced, as it inevitably will be, with bias.

How are these difficulties to be overcome? In the short term, they are not. In the short term, we will have to face up to the lack of evidence of efficacy and even evidence of lack of efficacy.

It seems to me that the arguments about complementary therapies, for pain or any other indication, have become stereotyped. They suffocate thought. Rather than argue endlessly about how poorly complementary therapies do in clinical trials, perhaps we should be asking ourselves why it is that mainline interventions appear in such an unflattering light. Perhaps many of the trial designs lack sensitivity, though in general they do appear to mirror, if faintly, clinical practice. Where quality, validity and size are adequate, then clinical trials and clinical practice give the same results, both for efficacy and for harm.

What we need is some original thought, lateral thinking, something from left field (a baseball term that appears to mean something wildly unrelated to the subject being discussed). Less heat, more light. This book, with its impassioned overview of the evidence, might just help to start that process.

Andrew Moore
Oxford, 2006

REFERENCES

1. Breivik H, Collett B, Ventafridda V, Cohen R, Gallacher D. Survey of chronic pain in Europe: prevalence, impact on daily life, and treatment. Eur J Pain 2006;10:287–333
2. Elliott AM, Smith BH, Penny KI, Smith WC, Chambers WA. The epidemiology of chronic pain in the community. Lancet 1999;354:1248–1252
3. Stannard C, Johnson M. Chronic pain management – can we do better? An interview-based survey in primary care. Curr Med Res Opin 2003;19:703–706
4. Crichton B, Green M. GP and patient perspectives on treatment with non-steroidal anti-inflammatory drugs for the treatment of pain in osteoarthritis. Curr Med Res Opin 2002;18:92–96
5. Sprangers MA, de Regt EB, Andries F, van Agt HM, Bijl RV, de Boer JB, Foets M, Hoeymans N, Jacobs AE, Kempen GI, Miedema HS, Tijhuis MA, de Haes HC. Which chronic conditions are associated with better or poorer quality of life? J Clin Epidemiol 2000;53:895–907
6. Bjordal JM, Klovning A, Ljunggren AE, Slordal L. Short-term efficacy of pharmacotherapeutic interventions in osteoarthritic knee pain: a meta-analysis of randomised placebo-controlled trials. Eur J Pain 2006;11:125–138
7. Lakshminarayanan M, Niculescu L, Andrade L, Moore A, Singh G. Influence of age, gender, race, and body mass index on the efficacy of nonsteroidal anti-inflammatory drugs in osteoarthritis trials. APLAR J Rheumatol 2006;9(Suppl. 1):248

Preface

Most pain clinics today have adopted some form of complementary and alternative medicine (CAM).[1,2] The reasons for this move may well be patient demand[3] enhanced by the continuous promotion of CAM by the media.[4] When we, for instance, extracted from seven lay books on CAM the treatments which were promoted for specific pain syndromes we found that a confusing array of therapies were recommended, with little consensus among authors and even less basis in scientific evidence (Table 0.1).[5]

During recent years, CAM has become increasingly evidence-based. Today Medline holds about 4300 controlled clinical trials and the Cochrane database includes 71 systematic reviews of CAM. Recent analyses have shown that these publications are as good as[6] or better than,[7] in terms of methodological quality, studies of conventional treatments. Reviewing the evidence systematically, we found good or encouraging evidence for a range of CAM therapies in the management of pain (Table 0.2). Thus, there is little reason to ignore this evidence.

To find out how CAM is covered in textbooks on pain, electronic searches for books were conducted in the bibliographic databases Global Books in Print and WorldCat. Additional searches were carried out using Amazon and via leading medical publishers' websites. Our aim was to identify all books with 'pain' or 'pain management' in the title that were published in English between January 2004 and November 2005, and were first editions aimed at the academic or medical professional market. Hard copies of all books thus located were obtained and studied. Specifically we determined whether the book in question contained a

Table 0.1 **Data extracted from seven popular lay books on CAM. Figures depict the total number of different CAM therapies recommended for each of the listed conditions in these books**

Pain syndrome	Number of CAM therapies recommended
Arthritis	131
Back pain	65
Chronic pain	29
Dysmenorrhoea	33
Fibromyalgia	7
Headache	78
Labour pain	10
Menorrhagia	31
Migraine	32
Neuralgia	30
Pain	31
Sciatica	55
Sprains and strains	28

Table 0.2 **Examples of CAM therapies for pain supported by good or encouraging evidence***

Modality	Indication
Acupuncture	Various pain syndromes
Chiropractic	Back pain
Chondroitin	Osteoarthritis
Devil's claw (*Harpagophytum procumbens*)	Back pain
Feverfew (*Tanacetum parthenium*)	Prevention of migraine
Glusosamine	Osteoarthritis
Herbal medicines	Various pain syndromes
Hypnotherapy	Various pain syndromes
Massage	Back pain
Osteopathy	Various pain syndromes
Relaxation techniques	Various pain syndromes
Willow (*Salix* spp.)	Osteoarthritis

*Data extracted from Ernst et al.[16] and based on systematic reviews conducted for this book.

dedicated chapter on CAM or on a specific CAM therapy and whether this information was in depth and factually correct.

Our searches identified eight books.[8–15] Table 0.3 gives an overview of the information related to CAM in these books. None of the books completely ignored CAM. Three contained a dedicated chapter on CAM[10,14,15] and two had dedicated chapters on a specific CAM therapy, which was acupuncture in both cases.[9,12] The three books without a dedicated CAM chapter had short sections about CAM in other chapters.[8,11,13] Two of the books provided CAM information that seemed both relatively in depth and correct.[12,14] In other books, we found the information at least partly misleading[9,13] or outdated.[10]

While most modern pain books contain information on CAM, this information usually does not cover the wide range of CAM modalities for which evidence is available (Table 0.2).[5,16] Compared to the total volume of each book, the CAM information was extremely brief. Considering the prevalence of CAM use[3] this might be seen as a significant under-representation. The information provided is not always reliable. As many conventional health-care professionals know very little about CAM,[17] the need for more and accurate information is huge.

This book is aimed at filling this gap. It is structured along the lines of, and based on the same principles as, our *Desktop Guide to Complementary and Alternative Medicine*.[5,16] Our aim was to provide evidence-based information on the effectiveness and safety of CAM for conditions that are often associated with pain. The text was written with clinicians, particularly conventional health-care professionals, in mind. It is therefore concise, straightforward and avoids the often flowery language of CAM. As we wanted our book to be valuable not only to pain specialists but to all clinicians, we also included conditions that are not normally seen in pain clinics.

This book deviates from most textbooks in that it contains a methods section where we explain how we have conducted the research underpinning it. We hope that this enhances transparency, objectivity and reproducibility. It is essential that the reader reads both the *Methods* and the *How to use this book* chapters.

Table 0.3 **Information on CAM provided in eight textbooks of pain**

Book	General chapter on CAM?	Chapter on specific modality	Information correct?
Banks[10]	Yes (12 pages)	No, sections within other chapters (massage 5 pages)	Aims to provide 'overview of CAM therapies' yet only selects four modalities: Alexander technique, tai chi, qigong and acupuncture. Extremely brief with little emphasis on clinical evidence, often outdated
Gatchel[11]	No, section within chapter (4 pages)	No	Sensible overview of CAM issues but very little on specific clinical evidence and incomplete
Holdcroft[12]	No	Yes, acupuncture (7 pages)	Yes, in depth information, e.g. on mechanism of action and clinical evidence (but not all relevant CAM topics are covered)
Marcus[13]	No	No, but 3 paragraphs in other chapters	Information on efficacy is misleading: they quote survey data which 'failed to find any benefit' from a range of CAM without presenting any trial evidence, even though such data exist
McCarberg[14]	Yes (23 pages)	No, sections within CAM chapter	Yes, careful discussion of several issues related to CAM; sections dedicated to the value of a range of specific CAM interventions (but not all relevant CAM topics are covered)
Ross[8]	No	No	Only a brief sentence to cover CAM in chapter 'Acute pain management': 'Alternative medicine treatments, such as acupuncture and chiropractic care, can also be used. These treatments provide extremely effective analgesia but should be used for short periods only.'
Stannard[9]	No	Yes, acupuncture (1.5 pages)	Not always: 'There are few double-blind randomised controlled trials ... but uncontrolled series and comparisons ... suggest ... .' (In fact there are in excess of 100 trials of acupuncture for pain control)
Wallace[15]	Yes (4.5 pages)	No	Yes, but incomplete and extremely brief

We are confident that our book fills glaring omissions in the pain literature. It will guide clinicians by summarising the facts and pointing them to treatments which demonstrably do more good than harm and steering them away from other options which fail to fulfil this elementary criterion.

Edzard Ernst, Max H Pittler, Barbara Wider, Kate Boddy
Exeter, 2006

REFERENCES

1. Orpen M, Harvey G, Millard J. A survey of the use of self-acupuncture in pain clinics – a safe way to meet increasing demand? Acupunct Med 2004;22:137–140
2. Burden B, Herron-Marx S, Clifford C. The increasing use of reiki as a complementary therapy in specialist palliative care. Int J Palliat Nurs 2005;11:248–253
3. Barnes PM, Powell-Griner E, McFann K, Nahin RL. Complementary and alternative medicine use among adults: United States, 2002. Adv Data 2004;343:1–19
4. Ernst E, Weihmayr T. UK and German media differ over complementary medicine. BMJ 2000;321:707
5. Ernst E, Pittler MH, Stevinson C, White AR. The desktop guide to complementary and alternative medicine. Edinburgh; Mosby; 2001
6. Klassen TP, Pham B, Lawson ML, Moher D. For randomized controlled trials, the quality of reports of complementary and alternative medicine was as good as reports of conventional medicine. J Clin Epidemiol 2005;58:763–768
7. Lawson ML, Pham B, Klassen TP, Moher D. Systematic reviews involving complementary and alternative medicine interventions had higher quality of reporting than conventional medicine reviews. J Clin Epidemiol 2005;58:777–784
8. Ross E. Pain management. Philadelphia, PA: Hanley & Belfus; 2004
9. Stannard C, Booth S. Pain. Edinburgh: Churchill Livingstone; 2004
10. Banks C, Mackrodt T. Chronic pain management. London: Whurr; 2005
11. Gatchel R. Clinical essentials of pain management. Philadelphia, PA: American College of Physicians, 2005
12. Holdcroft A, Jaggar S. Core topics in pain. Cambridge: Cambridge University Press, 2005
13. Marcus DA. Chronic pain: a primary care guide to practical management. Totowa, NJ: Humana Press; 2005
14. McCarberg B, Passik SD. Expert guide to pain management. Philadelphia, PA: American College of Physicians; 2005
15. Wallace MS, Staats PS. Pain medicine and management; just the facts. New York: McGraw-Hill; 2005
16. Ernst E, Pittler MH, Wider B, Boddy K. The desktop guide to complementary and alternative medicine, 2nd edn. Edinburgh; Mosby; 2006
17. Botting DA, Cook R. Complementary medicine: knowledge, use and attitudes of doctors. Complement Ther Nurs Midwifery 2000;6:41–47

Glossary

DEFINITIONS OF GENERAL TERMS

Cochrane review Cochrane reviews are systematic summaries of evidence of the effects of health-care interventions prepared and maintained by the Cochrane Collaboration. The reviews employ specific methods, are prepared using REVIEW MANAGER (REVMAN) software, adhere to a structured format and are regularly updated (http://www.cochrane.org).

Confidence interval (CI) Quantifies the uncertainty in measurement. Usually reported as 95% CI, which is the range of values within which one can expect to find the true value in 95% of cases.

Controlled clinical trial (CCT) Control is a standard against which experimental observations may be evaluated. In clinical trials, one group of participants is given an experimental intervention, while another group (i.e. the control group) is given either a standard treatment for the disease, a placebo or no treatment at all.

Cross-over Participants in the intervention group receive the control treatment upon completion of the treatment cycle. Similarly those in the control group 'cross over' and receive the experimental intervention.

Double-blind trial A clinical trial design in which neither the participating individuals nor the study staff know which participants are receiving the experimental treatment and which are receiving the control treatment or placebo. Double-blind trials are thought to produce objective results, because the expectations of the participant and study staff about the experimental drug do not affect the outcome.

Meta-analysis A quantitative statistical method to pool trial data in a single estimate; can be part of a systematic review.

P-value Probability that an observed difference between groups occurred by chance alone. A result is conventionally regarded as 'statistically significant' if the likelihood that it is the result of chance alone is less than five times out of 100 ($P < 0.05$).

Randomisation The process by which patients in a clinical trial are randomly assigned to experimental intervention or control treatment. Randomisation minimises the differences among groups by equally distributing participants with particular characteristics (known or unknown) among all the trial arms.

Randomised clinical trial (RCT) Study where participants are randomly allocated to receive experimental or control treatment.

Systematic review Review in which literature from multiple sources is systematically searched for, assessed and evaluated to answer clearly formulated questions.

ABBREVIATIONS OF FREQUENTLY USED TERMS

The following abbreviations are used throughout this book:

CAM	complementary and alternative medicine
CCT	controlled clinical trial
CI	confidence intervals (95% unless otherwise stated)
RCT	randomised clinical trial
g	gram(s)
mg	milligram(s)

μg   micrograms
h   hour(s)
m   metre(s)

DEFINITIONS OF PAIN TERMS

Analgesia   Absence of pain in response to stimulus that is normally painful.

Anaesthesia   Absence of all sensory modalities.

Central pain   Regional pain caused by a primary lesion or dysfunction in the central nervous system, usually associated with abnormal sensitivity to temperature and to noxious stimulation.

Complex regional pain syndrome (CRPS)   A term describing a variety of painful conditions following injury that appear regionally, have a distal predominance of abnormal findings, exceed in both magnitude and duration the expected clinical course of the inciting event, often result in significant impairment of motor function, and show variable progression over time. CRPS is a new term for disorders previously called reflex sympathetic dystrophy (RSD).

CRPS I (RSD)
- Type I is a syndrome that develops after an initiating noxious event.
- Spontaneous pain or allodynia/hyperalgesia occurs, is not limited to the territory of a single peripheral nerve, and is disproportionate to the inciting event.
- There is or has been evidence of oedema, skin blood flow abnormality or abnormal sudomotor activity in the region of the pain since the inciting event.
- This diagnosis is excluded by the existence of conditions that would otherwise account for the degree of pain and dysfunction.

CRPS II (causalgia)
- Type II is a syndrome that develops after a nerve injury. Spontaneous pain or allodynia/hyperalgesia occurs and is not necessarily limited to the territory of the injured nerve.
- There is or has been evidence of oedema, skin blood flow abnormality or abnormal sudomotor activity in the region of the pain since the inciting event.
- This diagnosis is excluded by the existence of conditions that would otherwise account for the degree of pain and dysfunction.

Chronic pain   Pain that persists beyond the course of an acute disease or a reasonable time for an injury to heal or that is associated with a chronic pathological process that causes continuous pain, or the pain recurs at intervals of months or years. Some investigators use a pain duration of ≥6 months to designate a pain as chronic.

Deafferentation pain   Pain as the result of a loss of sensory input into the central nervous system. This may occur with lesions of peripheral nerves, such as avulsion of the brachial plexus, or through pathology of the central nervous system.

Dysaesthesia   An unpleasant abnormal sensation, whether spontaneous or evoked.

Hyperalgesia   An increased response to a stimulus that is normally painful.

Hyperaesthesia   Increased sensitivity to stimulation; this excludes the special senses.

Hyperpathia   A painful syndrome, characterised by increased reaction to a stimulus, especially a repetitive stimulus, as well as increased threshold.

Hypoalgesia   Diminished sensitivity to noxious stimulation.

Hypoaesthesia   Diminished sensitivity to stimulation; this excludes the special senses.

Ischaemic pain   Pain caused by oxygen starvation of tissues; if the oxygen supply is not restored, cell death (necrosis) will ensue.

Neuritis   Inflammation of a nerve or nerves. (Not to be used unless inflammation is thought to be present.)

Neurogenic pain   Pain initiated or caused by a primary lesion, dysfunction or transitory perturbation in the peripheral or central nervous system.

Nociceptive pain Pain caused by activation of nociceptive afferent fibres. This type of pain satisfies the criteria for pain transmission, i.e. transmission to the spinal cord, thalamus and then to the cerebral cortex.

Nociceptor A receptor preferentially sensitive to a noxious stimulus or to a stimulus that would become noxious if prolonged.

Noxious stimulus A stimulus that is actually or potentially damaging to body tissue.

Pain An unpleasant sensory and emotional experience associated with actual or potential tissue damage, or described in terms of damage.

Pain threshold The least experience of pain that a subject can recognise.

Pain tolerance level The greatest level of pain that a subject is prepared to tolerate.

Pain of psychological origin

> *Delusional* or *hallucinatory*: pain of psychological origin and attributed by the patient to a specific delusional cause.
>
> *Hysterical, conversion* or *hypochondriacal*: pain specifically attributable to the thought process, emotional state, or personality of the patient in the absence of an organic or delusional cause or tension mechanism.

Paraesthesia An abnormal sensation, whether spontaneous or evoked. NB Paraesthesia is an abnormal sensation that is not unpleasant while dysaesthesia is an abnormal sensation that is considered unpleasant. Dysaesthesia does not include all abnormal sensations, but only those that are unpleasant.

Radicular pain Pain perceived as arising in a limb or the trunk wall caused by ectopic activation of nociceptive afferent fibres in a spinal nerve or its roots or other neuropathic mechanisms. The pain is usually lancinating and travels in a narrow band. Aetiological causes include anatomic lesions affecting the spinal nerve and dorsal root ganglion including herniated intervertebral disc and spinal stenosis.

Radiculopathy Objective loss of sensory and/or motor function as a result of a conduction block in the axons of a spinal nerve or its roots. Symptoms include numbness and weakness in the distribution of the affected nerve. Neurological examination and diagnostic tests confirm the neurological abnormality. NB Radicular pain and radiculopathy are not synonymous. The former is a symptom caused by ectopic impulse generation. The latter relates to objective neurological signs as a result of a conduction block. The two conditions may coexist and may be caused by the same lesion.

Referred pain Pain perceived as occurring in a region of the body topographically distinct from the region in which the actual source of pain is located.

Somatic Derived from the Greek word for 'body'. Although somatosensory input refers to sensory signals from all tissues of the body including skin, viscera, muscles and joints, it usually signifies input from body tissue other than the viscera.

Visceral pain Pain carried by the sympathetic fibres: this pain is diffuse and poorly localised.

SOURCE

Raja SN, Molloy RE, Liu S, Fishman SM, Benzon HT. Essentials of pain medicine and regional anesthesia. Edinburgh: Churchill Livingstone; 2004

PATIENTS' LANGUAGE OF PAIN

Ache A usually dull persistent pain; to become distressed or disturbed (as with anxiety or regret).
> Origin: from Old English *acan* 'to ache, suffer pain', perhaps imitative of groaning.

Afflict Cause pain or suffering to.
> Origin: from Latin *afflictare* 'knock about, harass', or *affligere* 'knock down, weaken'.

Aggrieve To give pain or trouble to; to inflict injury on.
> Origin: from Old French *agrever* 'bear heavily on', from Latin *aggravare* 'make heavier'.

Agony Extreme suffering; intense pain of mind or body; the struggle that precedes death.
 Origin: 'mental suffering' (especially that of Christ in the Garden of Gethsemane), from Greek *agonia* 'a (mental) struggle for victory', originally 'a struggle for victory in the games', from *agon* 'assembly for a contest'.
Anguish Severe mental or physical pain or suffering.
 Origin: from Old French *anguisse* 'choking sensation', from Latin *angustia* 'tightness, distress', from *ang(u)ere* 'to throttle, torment'.
Anxious Experiencing worry or unease.
 Origin: from Latin *anxius* 'solicitous, uneasy, troubled in mind', from *ang(u)ere* 'choke, cause distress'.
Awe Dread mixed with veneration; feeling of great respect mixed with fear.
 Origin: from Old Norse *agi* 'fright', current sense is through its biblical use with reference to the Supreme Being.
Chagrin Disquietude or distress of mind caused by humiliation, disappointment or failure.
 Origin: from French *chagrin* 'sad, melancholy', possibly from Old North French *graignier* 'to sorrow'.
Discomfort Slight pain; slight anxiety or embarrassment; cause discomfort to.
 Origin: from Old French *desconfort*, originally 'to deprive of courage'.
Disquiet A feeling of anxiety; make anxious.
 Origin: Quiet is from Old French *quiete*, from Latin *quies* 'rest, quiet'.
Distress Extreme anxiety or suffering; a state of physical strain, especially difficulty in breathing; cause distress to.
 Origin: from Old French *destresce*, from Latin *distringere* 'draw apart, hinder'.
Dolor A state of great sorrow or distress.
 Origin: from Latin *dolor* 'pain, grief '.
Excruciate To inflict intense pain on; to subject to intense mental distress.
 Origin: from Latin *excruciates* 'to torture, torment', from *ex-* 'out, thoroughly' and *cruciare* 'cause pain or anguish to, to crucify', from *cruc-*, *crux* 'cross'.
Grief/grieve Intense sorrow, especially caused by someone's death; trouble or annoyance.
 Origin: from Old French *grever* 'to burden'.
Gripe Express a trivial complaint, grumble; affect with stomach or intestinal pain.
 Origin: from Old English, 'grasp, clutch', related to grip and grope.
Hurt Cause or feel physical pain or injury; cause or feel mental pain or distress; injury or pain, harm.
 Origin: from Old French *hurter* 'to strike'.
Misery A state of suffering and want that is the result of poverty or affliction; a circumstance, thing or place that causes suffering or discomfort; a state of great unhappiness and emotional distress.
 Origin: from Old French *miserie*, from Latin *miseria* 'wretchedness', from *miser* meaning 'bodily pain' from 1825, American English.
Pang A sudden sharp pain or painful emotion.
 Origin: unknown, perhaps related to prong 'pointed tool'.
Smart Give a sharp, stinging pain; feel upset and annoyed.
 Origin: from Old English *smeortan* 'be painful', from West Germanic *smert-*, German *schmerzen* 'to pain', originally 'to bite', Latin *mordere* 'to bite'.
Sore Painful or aching; suffering pain; upset and angry; a raw or painful place on the body; a source of distress or annoyance.
 Origin: from Old English *sar* 'painful, grievous, aching', influenced in meaning by Old Norse *sarr* 'sore, wounded'.
Sting A small sharp-pointed organ of an insect, capable of inflicting a painful wound by injecting poison; a wound from a sting; a sharp tingling sensation or hurtful effect; to wound with a sting; produce a stinging sensation; hurt, upset.

Origin: from Old English *stingan* 'to prick with a small point' (of weapons, insects, plants, etc.).

Stitch A sudden sharp pain in the side of the body, caused by strenuous exercise.
Origin: from Old English *stice* 'a prick, puncture', from the root of stick; the sense of 'sudden, stabbing pain in the side' was used in late Old English.

Suffer Experience or be subjected to something bad or unpleasant; be affected by or subject to an illness or ailment.
Origin: from Latin *sufferre*, from *ferre* 'to bear'.

Throe Pang, spasm; pain of childbirth, agony of death; a hard or painful struggle.
Origin: from Middle English *thrawe, throwe* 'pain, pang of childbirth, agony of death', possibly from Old English *thrawan* 'twist, turn, writhe', or altered from Old English *threa* 'affliction, pang, evil, threat'.

Torment Severe physical or mental suffering.
Origin: 'inflicting of torture', also 'state of great suffering', from Old French *tourment*, Latin *tormentum* 'instrument of torture', from *torquere* 'to twist'.

Torture The infliction of severe pain as a punishment or a forcible means of persuasion; great suffering or anxiety.
Origin: from Middle French *torture* 'infliction of great pain, great pain, agony', Latin *tortura* 'twisting, writhing, torture, torment', from *torquere* 'to twist'.

Trouble Cause distress, pain or inconvenience to; showing or experiencing problems or anxiety.
Origin: from Old French *truble*, from Latin *turba* 'crowd, disturbance'.

Twinge A sudden, sharp localised pain; a brief, sharp pang of emotion.
Origin: from obsolete verb twinge 'to pinch, tweak', from Old English *twengan* 'to pinch,' of uncertain origin.

Unease Mental or spiritual discomfort.
Origin: ease is from Old French *aise* 'comfort, pleasure' of unknown origin; the earliest senses in French appear to be 'elbow-room' and 'opportunity'.

Vex To bring trouble, distress or agitation to; make annoyed or worried.
Origin: from Middle French *vexer*, from Latin *vexare* 'to shake, disturb'.

Woe Used to express grief, regret or distress.
Origin: from Middle English *wa, wo*, from Old English *wa*; akin to Old Norse *vei* 'interjection, woe', Latin *vae*.

Wretchedness Deeply afflicted, dejected or distressed in body or mind; extremely or deplorably bad or distressing.
Origin: from Old English *wrecca* 'outcast, exile'; akin to Old High German *hrechjo* 'fugitive'.

Using the book

THE BOOK AT A GLANCE

- The purpose of *Complementary Therapies for Pain Management* is to present relevant, reliable, thorough and up-to-date information on complementary and alternative medicine in a clear concise format with a focus on clinical evidence relating to various forms of pain.
- The clinical evidence was retrieved through systematic searches in six general and specialist literature databases carried out up to March 2006 (see *Methods* p. 3).
- Studies were selected according to the following priority order: systematic reviews and meta-analyses, randomised clinical trials, controlled clinical trials, uncontrolled trials (see *Methods* p. 3).
- Assessment of trials was a combination of the methodological quality of the body of evidence, the level of evidence and the volume of evidence resulting in an indication of the weight of the evidence (low O to high OOO) and the direction of the evidence (clearly positive ↑ to clearly negative ↓) (see *How to use this book* pp. 13–14).
- Key information and an application of judgement are presented in the *Risk–benefit assessments* (Sections 3 and 4), in the *Overall recommendation* (Section 5), and in the *Summary of evidence* tables (see *How to use this book* p. 5).
- Absence of evidence of effectiveness does not imply absence of effectiveness.
- For safety issues the precautionary principle has been applied, so a treatment is not considered risk-free unless evidence suggests otherwise. A simple Yes/No descriptor alerts the reader in a general way to the existence (however rare) of potentially serious safety concerns (see *Methods* p. 4).
- Pregnancy and lactation are cited as contraindications for all medicines included in this book unless there is positive evidence of safety in these situations (see *Methods* p. 4).

METHODS

The intention of this book is to provide relevant, reliable, thorough and up-to-date information in a clear, concise format. To achieve this, a systematic approach was used to locate, select, appraise and present information. The concept and format of the book are based on our highly acclaimed *Desktop Guide to Complementary and Alternative Medicine*.[1] This chapter describes the procedures followed.

DEFINITION OF COMPLEMENTARY AND ALTERNATIVE MEDICINE

For the purposes of this book complementary and alternative medicine (CAM) was defined as 'diagnosis, treatment and/or prevention which complements mainstream medicine by contributing to a common whole, satisfying a demand not met by orthodoxy, or diversifying the conceptual framework of medicine'.[2] What constitutes CAM may vary according to national differences and individual viewpoints. The list below indicates many of the treatments that we considered mainstream rather than CAM and that were therefore not generally covered in this book. However, some of these treatments are mentioned in Section 5 (Pain syndromes) for particular non-mainstream indications.

- Behavioural therapy
- Cognitive therapy
- Counselling
- Diets and nutritional advice
- Electromagnetic therapy

- Electrotherapy
- Exercise
- Lifestyle approaches
- Low-dose laser therapy
- Transcranial magnetic stimulation
- Transcutaneous electrical nerve stimulation (TENS)
- Ultrasound
- Vitamins and minerals.

SELECTION OF TOPICS

Sections 3 and 4 cover CAM treatments (therapies and medicines) that are popular with pain patients. Treatments for which evidence relating to effectiveness is available are the subject of individual chapters. Other treatments where there is only some evidence of effectiveness are covered in tables.

The pain syndromes included in Section 5 are those that are commonly seen by clinicians, that are frequently treated with CAM and for which the most evidence relating to effectiveness is available. Conditions for which insufficient evidence is available (for instance phantom pain) are not normally covered in separate chapters.

Provisional lists of potential topics for chapters and tables were produced during discussion and amended after inspecting the results of literature searches (see *Literature searches* below) and internal review (see *Review process* below).

SOURCES AND REFERENCING

A number of sources were used to compile information for this book. These included reference books, our own files, contact with other experts, and systematic literature searches (see *Literature searches* below). Since a considerable amount of information is compressed into each chapter it was decided to keep referencing to a minimum. Comprehensive referencing would involve lengthy and repetitive reference lists, which would distract the reader from quick access to clear information. For example, the information on risks presented in Sections 3 and 4 is largely based on a vast number of case reports and individual referencing would have been more of a hindrance than a help to the reader. Therefore, a bibliography of the main reference sources for the book is provided at the end of this section. The exception to this is information relating to clinical evidence, which provides the major focus of this book. In Sections 3, 4 and 5 key references are provided for the evidence cited at the end of each chapter, to allow the interested reader to trace the source.

LITERATURE SEARCHES FOR CLINICAL EVIDENCE

Systematic searches were carried out in the databases Medline, Embase, Amed, Scopus, the Cochrane Database of Systematic Reviews, Natural Standard and the Natural Medicines Comprehensive Database. Each database was searched from its respective inception until March 2006. The search strategy used to locate relevant literature was developed and refined. In addition, our own files, the bibliographies of relevant papers and the contents pages of all issues of the review journal *FACT* (*Focus on Alternative and Complementary Therapies*; London: Pharmaceutical Press, www.pharmpress.com/fact) were searched for further studies. No language restrictions were imposed. Studies in languages other than English were translated in-house.

SELECTION OF CLINICAL EVIDENCE

Each author selected relevant studies on a particular topic by scrutinising the abstracts. Systematic reviews and meta-analyses of clinical trials were given priority and copies of originals were obtained. Where systematic reviews or meta-analyses were not located, the evidence from randomised clinical trials and controlled clinical trials was considered next. In their absence, uncontrolled studies were considered. In most cases, original reports were obtained.

APPRAISAL OF CLINICAL EVIDENCE

All authors were familiar with critical appraisal and systematic reviews. They consistently evaluated the methodological quality of the studies by assessing important criteria such as randomisation, blinding and description of withdrawals and dropouts in an informal review process. For systematic reviews and meta-analyses, the assessment of the methodological quality of included trials by the original authors was accepted. The quality of the review itself was assessed informally. In the *Summary of clinical evidence* tables (Section 5), the methodological quality of the body of evidence of a particular treatment for a particular condition was combined with the level of the evidence and the volume of the evidence to produce a measure of 'weight'. This is intended to indicate the degree of confidence that can be placed on the evidence. Details are given in *How to use this book* (see pp. 13–14).

APPLICATION OF JUDGEMENT

Clinical judgement was used by the authors in two specific areas: the *Risk–benefit assessment* of each treatment (Sections 3 and 4) and the *Overall recommendation* (Section 5). These judgements are based on experience and current medical practice as well as on the evidence. In an attempt to minimise bias and achieve standardisation, the process was subjected to internal and external review (see *Review process* below). It should be noted that stating that there is a lack of compelling evidence for a treatment does not imply that the treatment is ineffective.

PRESENTATION OF INFORMATION

In most parts of each chapter, the information is presented in a concise narrative form in a predefined format (see *How to use this book*, pp. 6–13). However, for *Clinical evidence* in Section 5, key information is displayed in the *Summary of evidence* tables. Additionally, the most authoritative systematic review or meta-analysis on a subject has been abstracted into a box. Selected clinical trials are sometimes presented in standardised tables; usually these are the most scientifically rigorous or clinically relevant. Data have been extracted according to predefined criteria into tables, which also provide additional information or a critical comment. Treatments and pain syndromes that are not covered in separate chapters within Sections 3, 4 and 5 can be found in the tables at the end of the respective sections. At the end of Sections 3 and 4, tables are presented containing brief information on other treatments for which some evidence of effectiveness is available or which are used frequently but were not included as full chapters. The table at the end of Section 5 lists other frequently used treatments for specific conditions lacking sound evidence and pain syndromes for which no sufficient evidence is available.

INFORMATION ON SAFETY

Information on safety is central to the assessment of a treatment's value. Hence this material is an important component of the book. Unfortunately, there is often only fragmentary knowledge on safety in CAM. The treatment chapters (Sections 3 and 4) address risks as fully as is possible from the available data. In general, the precautionary principle has been applied, so a treatment is not considered risk-free unless evidence suggests otherwise. In our view, this is prudent and follows the most important axiom of medicine: *primum nihil nocere* – first do no harm. Unless there is positive evidence for safety, pregnancy and lactation are cited as contraindications for all medicines included in this book. Allergic reactions have been mentioned where they have been reported but should be assumed possible for all herbs and many supplements, with the potential to be serious. Mind–body medicines carry the risk of aggravating or causing psychosis in predisposed individuals.

For the *Summary of clinical evidence* tables in Section 5, many different ways of summarising safety data were considered but it proved impossible to provide sufficient useful detail. It was therefore decided to use a simple Yes/No descriptor to alert the reader in a general way to the existence (however rare) of potentially serious safety concerns, cross-referencing to the sections providing specific details (see *How to use this book*, p. 13). Even when a treatment is apparently innocuous, the table entry is 'Yes' if there is insufficient information available to establish safety and serious risks are considered possible. This applies to all herbs and some supplements. Other supplements are marked 'Yes' because overdose is associated with serious consequences. Most products derived from natural sources carry the risk of allergic reactions (see above). In the case of homeopathic remedies, this is unlikely at non-material dilutions, hence homeopathy is marked 'No'. Aromatherapy, on the other hand, is marked 'Yes' because of the allergic reactions that are possible with essential oils. Therapies marked 'Yes' that cannot be cross-referenced to a specific chapter or table are hydrotherapy (for which cardiorespiratory decompensation and bacterial infections have been reported), exercise (where sudden death has been recorded), electrotherapy (for which psychological disturbance and local injury from electrodes are possible) and fasting and particular diets (where malnutrition can occur). Our intention is not to be alarmist, but clearly the priority must be to minimise all possible risks for the patient.

REVIEW PROCESS

All information presented in this book was subjected to an internal review by all four editors. Chapters were revised accordingly and additional information was incorporated. Regular consensus conferences were held to ensure a standardised approach. This was performed particularly with a view to minimising bias in areas where a degree of personal judgement was introduced (see *Application of judgement* above). Any disputes that appeared during the consensus conferences were resolved through discussion.

As the book is based on the format and style of the *Desktop Guide to Complementary and Alternative Medicine*,[1] criticism and praise from book reviews, the professional organisations of complementary therapies and any other feedback received on the *Desktop Guide* were collated, internally discussed and, where appropriate, applied to *Complementary Therapies for Pain Management*. The ultimate review, however, remains with you, the reader.

REFERENCES
1. Ernst E, Pittler MH, Wider B, Boddy K. The desktop guide to complementary and alternative medicine, 2nd edn. Edinburgh: Mosby; 2006
2. Ernst E, Resch KL, Mills S, Hill R, Mitchell A, Willoughby M, White A. Complementary medicine – a definition. Br J Gen Pract 1995;309:107–111

HOW TO USE THIS BOOK

This book is divided into four main sections:

- general topics
- therapies
- herbal and non-herbal medicines
- pain syndromes.

The first of these sections covers general topics such as epidemiology of pain, pain measurement and a general introduction to CAM. For the chapters presenting different concepts of pain, we have invited experts in these fields to write about how pain is viewed according to the principles of their respective CAM system or therapies. They are intended to contrast with the current medical and psychological concepts of pain and represent the views of the respective chapter authors.

For the chapters within the sections on *Therapies*, *Herbal and non-herbal medicines* and *Pain syndromes*, standardised structures have been adopted. To help the reader understand and make the best use of the information in the individual chapters, brief explanations of the material provided under each subheading are given below, with the help of examples taken from the book.

For further details on the methods employed for writing these sections, see p. 2.

SECTION 3 THERAPIES

This section includes chapters on forms of CAM that are identified as therapeutic modalities and excludes medicines such as herbs or food supplements. Chapters are presented in alphabetical order and are subdivided according to the headings shown in the example below (aromatherapy).

TABLE

Other therapies for which some evidence of effectiveness is available or which are used frequently but were not included as full chapters are presented in a table at the end of this section. Brief information is provided for each one, including a description, its main uses and any concerns about its safety.

AROMATHERAPY **104**

AROMATHERAPY

Other forms of treatment that share important features with the therapy

DEFINITION

The controlled use of plant essences for therapeutic purposes.

RELATED TECHNIQUES

Massage.

Brief introduction to the origins of the therapy, its cultural context and historical development

BACKGROUND

The medicinal use of plant oils has a long history in ancient Egypt, China and India. The development of modern aromatherapy is attributed to the French chemist René Gattefosse, who burned his hand while working in a perfume laboratory and immediately doused it in some nearby lavender oil. The burn healed quickly without scarring, leading him to study the potential curative powers of plant oils. He coined the term aromatherapy in 1937.

TRADITIONAL CONCEPTS

Essential oils can be applied directly to the skin through massage or a compress, added to baths, inhaled with steaming water or spread throughout a room with a diffuser. The oils are believed to have effects at the psychological, physiological and cellular levels. These effects are claimed to be relaxing or stimulating depending on the chemistry of the oil and the previous associations of the individual with a particular scent.

Summary of the underlying principles of the therapy.
NB Not all practitioners use the traditional concepts

SCIENTIFIC RATIONALE

The scent from the oil activates the olfactory sense. This triggers the limbic system, which governs emotional responses and is involved with the formation and retrieval of learned memories. Essential oils are also absorbed through the skin. Laboratory studies suggest that molecules of the oil can affect organ function, although the clinical relevance of these findings is not clear.

Evaluation of the principles of the therapy and mechanism of action from a scientific perspective

PRACTITIONERS

In most countries aromatherapy is largely unregulated. In the UK it is currently in the process of becoming regulated. Various associations offer courses with the number of hours of training required ranging from 180 to 500. Many nurses and other health-care professionals seek aromatherapy qualifications.

CONDITIONS FREQUENTLY TREATED

Headaches, musculoskeletal pain, insomnia, anxiety and other conditions. Some therapists recommend regular aromatherapy as a means of maintaining general health and well-being. A US survey suggests that stress, musculoskeletal problems and pain are the most common conditions treated by aromatherapists.[1]

TYPICAL SESSION

During an initial session the aromatherapist takes the client's medical history and asks which aromas are liked or disliked. The therapist then selects essential oils deemed appropriate for the client. Treatment usually consists of an aromatherapy massage and advice may be given about home treatments involving the use of oils in baths or a diffuser. The initial session may last up to 2 hours. Subsequent sessions would typically last 1 hour.

Persons employing the therapy. Patients should ensure that any therapist used is a member of a recognised body or association, holds professional liability insurance cover and that the recognised body has a code of ethics and conduct and a complaints and disciplinary procedure.
NB Many therapies are practised by more than one professional group

COURSE OF TREATMENT

For chronic conditions, one weekly session would be recommended for several weeks, with fortnightly or monthly follow-ups.

CLINICAL EVIDENCE

A Cochrane review focused on aromatherapy and massage for symptom relief in patients with cancer. It included 10 RCTs and found that 'massage and aromatherapy confer short-term benefits on psychological well-being, with the effect on anxiety supported by limited evidence'.[2] A systematic review of CAM for labour pain found one RCT of aromatherapy; its results did not demonstrate that baths with essential oil of ginger or lemongrass reduced analgesic consumption.[3] Other RCTs fail to show benefit in terms of symptom control in cancer patients,[4] or pain control, anxiety or quality of life in hospice patients.[5] More recent controlled clinical trials (CCTs) or RCTs suggest that aromatherapy can reduce the pain of arthritis.[6] An RCT tested whether the mere olfactory absorption of lavender or rosemary essential oils affected pain sensitivity in healthy volunteers ($n = 26$); no such effect was demonstrated.[7]

Evidence-based summary of the data relating to the effectiveness of the therapy. In cases where a considerable amount of evidence exists, only the most important is presented. Priority is given to systematic reviews/meta-analyses and RCTs

SECTION ONE

SECTION THREE

105 THERAPIES

Safety issues specific to the therapy. NB For a general discussion of CAM safety, see p. 24

RISKS

CONTRAINDICATIONS

Pregnancy, contagious diseases, epilepsy, local venous thrombosis, varicose veins, broken skin, recent surgery, circulatory disorders.

PRECAUTIONS/WARNINGS

Essential oils should not be taken orally or used undiluted on the skin. Some oils cause photosensitive reactions and some have carcinogenic potential. Allergic reactions are possible with all oils. Aromatherapy should generally be considered an adjunctive treatment, not an alternative to conventional care.

ADVERSE EFFECTS

Allergic reactions, phototoxic reactions, nausea, headache.

INTERACTIONS

Many essential oils are believed to have the potential to either enhance or reduce the effects of prescribed medications including antibiotics, tranquillisers, antihistamines, anticonvulsants, barbiturates, morphine, quinidine.

QUALITY ISSUES

Products marketed as 'aromatherapy oils' may be synthetic or adulterated rather than the pure essential oil.

An evidence-based judgment on whether the therapy does more good than harm.
NB A lack of compelling evidence is not the same as ineffectiveness

RISK–BENEFIT ASSESSMENT

The trial evidence on aromatherapy is contradictory. Aromatherapy appears to have some benefits as a palliative or supportive treatment, particularly in reducing anxiety. In the hands of a responsible therapist there seem to be few risks. Aromatherapy may thus be worth considering as an adjunctive treatment for chronically ill patients or individuals with psychosomatic illness.

REFERENCES

1. Osborn CE, Barlas P, Baxter GD, Barlow JH. Aromatherapy: a survey of current practice in the management of rheumatic disease symptoms. Complement Ther Med 2001;9:62–67
2. Fellowes D, Barnes K, Wilkinson S. Aromatherapy and massage for symptom relief in patients with cancer. The Cochrane Database of Systematic Reviews 2004, Issue 3. Art. No.: CD002287
3. Huntley AL, Coon JT, Ernst E. Complementary and alternative medicine for labor pain: a systematic review. Am J Obstet Gynecol 2004;191:36–44
4. Wilcock A, Manderson C, Weller R, Walker G, Carr D, Carey AM, Broadhurst D, Mew J, Ernst E. Does aromatherapy massage benefit patients with cancer attending a specialist palliative care day centre? Palliat Med 2004;18:287–290
5. Soden K, Vincent K, Craske S, Lucas C, Ashley S. A randomized controlled trial of aromatherapy massage in a hospice setting. Palliat Med 2004;18:87–92
6. Kim MJ, Nam ES, Paik SI. The effects of aromatherapy on pain, depression, and life satisfaction of arthritis patients. [In Korean] Taehan Kanho Hakhoe Chi 2005;35:186–194
7. Gedney JJ, Glover TL, Fillingim RB. Sensory and affective pain discrimination after inhalation of essential oils. Psychosom Med 2004;66:599–606

SECTION 4 HERBAL AND NON-HERBAL MEDICINE

This section includes chapters on forms of CAM that are considered medications such as herbal and non-herbal supplements. Vitamins and minerals are not included (see p. 2). Chapters are presented in alphabetical order according to the common name and are subdivided according to the headings in the example below (comfrey). It was decided to use the common name of herbs because of the frequent uncertainties of terminology in the original articles. Exact taxonomic names is an area that requires attention in future studies.

TABLE

Other herbs and non-herbal supplements for which some evidence of effectiveness is available or which are used frequently but were not included as full chapters are presented in a table at the end of this section. Brief information is provided, including a description, main uses and safety concerns.

COMFREY **188**

| COMFREY | (*Symphytum officinale*) |

Plant taxonomy according to Germplasm Resources Information Network (GRIN) (see p. 16)

SOURCE
Leaf, rhizome, root.

In alphabetical order

MAIN CONSTITUENTS
Allantoin, derivatives of rosmarinic acids, saponins, tannins.

BACKGROUND
Comfrey is a perennial herb of the Boraginaceae family and is native to Europe and Asia. Its name is derived from the Latin word for 'grow together'. Comfrey has been cultivated since about 400 BCE as a medicinal herb for wound healing and broken bones and to stop bleeding. There are concerns about its toxicity, caused by pyrrolizidine alkaloids, so it is recommended for external use only.

For herb: brief description of historical background, etymology and botany. For supplement: rationale for its use

EXAMPLES OF TRADITIONAL USES
Angina, bloody urine, bronchitis, cancer, diarrhoea, excessive menstrual flow, gum disease, persistent cough, pharyngitis, pleuritis, rheumatism and ulcers.

PHARMACOLOGICAL ACTION
Analgesic, anti-inflammatory, anti-oedematous, wound healing.

Conditions and purposes for which the medicine was traditionally used in alphabetical order. NB May be unsupported or even contraindicated by current evidence

CONDITIONS FREQUENTLY TREATED
Bruises and sprains, fractures, ulcers and wounds.

CLINICAL EVIDENCE
Topically applied comfrey in the treatment of ankle distortions was tested in several RCTs. One single-blind RCT ($n = 164$) found comfrey ointment to be non-inferior to diclofenac with regards the pain reaction to pressure on the injured area, swelling and pain at rest and at movement.[1] The same comfrey ointment was found to be superior to placebo in a double-blind RCT ($n = 142$) in reducing pain, ankle oedema and in increasing ankle mobility.[2] Two different concentrations of comfrey were compared in a double-blind RCT ($n = 104$), which found the higher concentration to be far more effective than the lower one at decreasing pain and improving functional impairment.[3] One double-blind RCT compared two concentrations of a topical comfrey product with placebo in the treatment of myalgia patients and found better overall efficacy and faster onset of effects with the high-concentration product on pain in the lower and upper back.[4]

Pharmacologic effects demonstrated. NB Mention is made of mechanisms only if considered relevant

In alphabetical order

DOSAGE
Ointments and other external preparations are commonly made with 5–20% of comfrey.

Evidence-based summary of the data relating to the effectiveness of the medicine. In cases where a considerable amount of evidence exists, only the most important is presented. Priority is given to systematic reviews/meta-analyses and RCTs

Usual therapeutic dose, where possible based on clinical trial data. NB Due to scarce data, no attempt is made to suggest optimum duration of treatment. The effects of some herbs may take several weeks to appear. There is generally a lack of adequate data regarding long-term use

SECTION ONE

SECTION FOUR

Safety issues specific to the medicine. NB For a general discussion of CAM saftey, see p. 24

189 HERBAL AND NON-HERBAL MEDICINE

RISKS

CONTRAINDICATIONS
Broken skin, pregnancy and lactation (see p. 4).

PRECAUTIONS/WARNINGS
Products, particularly those prepared from the roots, may contain liver-toxic pyrrolizidine alkaloids and are not recommended for internal use. Should not be used for more than 6 weeks a year.

ADVERSE EFFECTS
Veno-occlusive disease, liver damage (oral usage).

OVERDOSE
Daily use should not exceed 100 μg of the pyrrolizidine alkaloids.

INTERACTIONS
Risk of additive toxicity with concomitant use of other pyrrolizidine alkaloid-containing herbs.

QUALITY ISSUES
Only products with reduced toxicity levels should be used. Some products labelled comfrey or *Symphytum officinale* instead contain the more toxic prickly comfrey.

An evidence-based judgement on whether the medicine does more good than harm. NB A lack of compelling evidence is not the same as ineffectiveness

RISK–BENEFIT ASSESSMENT

There is encouraging yet limited evidence for the effectiveness of comfrey ointment in the treatment of ankle distortions. Cautiously used on unbroken skin only, it might be a useful adjunct in this indication but further evidence is required to make any firm recommendations.

REFERENCES
1. Predel HG, Giannetti B, Koll R, Bulitta M, Staiger C. Efficacy of a comfrey root extract ointment in comparison to a diclofenac gel in the treatment of ankle distortions: results of an observer-blind, randomized, multicenter study. Phytomedicine 2005;12:707–714
2. Koll R, Buhr M, Dieter R, Pabst H, Predel HG, Petrowicz O, Giannetti B, Klingenburg S, Staiger C. Efficacy and tolerance of a comfrey root extract (Extr. Rad. Symphyti) in the treatment of ankle distorsions: results of a multicenter, randomized, placebo-controlled, double-blind study. Phytomedicine 2004;11:470–477
3. Kucera M, Barna M, Horacek O, Kovarikova J, Kucera A. Efficacy and safety of topically applied Symphytum herb extract cream in the treatment of ankle distortion: results of a randomized controlled clinical double blind study. Wien Med Wochenschr 2004;154: 498–507
4. Kucera M, Barna M, Horacek O, Kalal J, Kucera A, Hladikova M. Topical symphytum herb concentrate cream against myalgia: a randomized controlled double-blind clinical study. Adv Ther 2005;22:681–692

SECTION 5 PAIN SYNDROMES

This section includes chapters on pain syndromes commonly seen by clinicians for which CAM is popular. Chapters are presented in alphabetical order and are subdivided according to the subheadings shown in the example below (headache).

TABLE

Other frequently used treatments for specific conditions lacking sound evidence and pain syndromes for which no sufficient evidence is available are presented in a table at the end of this section.

HEADACHE **263**

HEADACHE

SYNONYMS/SUBCATEGORIES
Tension headache, chronic or episodic tension-type headache, cephalodynia, cephalalgia, cephalea, cerebralgia, encephalalgia, encephalodynia, cervicogenic headache (formerly muscle tension headache). For migraine see p. 275.

> Quoted from BMJ Clinical Evidence (see p. 16) where availabe

DEFINITION
The 1988 International Headache Society criteria for chronic tension-type headache are headaches on 15 or more days a month (180 days/year) for at least 6 months; pain that is bilateral, pressing or tightening in quality, of mild or moderate intensity, which does not prohibit activities and is not aggravated by routine physical activity; presence of no more than one additional clinical feature (nausea, photophobia or phonophobia) and no vomiting. Episodic tension-type headache can last for 30 minutes to 7 days and occurs for fewer than 180 days a year.

> Information on the use of CAM by patients with the condition

CAM USAGE
Thirty-two per cent of Americans with headache have used CAM in the previous 12 months, most frequently relaxation and chiropractic.[1] Many other therapies are also popular, especially herbal medicine, homeopathy, acupuncture and reflexology.

RELATED CONDITIONS
Migraine (see p. 275).

> An evidence-based summary of the data relating to the effectiveness of different forms of CAM for the condition. Priority is given to systematic reviews/meta-analyses and RCTs. Treatments are listed in alpabetical order (except Other therapies; see below)

CLINICAL EVIDENCE
A Cochrane review[2] found encouraging evidence for spinal manipulation, therapeutic touch, electrotherapy and transcutaneous electrical nerve stimulation (TENS) for treating tension-type headaches. It also noted that spinal manipulation and exercise are promising for cervicogenic headache.

ACUPUNCTURE
Three good-quality studies were included in a systematic review.[3] It concluded that acupuncture might have a role to play in idiopathic headache but the current evidence was insufficient to make firm recommendations. Since then, results of RCTs have been mixed. Three placebo-controlled RCTs ($n = 69$, $n = 37$ and $n = 50$) suggested positive effects of acupuncture on pain or quality of life.[4–6]

> Brief overview of the evidence relating to a treatment for the condition

AUTOGENIC TRAINING
In one study, 146 patients with tension headache were randomised to autogenic training, hypnotherapy or waiting list control.[13] Autogenic training (but not hypnotherapy) was better than waiting list for symptom control.

BIOFEEDBACK
A systematic review[14] (Box 5.21) concluded that both relaxation and biofeedback (either on its own or in combination with relaxation) were superior to no treatment and to placebo therapy. Subsequent RCTs[15–17] (Table 5.16) tested biofeedback in adolescents and adults, mainly in comparison with relaxation. The majority found that biofeedback was more effective.

EXERCISE
A small ($n = 53$) RCT suggested that workplace physical exercise reduces headaches during a 4-week period.[20]

HERBAL MEDICINE
In an RCT involving 41 adults with a history of tension headache, 164 acute headache episodes were treated with either peppermint oil or placebo oil locally and either paracetamol (acetaminophen) or placebo tablet orally.[21] Peppermint oil was superior to placebo and not different from the analgesic drug in reducing headache.

HOMEOPATHY
One rigorous RCT with 98 subjects included patients with tension-type headache as well as those with migraine and found no benefit from 12 weeks of individualised homeopathy compared with placebo.[23] The results were similar after 1 year of follow-up.[24]

HYPNOTHERAPY
Like other forms of therapy involving regular relaxation, self-hypnosis appears to be more effective than waiting list control.[25]

Summary details of any authoritative systematic review/meta-analysis on a subject

Optional standardised tables of RCTs.
NB When several exist, only a few examples appear in the table, selected for their rigour or clinical relevance

264 PAIN SYNDROMES

Box 5.21 *Meta-analysis: biofeedback and relaxation for headache*[14]

- All prospective investigations, including uncontrolled studies
- Seventy-eight studies were included in the review, involving 2866 patients
- Mean (SD) effect size from 29 studies of EMG biofeedback was 47% (26%)
- Mean (SD) effect size from 38 studies of relaxation was 36% (20%)
- For comparison, mean (SD) effect size from pharmacological treatment was 39% (23%) and for placebo treatment was 20% (38%)
- **Conclusion**: biofeedback is likely to be an effective option for headache

Table 5.15 **Parallel-arm RCTs of biofeedback for headache**

Reference	Sample size	Interventions (regimen)	Result	Comment
Arena[15]	26	(A) Frontal EMG biofeedback [12 sessions] (B) Trapezius EMG biofeedback [12 sessions] (C) Relaxation [seven sessions]	B better than A or C at 3 months	
Bussone[16]	35	(A) Biofeedback relaxation [10 sessions in 5 weeks] (B) Relaxation placebo	A better than B at 1 year	Adolescents
Kroner-Herwig[17]	50	(A) Biofeedback [12 30-minute sessions in 6 weeks] (B) Relaxation [six 1-hour sessions in 6 weeks] (C) Untreated control	No difference between A and B. Both better than C for some outcomes	Children; parental involvement had no influence

However, it is not clear whether it is superior to other forms of relaxation. Several trials have compared different combinations of therapies including hypnotherapy with various control interventions.[13,26] Subjects who are highly hypnotisable tend to show a greater reduction of headaches than those who are less easily hypnotised.[13]

RELAXATION

A systematic review[14] of biofeedback and relaxation (Box 5.21) concluded that relaxation is effective, with a mean effect size of 36%. In children and adolescents, RCTs indicate that relaxation has a positive effect on tension headache, though the size of the effect is often modest. More than two-thirds of the children in one study ($n = 26$) recorded at least 50% improvement at follow-up after 6 months, compared with only a quarter of controls.[27]

SPINAL MANIPULATION

The most recent and authoritative systematic review[30] of spinal manipulation found that, because of the small number and poor quality of the primary data, it is not possible to draw valid conclusions about the effectiveness of this approach (Box 5.22). An independent research group reached similar conclusions regarding both spinal manipulation and mobilisation.[31]

OTHER THERAPIES

Cranial electrotherapy applies a high-frequency, low-intensity current transcranially. It was found to be more effective in treating acute headache than placebo in a multicentre RCT of 100 patients, reducing headache scores by 35% after 20 minutes compared with 18% in the placebo group.[32]

Imagery was used as an adjunct to standard medical treatment in an RCT of 260 adults with chronic tension headache with or without migraine.[33] The intervention group received an imagery tape to listen to every day for 1 month and controls received standard medical treatment alone. Imagery was superior in global assessment and some quality of life measures.

HEADACHE **265**

Box 5.22 *Systematic review: spinal manipulation for tension-type headache*[30]

- Four RCTs were included
- Three studies were of chiropractic, one of osteopathic techniques
- Overall methodological quality was poor
- Best evidence synthesis generated no convincing evidence for spinal manipulation
- Few adverse events were reported
- **Conclusion**: the evidence is insufficient

OVERALL RECOMMENDATION

The evidence is not convincing that any particular CAM therapy is more effective than placebo in preventing tension headaches. However, in the absence of genuinely safe and effective conventional preventive measures, patients may benefit from treatments involving relaxation. Relaxation in various forms, including muscular and mental relaxation, hypnotherapy and autogenic training, is simple, relatively safe and beneficial compared with no treatment. The addition of biofeedback may increase the benefit compared with simple relaxation alone. In the treatment of acute headache, preliminary evidence supports the use of tiger balm or peppermint oil locally, and possibly electrotherapy. It seems unlikely, however, that these options are superior to conventional treatments.

> An evidence-based judgement evaluating the benefits and risks of CAM for the condition in relation to conventional treatments. NB A lack of compelling evidence is not the same as ineffectiveness

Table 5.16 **Summary of clinical evidence for headache**

Treatment	Weight of evidence	Direction of evidence	Serious safety concerns
Acupuncture	OO	→	Yes (see 96)
Autogenic training	O	↗	Yes (see 106)
Biofeedback	OOO	↗	No (see 110)
Herbal medicine			
Peppermint oil (local)	O	↑	Yes (see 209)
Tiger balm (local)	O	↗	Yes (see 4)
Homeopathy	O	↓	No (see 124)
Hypnotherapy	OO	↗	Yes (see 130)
Relaxation	OO	↗	No (see 158)
Spinal manipulation	OO	→	Yes (see 112)

> For each treatment, the totality of available evidence is assessed and presented according to three criteria: 1) weight of evidence; 2) direction of evidence; 3) serious safety concerns (see p. 5 for explanations)

REFERENCES

1. Eisenberg DM, Davis R, Ettner SL, Appel S, Wilkey S, Rompay MV. Trends in alternative medicine use in the United States, 1990–1997. JAMA 1998;280:1569–1575

2. Bronfort G, Nilsson N, Haas M, Evans R, Goldsmith CH, Assendelft WJJ, Bouter LM. Non-invasive treatments for chronic/recurrent headache. The Cochrane Database of Systematic Reviews 2004, Issue 3. Art No.: CD001878

SIGNIFICANCE LEVELS

When reporting research results, only differences that are statistically significant ($P < 0.05$) are mentioned; P values and the term 'significant' are omitted for conciseness.

WEIGHT OF EVIDENCE

The weight of the evidence refers to the level of confidence (see p. 4) that can be placed on it. There are three discrete categories of weight:

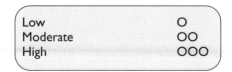

The judgement of weight is based on a combination of three largely independent factors:

● the level of evidence (the highest level being systematic review/meta-analysis, followed by randomised clinical trial, controlled clinical trial and uncontrolled study)
● the methodological quality of the investigations (the validity and reliability of the studies)
● the volume of information (the number of studies and their sample sizes).

Judgements take into account all three of these dimensions of weight. Therefore a treatment for which volume and level are high (e.g. a meta-analysis of 50 studies) will not necessarily receive a high weight if the quality is low (e.g. methodologically flawed studies). Similarly, even if quality and level are high (e.g. a rigorous randomised clinical trial), weight can only be considered low if there is a low volume of evidence (only a single trial).

DIRECTION OF EVIDENCE

The direction of the evidence refers to the collective positive or negative outcome of the studies for that treatment. Direction can be reported in one of five ways:

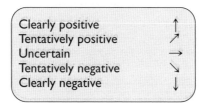

Direction is largely judged independently of weight of evidence. The reader must interpret the direction of the evidence in the light of its weight. For example, a clearly positive result based on evidence with low weight (e.g. a single, small, non-randomised trial) may not be as informative as a tentatively positive finding backed by a body of evidence with high weight (e.g. a systematic review of randomised clinical trials).

SERIOUS SAFETY CONCERNS

Cases where a treatment has been, or may potentially be, associated with life-threatening consequences, hospitalisation or sustained harm, are indicated even if rare.

● 'No' indicates that reports of serious events were not located and are considered unlikely.
● 'Yes' indicates that serious events have been reported or are considered possible.

Whenever possible, page references are provided for the treatment's own chapter or relevant table. In some cases, information is not available about safety. The general principle is to err on the side of caution; so when in doubt, a treatment is marked 'Yes'. This applies to all herbs and some supplements (see *Methods*, p. 5).

NB. It is imperative that the reader refers to the treatment chapter or table. Even where a treatment is marked 'No', there may be contraindications and precautions that, if ignored, could have potentially serious consequences.

Even where a therapy is not associated with serious complications, indirect risks may exist and could have serious consequences. CAM practitioners may not be medically qualified and should not therefore be expected to have competence in orthodox medical diagnostics or management.

Many of the reported serious adverse events are avoidable through good clinical practice. For a general discussion of CAM safety, see p. 24.

BIBLIOGRAPHY OF MAIN REFERENCE SOURCES

SECTION 3 THERAPIES

Barnett H. The Which? guide to complementary therapies. London: Which?; 2002

Callahan D, ed. The role of complementary and alternative medicine. Washington: Georgetown University Press; 2002

Freeman L. Mosby's complementary and alternative medicine evidence-based approach. St Louis: Mosby; 2001

Fugh-Berman A. Alternative medicine: what works. Tucson: Odonian; 1996

Jonas WB, Levin JS, eds. Essentials of complementary and alternative medicine. Baltimore: Lippincott Williams and Wilkins; 1999

Kelner MJ, Wellman B, Saks M, eds. Complementary and alternative medicine: challenge and change. Reading: Harwood Academic Publishers; 2000

Lewith G, Jonas WB, Walach H. Clinical research in complementary therapies. Edinburgh: Churchill Livingstone; 2001

MacBeckner W, Berman BM. Complementary therapies on the internet. St Louis: Churchill Livingstone, USA; 2003

Micozzi, MS. Fundamentals of complementary and alternative medicine. Edinburgh: Churchill Livingstone; 2000

Novey DW, ed. Clinician's complete reference to complementary and alternative medicine. St Louis: Mosby; 2000

Peters D, Woodham A. The complete guide to integrated medicine: the best of complementary and conventional care. New York: Dorling Kindersley; 2000

Schimmel KC, ed. Lehrbuch der Naturheilverfahren. Stuttgart: Hippokrates; 1990

Spencer JW, Jacobs J. Complementary and alternative medicine: an evidence-based approach, 2nd edn. St Louis: Mosby; 2003

Stone J. An ethical framework for complementary and alternative therapies. London: Routledge; 2002

Yuan CS, Bieber EJ. Textbook of complementary and alternative medicine. London: Parthenon; 2003

Zollman C, Vickers A. ABC of complementary medicine. London: BMJ Books; 2000

SECTION 4 HERBAL AND NON-HERBAL MEDICINES

Barnes J, Anderson LA, Phillipson JD. Herbal medicines, 2nd edn. London: Pharmaceutical Press; 2002

Basch E, Ulbricht C E, eds. Natural standard herb and supplement handbook: the clinical bottom line. St Louis: Elsevier Mosby; 2005

Blumenthal M, ed. The ABC clinical guide to herbs. Austin: American Botanical Council; 2003

Blumenthal M, Goldberg A, Brinckmann J, eds. Herbal medicine: expanded commission E monographs. Austin: American Botanical Council; 2000

Boon H, Smith M. The botanical pharmacy. Kingston: Quarry Press; 1999

Boon H, Smith M. The complete natural medicine guide to the 50 most common medicinal herbs. Toronto: Robert Rose; 2004

Bratman S, Gitman AM. Mosby's handbook of herbs and supplements and their therapeutic uses. St Louis: Mosby; 2003

Braun L, Cohen M. Herbs and natural supplements. An evidence-based guide. Sydney: Elsevier; 2005

Brinker F. Herb contraindications and drug interactions. Sandy: Eclectic Medical Publications; 1998

Capasso F, Gaginella TS, Grandolini G, Izzo AA. Phytotherapy: a quick reference to herbal medicine. Berlin: Springer-Verlag; 2003

Cupp MJ. Toxicology and clinical pharmacology of herbal products. Totowa, NJ: Humana Press; 2000

Dukes MNG, Aronson JK, eds. Meyler's side effects of drugs, 14th edn. Amsterdam: Elsevier; 2000

Ernst E. Herb–drug interactions – an update. Perfusion 2003;16:175–194

Fetrow C, Avila J. The complete guide to herbal medicines. Springhouse: Springhouse Corporation; 2000.

Fetrow CW, Avila JR. Professional's handbook of complementary and alternative medicines. Springhouse, PA: Springhouse; 1999

Fugh-Berman A. Herb–drug interactions. Lancet 2000;355:134–138

Fugh-Berman A. The 5-minute herb and dietary supplement consult. Philadelphia: Lippincott Williams & Wilkins; 2003

Hänsel R, Keller K, Rimpler H, Schneider G. Hagers Handbuch der pharmazeutischen Praxis. Berlin: Springer; 1994

Harkness R, Bratman S. Mosby's handbook of drug–herb and drug–supplement interactions. St Louis: Mosby; 2003

Hildebrandt H, ed. Pschyrembel Wörterbuch Naturheilkunde und alternative Heilverfahren. Berlin: deGruyter; 1996

Lininger SW, ed. A–Z guide to drug–herb–vitamin interactions. Rocklin; CA: Prima; 1999

Mahady GB, Fong HHS, Farnsworth NR. Botanical, dietary supplements: quality, safety and efficacy. Rotterdam: AA Balkema Publishers; 2001

Mason P. Dietary supplements, 2nd edn. London: Pharmaceutical Press; 2001. Available online: http://www.medicinescomplete.com/mc/

Meletis CD, Jacobs T. Interactions between drugs and natural medicines. Sandy: Eclectic Medical Publications; 1999

Murray MT. Encyclopedia of nutritional supplements. Rocklin: Prima; 1996

Jellin JM, ed. Natural Medicines Comprehensive Database. Available online: www.naturaldatabase.com

Natural Standard Database. Available online: www.naturalstandard.com

Rapport L, Lockwood B. Nutraceuticals. London: Pharmaceutical Press; 2002

Reynolds Sweetman SJEF, ed. Martindale: the complete drug reference. Martindale: the extra pharmacopoeia. London: Pharmaceutical Press; 2005. Available online: http://www.medicinescomplete.com/mc/

Ross IA. Medicinal plants of the world, Vol. 2. Totowa, NJ: Humana Press; 2001

Rotblatt M, Ziment I. Evidence-based herbal medicine. Philadelphia: Hanley & Belfus; 2002

Royal Pharmaceutical Society of Great Britain, ed. British national formulary. London: Pharmaceutical Press; 2005. Available online: http://www.medicinescomplete.com/mc/

Schulz V, Hänsel R, Blumenthal M, Tyler VE. Rational phytotherapy: a reference guide for physicians and pharmacists, 5th edn. Berlin: Springer Verlag; 2004

Skidmore-Roth L. Mosby's handbook of herbs & natural supplements. St Louis: Mosby; 2001

Stockley IH, ed. Stockley's interaction alert. London: Pharmaceutical Press; 2005. Available online: http://www.medicinescomplete.com/mc/

Ulbricht CE, Basch E, eds. Natural standard herb and supplement reference: evidence-based clinical reviews. St Louis: Elsevier Mosby; 2005

USDA, ARS, National Genetic Resources Program. Germplasm Resources Information Network (GRIN) Online Database. Beltsville, MD: National Germplasm Resources Laboratory. Available online: http://www.ars-grin.gov2/cgi-bin/npgs/html/index.pl

Wichtl M, ed. Herbal drugs and phytopharmaceuticals, 3rd edn. Stuttgart: Medpharm Scientific Publishers; 2004

World Health Organization. Monographs on selected medicinal plants. Geneva: WHO; 1999

SECTION 5 PAIN SYNDROMES

Banks C, Mackrodt T. Chronic pain management. London: Whurr; 2005

British Medical Journal. Clinical evidence. British Medical Journal Publishing Group; 2005. Available online: http://www.clinicalevidence.com

Gatchel R. Clinical essentials of pain management. Philadelphia: American College of Physicians; 2005

Holdcroft A, Jaggar S. Core topics in pain. Cambridge: Cambridge University Press; 2005

Marcus DA. Chronic pain: a primary care guide to practical management. Totowa, NJ: Humana Press; 2005

McCarberg B, Passik SD. Expert guide to pain management. Philadelphia: American College of Physicians; 2005

McMahon SB, Koltzenburg M, eds. Wall and Melzack's textbook of pain, 5th edn. Churchill Livingstone; 2006

Raja SN, Molloy RE, Liu S, Fishman SM, Benzon HT. Essentials of pain medicine and regional anesthesia. Edinburgh: Churchill Livingstone; 2004

Ross E. Pain management. Philadelphia: Hanley & Belfus; 2004

Stannard C, Booth S. Pain. Edinburgh: Churchill Livingstone; 2004

Stedman T. Stedman's medical dictionary, 27th edn. Baltimore: Williams and Wilkins; 2003

Wallace MS, Staats PS. Pain medicine and management; just the facts. New York: McGraw-Hill; 2005

General topics

COMPLEMENTARY AND ALTERNATIVE MEDICINE – AN OVERVIEW

PREVALENCE

The understanding of what precisely constitutes complementary and alternative medicine (CAM) differs considerably between countries. Not surprisingly then, there are many definitions of CAM (Table 2.1). As the result of different historical developments and traditions, therapies such as herbal medicine, hydrotherapy and massage are firmly established in the mainstream medicine of many continental European countries, while they are often classified as CAM elsewhere. Regardless of these national differences, there is consensus that the use of and demand for CAM is high (Table 2.2) and most experts agree that it is increasing.

REASONS FOR HIGH PREVALENCE

EXPLANATIONS FOR CAM USE

Furnham[2] summarised the main hypotheses relating to why people use CAM (Box 2.1). The 'push' factors include dissatisfaction with or outright rejection of orthodox medicine through

Table 2.1 **A selection of currently used definitions of CAM**

Definition	Source
'A group of diverse medical and health-care systems, practices and products that are not presently considered to be part of conventional medicine.'	National Center of Complementary and Alternative Medicine, USA http://nccam.nih.gov/health/whatiscam/#1
'A broad set of health-care practices that are not part of a country's own tradition and not integrated into the dominant health-care system. Other terms sometimes used to describe these health-care practices include "natural medicine", "non-conventional medicine" and "holistic medicine".'	World Health Organization. Guidelines on developing consumer information on proper use of traditional, complementary and alternative medicine. Geneva: World Health Organization; 2004:xiii
'Refers to a group of therapeutic and diagnostic disciplines that exist largely outside the institutions where conventional health care is taught and provided.'	Zollman C, Vickers A. What is complementary medicine? BMJ 1999;319:693–696
'A broad domain of healing resources that encompasses all health systems, modalities and practices and their accompanying theories and beliefs, other than those intrinsic to the politically dominant health systems of a particular society or culture in a given historical period.'	Cochrane Collaboration http://www.compmed.umm.edu/Cochrane/
'Diagnosis, treatment and/or prevention which complements mainstream medicine by contributing to a common whole, satisfying a demand not met by orthodoxy, or diversifying the conceptual framework of medicine.'	Ernst E, Resch KL, Mills S, Hill R, Mitchell A, Willoughby M, White A. Complementary medicine – a definition. Br J Gen Pract 1995;309:107–111

Table 2.2 **One-year prevalence of CAM in general population samples***

Country	Year of publication	Year of sampling	Sample n	Prevalence %
Australia	1996	1993	Random 3004	48.5
Canada	1997	1995	Representative 17,626	15
Finland	1993	1982	Random 1618	23
France	1990	1985	Representative 1000	49
Germany	2004	2002	Representative 1750	62.3
Hungary	2002	1999	2357	13
Israel	2004	2000	Representative 2505	10
Italy	2002	1997–99	Representative 70,898	15.6
Japan	2002	2001	Random 1000	76
United Kingdom	2004	2001	Representative 1794	10
United States	2004	2002	Representative 31,044	62 (incl prayer)

* Data extracted from Harris.[1]

Box 2.1 *Possible factors contributing to CAM use*

Push factors
- Dissatisfaction with orthodox medicine
  - ineffective
  - adverse effects
  - poor communication with doctor
  - insufficient time with doctor
  - waiting lists
- Rejection of orthodox medicine
  - anti-science or anti-establishment attitude
- Desperation
- Cost of private orthodox medical care

Pull factors
- Philosophical congruence
  - spiritual dimension
  - emphasis on holism
  - active role of patient
  - explanation intuitively acceptable
  - natural treatments
- Personal control over treatment
- Good relationship with therapist
  - on equal terms
  - time for discussion
  - allows for emotional factors
- Accessible
- Increased well-being

previous negative experiences or a general anti-establishment attitude. 'Pull' factors include compatibility between the philosophy of certain therapies and a patient's own beliefs and a greater sense of control over one's own treatment.

Three of these hypotheses were tested by Astin in a preliminary attempt to develop explanatory models that account for the increasing use of CAM.[3] He predicted that dissatisfaction with conventional care, need for personal control over treatment and philosophical congruence with own beliefs would distinguish CAM users from non-users.

THE PERSUASIVE APPEAL OF CAM

Persuaded for instance by the media,[4] or by past experience, many consumers are convinced that CAM is effective[5-8] and improves psychosocial functioning.[9] Kaptchuk & Eisenberg[10] suggest that certain fundamental premises of most forms of CAM contribute to its persuasive appeal. One of these is the perceived association of CAM with nature. It is inextricably linked with certain terminology: natural rather than artificial; pure versus synthetic; and organic as opposed to processed.[11] Natural is often somewhat naively equated with safe.[12] Another fundamental component of CAM is vitalism. The enhancement or balancing of 'life forces', '*qi*', 'psychic energy', etc. is central to many forms of CAM. For patients, there is an intuitive appeal in this non-invasive notion of healing from within. Many therapies have long intellectual traditions and sophisticated philosophies, with training involving many years of study of complex systems and concepts. This contributes to the credibility and authority of the scientific label. The science of CAM is less dependent on the principles of objectivity and clinical experimentation than positivist science. The approach tends to be person-centred, relying on observation, self-knowledge and human awareness. The language is one of unity and holism in contrast to the distant, reductionist terminology of normative science.[13] Human experience, rather than being marginalised, is the central element of CAM science. A further element in the appeal of CAM is spirituality. This bridges the gap between the domain of medical science, with its search for truth and strict causality, and the domain of religion, with its moral freedom and self-chosen values. CAM offers a satisfying unification of the physical and spiritual.[14]

UNDERLYING MOTIVES

Other proposed explanations for the use of CAM refer to underlying reasons rather than deliberate patient motives. One of these is that CAM users are essentially neurotic and therefore drawn towards the 'touchy-feely' approach of many therapies. However, this may be nothing more than a reflection of the nature of the conditions being treated. CAM practitioners often see patients with chronic or incurable disorders in whom the incidence of neurosis is likely to be high. Significant associations have also been found between CAM use and specific domains of personality, coping strategies and social support.[15] Patients with a better understanding of the workings of the human body might be attracted to CAM therapists because diagnosis and treatment involve more discussion and explanation than are offered by orthodox medical practitioners. This does not prove a causal relationship, however. Furthermore, better understanding of the human body may simply be a reflection of the higher levels of education that have been consistently reported for CAM users.

DIRECT INVESTIGATIONS OF PATIENT MOTIVES

Numerous surveys have investigated why patients use CAM and have suggested the following motives:

- incorporates mind, body and spirit
- desire to take control of own health
- desire for an effective treatment

- perception that their condition was not serious and did not require medical treatment
- belief that CAM is safe while drugs are dangerous
- perception of CAM as an effective and easily accessible option, compared with lack of confidence in, and barriers to, orthodox medical care
- following doctor's advice.

Patients who turned to CAM as a last resort could be clearly differentiated from those who embraced CAM for its compatibility with their own beliefs in a UK-based study.[16] Interview and questionnaire data from 38 patients attending a CAM centre suggested two discrete patient types. Those who sought CAM as a last resort because no conventional treatments had proved effective for their complaint had similar scores to the general population on locus of control. They also maintained faith in the principles of orthodox medicine and displayed little initial commitment to the values or philosophies of CAM. The other type of patients chose CAM because it matched their beliefs about health and illness. These individuals showed a greater internal locus of control and scepticism about orthodox methods, as well as commitment to CAM.

These notions were partly confirmed by an interview study of 46 Hawaiian breast cancer patients[16] and a survey of elderly US cardiac patients.[17] A strong theme from a study of young people with inflammatory bowel disease was the hope of receiving benefit from using CAM.[18]

THE ROLE OF THE THERAPEUTIC RELATIONSHIP

Sixty-eight per cent of patients reported a better relationship with the CAM practitioner than with their own general practitioner (GP), and this finding was not related to their commitment to CAM.[16] CAM practitioners were perceived as friendlier and more personal, treated the relationship more like a partnership and provided more time for the consultation. Satisfaction with the therapeutic encounter was also greater with CAM practitioners than GPs in a survey of arthritis sufferers in the UK,[19] although 'friendliness' was rated higher for GPs. Again, satisfaction with the time spent on the patient was higher with CAM practitioners, as it also was in a Spanish study of CAM use by patients with somatoform disorder.[20] The duration of CAM consultations is invariably longer than with orthodox medicine. A comparison of physicians using homeopathy with those practicing conventional medicine reported that the former spent more than twice as long on patient consultations.[21] As well as leading to greater satisfaction of patients, this may be one of the key factors in the success of CAM. A clinical trial of homeopathy for premenstrual syndrome reported a response rate of 47% in a pre-treatment placebo wash-out phase,[22] which the authors suggested may have been largely the result of the depth and intimacy of the homeopathic interview.

SHOPPING FOR HEALTH

Rather than replacing orthodox medical care, CAM usually serves as a substitute in some particular situations and as an adjunct in others, while being disregarded when not considered appropriate for the condition in question. This has led to CAM use being described as 'shopping for health'.[2] Rather than being specifically 'pushed' or 'pulled' towards CAM, patients simply perceive it as one of a range of treatment options available to them and exercise their freedom of choice accordingly. The desire to try all available options may be for some an attempt to leave no stone unturned as they become increasingly desperate for an effective treatment. However, for others, it may simply reflect opportunism, a desire for experimentation or what is aptly expressed in the advertising slogan 'because you are worth it'. The finding that CAM use is associated with higher levels of income may support the concept of CAM as a commodity for those that can afford it. Intriguingly, a strong positive

Box 2.2 *Reasons for not using or abandoning CAM*

Not using CAM
- Never considered it
- Not enough information
- Too expensive
- Satisfied with conventional treatment
- No belief in its effectiveness
- Doctor advised against it
- Religious/moral reasons
- Not available
- Too embarrassing

Terminating CAM use
- Not helpful
- No longer affordable
- Experienced adverse effects
- Doctor advised against it

correlation was reported between sale data of BMW cars (a possible measure of affluence) and the use of herbal remedies in the US and the UK.[23]

BARRIERS TO CAM

Why do some people choose not to use CAM? Cost and lack of information were the most common barriers stated, with fear of harm, lack of time and lack of access also cited.[24–26] Only a small percentage reported fear of their physician's disapproval as a barrier. Studies of US patients suggested intriguing reasons for abandoning or not using CAM[27,28] (Box 2.2).

IMPORTANT SAFETY ISSUES

Throughout this book we place much emphasis on safety issues. In particular, we have alerted the reader to the risks associated with specific therapies. Direct toxicity, interactions, contraindications, etc. have therefore been given a prominent place. The following discussion is aimed at more general aspects of the safety issues related to CAM.

PROBLEMS WITH UNREGULATED FOOD SUPPLEMENTS

In many countries, herbal medicinal products (HMPs) are marketed as food supplements. Rigorous regulation comparable to the pharmaceutical sector therefore does not apply. In particular, the necessity for a manufacturer to demonstrate safety and quality of the marketed product is far less. In Europe, this situation will change through the 'EU Traditional Use Directive' but, for the near future, unlicensed HMPs will remain on most national markets.[29,30]

A particular concern has been the quality of unlicensed HMPs. Table 2.3 shows some of the contaminants that have been found in HMPs and that have obvious safety implications. Contamination of Asian and other HMPs with heavy metals and other toxins is a continuous issue in many parts of the world.[31–35] Adulteration of HMPs with non-declared herbs or conventional drugs is a further problem with unregulated HMPs of dubious quality. It pertains in particular to Asian HMPs[36] and is a problem that is regularly reported from many regions.[37]

Underdosing is another problem with HMPs. Whenever herbal food supplements from the US market are analysed by independent experts, the findings reveal that, in a substantial

Table 2.3 **Contaminants that have been found in herbal medicines**

Type of contaminant	Examples
Micro-organisms	*Staphylococcus aureus*, *Escherichia coli* (certain strains), *Salmonella*, *Shigella*, *Pseudomonas aeruginosa*
Microbial toxins	Bacterial endotoxins, aflatoxins
Pesticides, herbicides	Chlorinated pesticides (e.g. DDT, DDE, HCH-isomers, HCB, aldrin, dieldrin, heptachlor), organic phosphates, carbamate insecticides and herbicides, dithiocarbamate fungicides, triazine, herbicides
Fumigation agents	Ethylene oxide, methyl bromide, phosphine
Radioactivity	^{134}Cs, ^{137}Cs, ^{103}Ru, ^{131}I, ^{90}Sr
Heavy metals	Lead, cadmium, mercury, arsenic

proportion of them, the active ingredient content differs marginally from label claims.[38] When 880 HMPs were purchased in the US, 37% of them proved to be not consistent with the information on the label or the label information was insufficient.[39]

PROBLEMS CAUSED BY CONVENTIONAL PROVIDERS OF HEALTH CARE

Numerous studies show that patients fail to inform their physician of their CAM use.[40–42] This is not merely the fault of patients but can also be seen as a failure of doctors who tend to omit asking about CAM use or documenting CAM use in patients' records.[43–45] It is self-evident that such behaviour can increase the risk of CAM use.

PROBLEMS CAUSED BY UNREGULATED PROVIDERS OF CAM

In most countries, the majority of CAM providers are not medically qualified. Most of these are probably adequately trained to do what they do. However, in the absence of adequate regulations, some providers will not adhere to adequate standards of clinical practice. There is little systematic research into the question of how frequently this causes health problems. Preliminary data suggest that there is sufficient reason for concern.[46]

Some CAM providers may delay or hinder access to potentially life-saving conventional treatment.[47,48] The best-researched example in this respect is probably the advice of some CAM providers against immunisation of any type.[49,50] Similar problems relate to CAM providers not screening for contraindications to treatment. If, for instance, a bleeding abnormality or advanced osteoporosis is a contraindication against chiropractic manipulation, how will the average chiropractor reliably exclude such abnormalities before treating a new patient?

Changing or omitting prescribed treatments might be another problem. A significant proportion of CAM providers seem to be doing this;[51] 3% of non-medically trained acupuncturists in the UK advise their patients to alter prescribed treatments.[52]

Some CAM providers may also be unable to adequately diagnose medical problems while patients are in their care. For instance, one could imagine a patient being treated for a headache that reveals increasingly clearer signs of a sinister underlying cause. If these signs are missed, valuable time for adequate, perhaps life-saving, treatment could be lost.

Another problem could be the use of diagnostic techniques that are either in themselves not risk-free or that are invalid. An example for the first scenario is the overt overuse of X-ray diagnosis by some chiropractors.[53] An example of the second scenario is the use of iridology, which would lead to a false-negative or false-positive diagnosis.[54]

SECTION TWO

A similar problem is the quality of the advice provided to consumers by health-food stores or other outlets of CAM. Surveys have repeatedly shown that such recommendations can border on the irresponsible.[55,56] Worryingly, many websites on CAM also issue information which, if followed, has the potential to harm patients.[57]

A further risk associated with CAM might lie in the plethora of lay books on CAM now available in every high-street bookshop. This lay literature has the potential to put the health of the reader at risk if the advice from these books is adhered to by seriously ill individuals.[58] A significant proportion of the UK daily press also reports about CAM in a much more favourable tone than about mainstream medicine.[59] This could lead to distrust in the latter, unjustified trust in the former or both and thus put the health of CAM users at risk. These concerns relate to the (lack of) competence or responsibility of CAM providers, sales people or authors.

PROBLEMS WITH USERS OF CAM

The attitudes of the consumer towards CAM may constitute risks that are independent of CAM providers. For instance, when users of HMPs were interviewed about their behaviour vis-à-vis an adverse effect of a herbal versus a synthetic 'over-the-counter' drug, the results suggested that about one-quarter would consult their doctor for a serious adverse effect of conventional medication while less than 1% would do the same in relation to a herbal remedy.[60] Other studies suggest that the majority of CAM users employ CAM with insufficient information.[61] Consumers want and need guidance on CAM. Survey data suggest that, foremost, they want information on the effectiveness and safety of treatments and that they would prefer it in a brochure rather than from a website.[62] It is thus very disappointing that even government-sponsored guides for CAM users fail to provide such information.[63]

IMPORTANT COST ISSUES

Even though estimates vary considerably as to the money spent on CAM, most experts agree that CAM is not cheap. Table 2.4 summarises recent survey data and highlights the heterogeneity of the information derived from such sources.[64–77]

A US analysis of insurance claims demonstrated that 'billed amounts for alternative services were about 2% of the overall medical bills for cancer patients'.[78] Studies from several countries suggest that CAM use is associated with higher rates of consultations in conventional medicine.[79–82] This implies that CAM use is unlikely to contribute to any overall cost savings. In other settings, however, CAM seems to be employed as a substitute for medical care.[83–85] Furthermore, it has been suggested that CAM use may save money on the costs of conventional drugs.[86] Much of the future of CAM will depend on the question of whether it saves money or causes extra expenditure. Yet CAM researchers have been slow to face the challenge of conducting rigorous cost analyses.

This is perhaps understandable – such projects can be exceedingly complex and are usually expensive (Table 2.4). Considering the fact that, in most countries, CAM has been paid for privately by its users,[64–88] there may not be a strong incentive for governments to change this situation. Thus, cost evaluations are difficult to fund through official channels. A further important complication is that the results of cost-evaluation studies, even if performed to a high standard, may not be transferable from one health-care system to another.

EXAMPLES OF RECENT STUDIES

Notwithstanding such formidable obstacles, several informative studies have recently emerged (Table 2.5).[89–96] This list serves as a reminder that cost evaluations typically address distinctly different research questions and use a range of research tools. It is therefore not surprising that their results fail to generate a uniform overall picture as to the question of whether CAM saves money or causes extra expenditure.

Table 2.4 **Recent estimates of costs associated with CAM use in defined populations**

First author and reference	Country	Cost included	Comment
Ernst[64]	UK	CAM users spent an average of £163 per year on CAM. This extrapolates to £1.6 billion per year for CAM use in the UK	Cost data were available only for 11% of the sample
Thomas[65]	UK	Out-of-pocket expenditure for acupuncture, chiropractic, homeopathy, hypnotherapy, herbalism, osteopathy was £450 million (£108 per user) per year	About 10% of the cost was paid for by the NHS
Harris[66]	UK	Out-of-pocket cost for CAM practitioners and money spent by cancer patients was £648 per patient per year	Large sample from Wales (which might not be representative for all of the UK)
Ramsey[67]	US	Older patients with osteoarthritis spent US$1127 per year on CAM	They spent a similar amount, US$1148, for orthodox therapies
Patterson[68]	US	Cancer patients spent an average of US$68 per year on CAM	356 patients with colon, breast or prostate cancer; range of expenditure was large (US$4–14,659)
Wasner[69]	Germany	Patients with amyotrophic lateral sclerosis spent an average of €4000 per year on CAM	Small sample ($n = 92$); most of the costs were reimbursed by insurance schemes
Marstedt[70]	Germany	Cost of 20,928 CAM interventions by physicians paid by one health insurer was DM6 million	Amount for CAM is ~1/7 of total medical cost
Schäfer[71]	Germany	Allergy patients spent an average of €205 for a complete series of CAM treatments	Different treatments had different average costs: bioresonance, €409; acupuncture, €363; homeopathy, €192; autologous blood therapy, €77
McKenzie[72]	Canada	Elderly Canadians spent an average of C$226 per year on vitamins, minerals and herbals	Small sample ($n = 128$)
Shenfield[73]	Australia	On average A$120 per year was spent on CAM for asthmatic children. Those who consulted CAM providers spent A$480 per year	Small sample ($n = 174$)

table continues

Yamashita[74]	Japan	A random sample of the population ($n = 1000$) spent Yen 19,080 per person annually on CAM	Costs were ~50% of costs for orthodox health care
Chrystal[75]	New Zealand	Cancer patients spent an average of NZ$102 on CAM (including visits and travel)	Small sample ($n = 200$), patients suffered from various types of cancer
Nielsen[76]	Denmark	88% of medical patients spent less than DKK500 per month; 55% spent less than DKK100 and 12% spent more than DKK500 per month	No group average supplied
Pucci[77]	Italy	Out-of-pocket expenditure for CAM by outpatients with multiple sclerosis was €483 per patient per year	Small sample ($n = 109$)

Table 2.5 **Examples of recent cost evaluations**

First author and reference	Country	Research question	Main result
Kominski[89]	US	Comparison of total outpatient costs of various approaches for treating back pain	Chiropractic care was 52% more expensive than medical care
UK BEAM trial[90]	UK	Assess cost-effectiveness of adding spinal manipulation, exercise classes, or manipulation followed by exercise to best care for back pain	Spinal manipulation is a cost-effective addition
Wonderling[91]	UK	Evaluate cost-effectiveness of acupuncture for chronic headache	Total 1-year costs were higher for acupuncture than standard care but mean health gain was greater with acupuncture. One QALY equalled £9180
Williams[92]	UK	Assessment of cost-utility of primary-care osteopathy for subacute back pain	Osteopathy plus usual GP care was more expensive but also more effective than GP care alone
Phelan[93]	US	Estimate cost from insurance database for musculoskeletal injuries	Costs associated with chiropractic care were lower than medical care; both of thesewere lower than combined care
Legorreta[94]	US	Retrospective comparison of expenditure of individuals with and without insurance cover for chiropractic care	Members with chiropractic insurance cover had lower total health-care expenditure (US$1463 vs US$1671 per member per year)

table continues

Korthals-de Bos[95]	Netherlands	Evaluation of cost-effectiveness of three approaches to neck pain care	Spinal manipulation is more cost-effective than physiotherapy or care by GPs
Stano[96]	US	Compare 1-year costs for back pain treated either medically or by chiropractors	Average costs of chiropractic were higher than for medical care (US$214 vs US$123)

Table 2.6 **Systematic reviews of cost evaluations**

First author	n	Type of studies included	Conclusion	Comment
White[97]	34	Any type of cost evaluation, including retrospective studies	Retrospective studies suggested savings, prospective studies suggested extra cost	Need for more rigorous studies was identified
Kernick[98]	5	Controlled trials of manipulation for back pain with basic economic evaluation	No clear indication that manipulation was associated with less cost than other treatments	Not strictly speaking a systematic review
Hulme[99]	19	Any form of cost evaluation	No conclusion regarding cost. A CAM-sensitive approach is required	Aim was to see whether existing methodologies are adequate for CAM
Thompson Coon[100]	28	Any type of prospective economic analysis	No firm conclusions are possible	Data set included 27 cost-effectiveness analyses
Canter[101]	4	UK cost-effectiveness studies	CAM in the UK probably represents an additional cost	Very limited data restricted to acupuncture and spinal manipulation only

n = number of studies included.

SYSTEMATIC REVIEWS

Systematic reviews could in principle overcome this confusion. Several such projects have recently become available (Table 2.6).[97–101] Canter et al.[101] indicate that CAM in the UK, when subjected to proper cost-effectiveness analysis, does represent an additional health-care cost. For acupuncture[91] and spinal manipulation[90,92] the cost per quality of life adjusted years (QALY) relative to usual care is between £6000 and £10,000 depending on the exact assumptions made. Policy-makers must judge whether the typically small increases in quality of life achieved are worth the extra expenditure. Even though cost per QALY may compare favourably with other more expensive treatments, such as surgery, there is a ceiling to the incremental quality of life that can be achieved with any modality. It should also be noted that cost-effectiveness studies are typically less rigorous than randomised controlled trials and do not use blinding and placebo controls. The effectiveness side of the equation may therefore include a hefty slice of non-specific effect.

SECTION TWO

Collectively, these reviews fail to bring sufficient clarity. They do, however, emphasise two important points: we need better quality data and we must focus our research questions.

REFERENCES

1. Harris P, Rees R. The prevalence of complementary and alternative medicine use among the general population: a systematic review of the literature. Complement Ther Med 2000;8:88–96
2. Furnham A. Why do people choose and use complementary therapies? In: Ernst E, ed. Complementary medicine: an objective appraisal. Oxford: Butterworth Heinemann; 1996
3. Astin J. Why patients use alternative medicine. Results of a national survey. JAMA 1998;279: 1548–1553
4. Passalacqua R, Caminiti C, Salvagni S, Barni S, Beretta GD, Carlini P, Contu A, Di Costanzo F, Toscano L, Campione F. Effects of media information on cancer patients' opinions, feelings, decision-making process and physician-patient communication. Cancer 2004;100:1077–1084
5. Harnack LJ, Rydell SA, Stang J. Prevalence of use of herbal products by adults in the Minneapolis/St Paul, Minn, Metropolitan area. Mayo Clin Proc 2001;76:688–694
6. Tough SC, Johnston DW, Verhoef MJ, Arthur K, Bryant H. Complementary and alternative medicine use among colorectal cancer patients in Alberta, Canada. Altern Ther 2002;8:54–64
7. Ernst E, White A. The BBC survey of complementary medicine use in the UK. Complement Ther Med 2000;8:32–36
8. Hartel U, Volger E. Use and acceptance of classical natural and alternative medicine in Germany – findings of a representative population-based survey. [In German.] Forsch Komplementärmed Klass Naturheilkd 2004;11:327–334
9. Jacobs JWG, Kraaimaat FW, Bijlsma JWJ. Why do patients with rheumatoid arthritis use alternative treatments? Clin Rheumatol 2001;20:192–196
10. Kaptchuk TJ, Eisenberg DM. The persuasive appeal of alternative medicine. Ann Intern Med 1998;129:1061–1065
11. Clement YN, Williams AF, Aranda D, Chase R, Watson N, Mohammed R, Stubbs O, Williamson D. Medicinal herb use among asthmatic patients attending a specialty care facility in Trinidad. BMC Complement Altern Med 2005;5:3
12. Giveon SM, Liberman N, Klang S, Kahan E. Are people who use "natural drugs" aware of their potentially harmful side effects and reporting to family physician? Patient Educ Couns 2004; 53:5–11
13. Richardson J. What patients expect from complementary therapy: a qualitative study. Am J Public Health 2004;94:1049–1053
14. Feldman RH, Laura R. The use of complementary and alternative medicine practices among Australian university students. Complement Health Pract Rev 2004;9:173–179
15. Honda K, Jacobson JS. Use of complementary and alternative medicine among United States adults: the influences of personality, coping strategies, and social support. Prevent Med 2005; 40:46–53
16. Finnigan MD. The Centre for the Study of Complementary Medicine: an attempt to understand its popularity through psychological, demographic and operational criteria. Complement Med Res 1991;5:83–88
17. Ai AL, Bolling SF. The use of complementary and alternative therapies among middle-aged and older cardiac patients. Am J Med Qual 2002;17:21–27
18. Heuschkel R, Afzal N, Wuerth A, Zurakowski D, Leichtner A, Tolia V, Bousvaros A. Complementary medicine use in children and young adults with inflammatory bowel disease. Am J Gastroenterol 2002;97:382–388
19. Resch KL, Hill S, Ernst E. Use of complementary therapies by individuals with 'arthritis'. Clin Rheumatol 1997;16:391–395
20. Garcia-Campayo J, Sanz-Carrillo C. The use of alternative medicines by somatoform disorder patients in Spain. Br J Gen Pract 2000;50:487–488
21. Jacobs J, Chapman EH, Crothers D. Patient characteristics and practice patterns of physicians using homeopathy. Arch Fam Med 1998;7:537–540
22. Chapman EH, Angelica J, Spitalny G, Strauss M. Results of a study of the homeopathic treatment of PMS. J Am Inst Homeopath 1994;87:14–21

23. Ernst E, Furnham A. BMWs and complementary/alternative medicine. Focus Altern Complement Ther 2000;5:253–254

24. Dimmock S, Troughton PR, Bird HA. Factors predisposing to the resort of complementary therapies in patients with fibromyalgia. Clin Rheumatol 1996;15:478–482

25. Boon H, Brown JB, Gavin A, Kennard MA, Stewart M. Breast cancer survivors' perceptions of complementary/alternative medicine (CAM): making the decision to use or not to use. Qual Health Res 1999;9:639–653

26. Boon H, Stewart M, Kennard MA, Gray R, Sawka C, Brown JB, McWilliam C, Gavin A, Baron RA, Aaron D, Haines-Kamka T. Use of complementary/alternative medicine by breast cancer survivors in Ontario: prevalence and perceptions. J Clin Oncol 2000; 18:2515–2521

27. Lewis D, Paterson M, Beckerman S, Sandilands C. Attitudes towards integration of complementary and alternative medicine with hospital-based care. J Altern Complement Med 2001; 7:681–688

28. Nayak S, Matheis RJ, Schoenberger NE, Shiflett SC. Use of unconventional therapies by individuals with multiple sclerosis. Clin Rehabil 2003;17:181–191

29. Dawson W. Herbal medicines and the EU Directive. J R Coll Physicians Edinb 2005; 35:25–27

30. De Smet PAGM. Herbal medicine in Europe – relaxing regulatory standards. N Engl J Med 2005;352:1176–1178

31. Caldas ED, Machado LL. Cadmium, mercury and lead in medicinal herbs in Brazil. Food Chem Toxicol 2004;42:599–603

32. Schilling U, Mück R, Heidemann E. Bleiintoxikation durch Einnahme ayurvedischer Arzneimittel. Med Klin 2004;99:476–480

33. Saper RB, Kales SN, Paquin J, Burns MJ, Eisenberg DM, Davis RB, Phillips RS. Heavy metal content of Ayurvedic herbal medicine products. JAMA 2004;292:2868–2873

34. Araujo J, Beelen AP, Lewis MD. Lead poisoning associated with Ayurvedic medications – five States, 2000–2003. MMWR 2004;53:582–584

35. Raman P, Patino LC, Nair MG. Evaluation of metal and microbial contamination in botanical supplements. J Agric Food Chem 2004;52:7822–7827

36. Ernst E. Toxic heavy metals and undeclared drugs in Asian herbal medicines. Trends Pharmacol Sci 2002;23:136–139

37. Wooltorton E. Several Chinese herbal products may contain toxic aristolochic acid. CMAJ 2004;171:449

38. Gurely BJ, Gardner ST, Hubbord MA. Content versus label claims in ephedra-containing dietary supplements. Am J Health Syst Pharm 2000;57:1–7

39. Garrard J, Harms S, Eberly LE, Matiak A. Variations in product choices of frequently purchased herbs. Arch Intern Med 2003;163:2290–2295

40. Crowe S, Lyons B. Herbal medicine use by children presenting for ambulatory anesthesia and surgery. Pediatric Anesthesia 2004;14:916–919

41. Tan M, Uzun O, Akçay F. Trends in complementary and alternative medicine in Eastern Turkey. J Altern Complement Med 2004;10:861–865

42. Kim S, Hohrmann JL, Clark S, Munoz KN, Braun JE, Doshi A, Radeos MS, Camargo CA. A multicenter study of complementary and alternative medicine usage among ED patients. Acad Emerg Med 2005;12:377–380

43. Kales HC, Blow FC, Welsh DE, Mellow AM. Herbal products and other supplements: use by elderly veterans with depression and dementia and their caregivers. J Geriatr Psychiatr Neurol 2004;17:25–31

44. Cockayne NL, Duguid M, Shenfield GM. Health professionals rarely record history of complementary and alternative medicines. Br J Clin Pharmacol 2004;59:254–258

45. Glintborg B, Andersen SE, Spang-Hanssen E, Dalhoff K. Disregarded use of herbal medical products and dietary supplements among surgical and medical patients as estimated by home inspection and interview. Pharmacoepidemiol Drug Safety 2005;14:639–645

46. Schmidt K. The World Wide Web as a medical information source for Internet users – benefits and boundaries. Focus Altern Complement Ther 2004;9:187–189

47. Coppes MJ, Anderson RA, Egeler RM, Wolff JEA. Alternative therapies for the treatment of childhood cancer. N Engl J Med 1998;339:846

48. Oneschuk D, Bruera E. The potential dangers of complementary therapy use in a patient with cancer. J Palliat Care 1999;15:49–52

49. Ernst E. Attitude against immunisation within some branches of complementary medicine. Eur J Pediatr 1997;156:513–515

50. Schmidt K, Ernst E. Aspects of MMR. BMJ 2002;325:597

51. Moody GA, Eaden JA, Bhakta P, Sher K, Mayberry JF. The role of complementary medicine in European and Asian patients with inflammatory bowel disease. Public Health 1998;112: 269–271

52. MacPherson H, Scullion A, Thomas KJ, Walters S. Patient report of adverse events associated with acupuncture treatment: a prospective national survey. Qual Saf Health Care 2004;13:349–355

53. Ernst E. Chiropractors' use of X-rays. Br J Radiol 1998;71:249–251

54. Ernst E. Iridology – not useful and potentially harmful. Arch Ophthalmol 2000;118: 120–121

55. Mills E, Singh R, Ross C, Ernst E, Wilson K. Impact of federal safety advisories on health food store advice. J Gen Intern Med 2004;19:269–272

56. Buckner KD, Chavez ML, Raney EC, Stoehr JD. Health food stores' recommendations for nausea and migraines during pregnancy. Ann Pharmacother 2005;39:274–279

57. Schmidt K, Ernst E. Assessing websites on complementary and alternative medicine for cancer. Ann Oncol 2004;15:733–742

58. Ernst E, Armstrong NC. Lay books on complementary/alternative medicine: a risk factor for good health? Int J Risk Safety Med 1998;11:209–215

59. Ernst E, Weihmayr T. UK and German media differ over complementary medicine. BMJ 2000;321:707

60. Barnes J, Mills S, Abbot NC, Willoughby M, Ernst E. Different standards for reporting ADRs to herbal remedies. Br J Clin Pharmacol 1998;45:496–500

61. Hyodo I, Amano N, Eguchi K, Narabayashi M, Imanishi J, Hirai M, Nakano T, Takashima S. Nationwide survey on complementary and alternative medicine in cancer patients in Japan. J Clin Oncol 2005;23:2645–2654

62. Kuo GM, Hawley ST, Weiss LT, Balkrishnan R, Volk RJ. Factors associated with herbal use among urban multiethnic primary care patients: a cross-sectional survey. BMC Complement Altern Med 2004;4:18

63. The Prince of Wales's Foundation for Integrated Health. Complementary Health Care: a guide for patients. London: The Prince of Wales's Foundation for Integrated Health; 2005. Online. Available: http://www.fihealth.org.uk/fs_publications.html 10 May 2005.

64. Ernst E, White AR. The BBC survey of complementary medicine use in the UK. Complement Ther Med 2000;8:32–36

65. Thomas KS, Nicholl JP, Coleman P. Use and expenditure on complementary medicine in England – a population-based survey. Complement Ther Med 2001;9:2–11

66. Harris P, Finlay IG, Cook A, Thomas KJ, Hood K. Complementary and alternative medicine use by patients with cancer in Wales: a cross sectional survey. Complement Ther Med 2003; 11:249–253

67. Ramsey SD, Spencer AC, Topolski TD, Belza B, Patrick DL. Use of alternative therapies by older adults with osteoarthritis. Arthritis Rheum 2001;45:222–227

68. Patterson RE, Neuhouser ML, Hedderson MM, Schwartz SM, Standish LJ, Bowen DJ, Marshall LM. Types of alternative medicine use by patients with breast, colon, or prostate cancer: predictors, motives, and costs. J Altern Complement Med 2002;8: 477–485

69. Wasner M, Klier H, Borasio GD. The use of alternative medicine by patients with amyotrophic lateral sclerosis. J Neurol Sci 2001;191:151–154

70. Marstedt G, Moebus S. Inanspruchnahme alternativer Methoden in der Medizin. In: Gesundheitsberichterstattung des Bundes Heft 9. Berlin: Verlag Robert Koch-Institut; 2002:1–32

71. Schäfer T, Riehle A, Wichmann HE, Ring J. Alternative medicine in allergies – prevalence, patterns of use, and costs. Allergy 2002;57:694–700

72. McKenzie J, Keller HH. Vitamin–mineral supplementation and use of herbal preparations among community-living older adults. Can J Pub Health 2001;92:286–290

73. Shenfield G, Allen H. Survey of the use of complementary medicines and therapies in children with asthma. J Paediatr Child Health 2002;38:252–257

74. Yamashita H, Tsukayama H, Sugishita C. Popularity of complementary and alternative medicine in Japan: a telephone survey. Complement Ther Med 2002;10:84–93

75. Chrystal K, Allan S, Forgeson G, Isaacs R. The use of complementary/alternative medicine by cancer patients in a New Zealand regional cancer treatment centre. New Zealand Med J 2003;116:1–8

76. Nielsen J, Hansen MS, Fink P. Use of complementary therapy among internal medical inpatients. Prevalence, costs and association with mental disorders and physical diseases. J Psychosom Res 2003;55:547–552

77. Pucci E, Cartechini E, Taus C, Giuliani G. Why physicians need to look more closely at the use of complementary and alternative medicine by multiple sclerosis patients. Eur J Neurol 2004;11: 263–267

78. Lafferty WE, Bellas A, Baden AC, Tyree PT, Standish LJ, Patterson R. The use of complementary and alternative medical providers by insured cancer patients in Washington State. Cancer 2004; 100:1522–1530

79. Murray J, Shepherd S. Alternative or additional medicine? An exploratory study in general practice. Soc Sci Med 1993;37:983–988

80. Fautrel B, Adam V, St-Pierre Y, Joseph L, Clarke AE, Penrod JR. Use of complementary and alternative therapies by patients self-reporting arthritis or rheumatism: results from a nationwide Canadian survey. J Rheumatol 2002;29:2435–2441

81. Ni H, Simile C, Hardy AM. Utilization of complementary and alternative medicine by United States adults. Med Care 2002;40:353–358

82. Al-Windi A. Determinants of complementary alternative medicine (CAM) use. Complement Ther Med 2004;12:99–111

83. Wolsko PM, Eisenberg DM, Davis RB, Ettner SL, Phillips RS. Insurance coverage, medical conditions, and visits to alternative medicine providers. Arch Intern Med 2002; 162:281–287

84. Sharples FMC, van Haselen R, Fisher P. NHS patients' perspective on complementary medicine: a survey. Complement Ther Med 2003;11:243–248

85. Metz RD, Nelson CF, LaBrot T, Pelletier KR. Chiropractic care: is it substitution care or add-on care in corporate medical plans? J Occup Environ Med 2004;46:847–855

86. Slade K, Chohan BPS, Barker PJ. Evaluation of a GP practice based homeopathy service. Homeopathy 2004;93:67–70

87. Resch KL, Hill S, Ernst E. Use of complementary therapies by individuals with 'Arthritis'. Clin Rheumatol 1997;16:391–395

88. Eisenberg DM, Davis RB, Ettner SL, Appel S, Wilkey S, Van Rompay M, Kessler RC. Trends in alternative medicine use in the United States, 1990–1997: results of a follow-up national survey. JAMA. 1998;280:1569–1575

89. Kominski GF, Heslin KC, Morgenstern H, Hurwitz EL, Harber PI. Economic evaluation of four treatments for low-back pain. Results from a randomized controlled trial. Med Care 2005;43: 428–435

90. UK BEAM Trial Team. United Kingdom back pain exercise and manipulation (UK BEAM) randomised trial: cost effectiveness of physical treatments for back pain in primary care. BMJ 2004;329:1381

91. Wonderling D, Vickers AJ, Grieve R, McCarney R. Cost effectiveness analysis of a randomised trial of acupuncture for chronic headache in primary care. BMJ 2004;328:747

92. Williams NH, Edwards RT, Linck P, Muntz R, Hibbs R, Wilkinson C, Russell I, Russell D, Hounsome B. Cost–utility analysis of osteopathy in primary care: results from a pragmatic randomized controlled trial. Fam Pract 2004;21:643–650

93. Phelan SP, Armstrong RC, Knox DG, Hubka MJ, Ainbinder DA. An evaluation of medical and chiropractic provider utilization and costs: treating injured workers in North Carolina. J Manipulative Physiol Ther 2004;27:442–448

94. Legorreta AP, Metz D, Nelson CF, Ray S, Chernicoff HO, DiNubile NA. Comparative analysis of individuals with and without chiropractic coverage. Arch Intern Med 2004;164:1985–1992

95. Korthals-de Bos IBC, Hoving JL, van Tulder MW, Rutten-van Mölken PMH, Adèr HJ, de Vet HCW, Koes BW, Vondeling H, Bouter LM. Cost effectiveness of physiotherapy, manual therapy, and general practitioner care for neck pain: economic evaluation alongside a randomised controlled trial. BMJ 2003;326:911

96. Stano M, Haas M, Goldberg B, Traub PM, Nyiendo J. Chiropractic and medical care costs of low back care: results from a practice-based observational study. Am J Manag Care 2002;8:802–809

97. White AR, Ernst E. Economic analysis of complementary medicine: a systematic review. Complement Ther Med 2000;8:111–118

98. Kernick D, White A. Applying economic evaluation to complementary and alternative medicine. In: Kernick D, ed. Getting health economics in practice. Oxford: Radcliffe Medical Press; 2002: 173–180

99. Hulme C, Long AF. Square pegs and round holes? A review of economic evaluation in complementary and alternative medicine. J Altern Complement Ther Med 2005;11: 179–188

100. Thompson Coon J, Ernst E. Economic evaluation of complementary and alternative medicine – a systematic review. Perfusion 2005;18:202–214

101. Canter PH, Thompson Coon J, Ernst E. Cost effectiveness of complementary medicine in the UK – a systematic review. BMJ 2005;331:880–881

THE EPIDEMIOLOGY OF PAIN   Edzard Ernst

PREVALENCE

Pain is a symptom of many medical conditions and therefore it is among the most common reasons for patients to consult complementary practitioners.[1] Incidence (a measure of disease onset, i.e. new cases within a given time period) and prevalence (a measure of disease state: existing cases as a proportion of the total population) data are bedevilled by a range of problems, e.g. sample selection, diagnostic criteria, time frame, recall bias, etc. It is therefore hardly surprising that figures relating to the prevalence of pain vary from 7 to 82%.[2] McQuay & Moore[3] published rough but useful estimates suggesting that about 10% of the general population suffer from acute pain for an average of about 3 days each year. As a result, there are 18 million acute pain days in the UK per year. Assuming that 10% of the 60 million people in Britain suffer from persistent pain, the total number of chronic pain days per year in the UK was estimated to be 2190 million. Others have estimated the point prevalence of persistent pain to be 22%.[4] The prevalence of chronic widespread pain ranges from 0 to 55%.[5]

These data highlight the overwhelming importance of chronic relative to acute pain in terms of human suffering, public health and economy. People enduring chronic pain use health services up to five times more frequently than the rest of the population.[6] Considerable differences exist, of course, in the prevalence and severity of specific pain syndromes. At least 600 identifiable pain syndromes have been described,[7] of which back pain and arthritis are generally believed to be the most prevalent.[8]

WHO IS AFFECTED?

Pain affects us all virtually on a daily basis. One problem with the epidemiology of pain is to decide what level of intensity or frequency is clinically relevant and what is not. Patients affected by specific conditions suffer pain that is dependent on the nature of their disease. For instance, 57% of cancer patients reported pain as a result of their illness and, in 69% of them, the pain was sufficiently severe to limit their ability to function.[2,9] Not many diseases are totally pain free but there are plenty of pain sufferers who do not report pain. For instance, only one in seven individuals with a new episode of back pain seem to report to their doctor.[10] Thus, the study of the epidemiology of pain often becomes the study of the epidemiology of the reporting of the pain.[11]

The ability to sense pain changes as neurophysiological function alters with age. Chronic pain is more frequent in older than younger individuals.[2] The elderly obviously experience degenerative conditions such as osteoarthritis more frequently.[12] Other pain syndromes (e.g. headache or abdominal pain) are more common in younger individuals.[2] The prevalence of recurrent abdominal pain in children ranges from 0.3 to 19%.[13] Some pain syndromes follow a pattern where prevalence increases up to middle age and decreases thereafter[11]

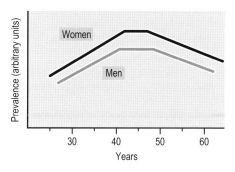

Figure 2.1 **Prevalence of pain according to age: this pattern is typical, for instance, for shoulder pain, low back pain and fibromyalgia.**

(Figure 2.1). Because of the relatively high prevalence of degenerative diseases, the net frequency of pain rises with age. Population-based studies have estimated that 25–50% of elderly individuals suffer from clinically important pain,[14] and this figure rises to 45–80% when considering populations living in nursing homes.[15]

Most pain syndromes are more prevalent in women than in men.[11,16] The pattern is, however, not uniform across all conditions. It crucially depends on the nature of the underlying disease. Generally speaking, women seem to experience and express pain more frequently than men.[17]

Ethnic differences in pain perception have not been extensively studied. Some differences seem to exist. For instance, studies have shown a lower pain tolerance in African compared to white Americans.[18]

PREDISPOSING FACTORS

Other factors predisposing to the experience of pain and determining its prevalence depend on the type of pain syndrome in question (Table 2.7). Unsurprisingly, nurses and other professions associated with regularly lifting heavy weights in non-ergonomic positions are at a higher risk of suffering from back pain than the general population.[19] Other risk factors for back pain include smoking, exposure to vibration and a mismatch between physical stress and strength.[20] Repetitive strain on weight-bearing joints (e.g. jogging or obesity) increases the risk of osteoarthritic pain.[21] Depending on the nature of the pain, a multitude of predisposing factors can be identified. Many patients perceive the weather to affect their pain but, in fact, the data are conflicting. For instance, a US cross-sectional survey of people living in different climates found no influence of the weather on pain perception.[22]

PREDICTORS OF CHRONICITY

There seems to be a link between self-reported sexual abuse of women and pain; sexual abuse may thus predict chronic pain.[23] Previous pain episodes increase the risk of experiencing pain later in life. Such associations could be because anxiety, depression, helplessness and psychological distress increase the risk and intensity of pain – which in turn increases distress thus giving rise to a vicious circle.[24,25]

Other predictive factors of pain chronicity include the intensity of the initial pain experience, fear avoidance behaviour and the ability to cope with pain.[26,27] As pain becomes chronic, the probability of successful treatment is reduced from 70% to 25%.[25] The use of CAM for chronic pain has been associated with high pain intensity.[27]

Table 2.7 **Prevalence figures for some pain syndromes***

Condition	1-year prevalence	Other time period prevalence
Abdominal pain		22% (1 month)
Dental/facial pain		27% (1 month)
Fibromyalgia		11–14% (life prevalence)
Headache	7% males	
	21% females	
Hip pain	14%	
Low back pain	18–50%	
Non-cardiac chest pain		14–23% (life prevalence)
Upper limb pain	7–61%	

*Data are extracted from reference 11.

CAM AND PAIN

Clinicians' trust in the efficacy of CAM treatments for pain control seems to correlate only loosely with the scientific evidence for or against these modalities.[28] Patients' trust in CAM for managing pain is often considerably stronger than that of their health-care professional.[29–32] In particular, patients believe that massage and heat are effective therapies for pain.[29,30] A US survey suggested that pain specialists rate acupuncture, biofeedback, relaxation, manipulation and hypnotherapy as the five most helpful CAM options for controlling pain.[33]

CONCLUSION

The epidemiology of pain is complex and crucially depends on the underlying condition. Many confounding factors have been identified. There is universal agreement that chronic pain patients are frequent users of health services – and that includes CAM.

REFERENCES

1. Braun CA, Bearinger LH, Halcon LL, Pettingell SL. Adolescent use of complementary therapies. J Adolesc Health 2005;37:76
2. Macrae WA. Epidemiology of pain. In: Holdcroft A, Jaggar S, eds. Core topics in pain. Cambridge: Cambridge University Press; 2005;99–102
3. McQuay HJ, Moore A. An evidence-based resource for pain relief. Oxford: Oxford University Press; 1998
4. Gureje O, Von Korff M, Simon GE, Gater R, Häusermann D. Persistent pain and well-being: a World Health Organization study in primary care. JAMA 1998;28:147–151
5. Gran JT. The epidemiology of chronic generalized musculoskeletal pain. Best Pract Res Clin Rheumatol 2003;17:547–561
6. Von Korff M, Wagner EH, Dworkin SF, Saunders KW. Chronic pain and use of ambulatory health care. Psychosom Med 1991;53:61–79
7. Merskey H, Bogduk N. Classification of chronic pain: descriptions of chronic pain syndromes and definitions of pain terms. Seattle: IASP Press; 1994
8. Elliott AM, Smith BH, Penny KI, Smith WC, Chambers WA. The epidemiology of chronic pain in the community. Lancet 1999;354:1248–1252
9. Larue F, Colleau SM, Brasseur L, Cleeland CS. Multicentre study of cancer pain and its treatment in France. BMJ 1995;310:1034–1037

10. Papageorgiou AC, Croft PR, Ferry S, Jayson MI, Silman AJ. Estimating the prevalence of low back pain in the general population. Evidence from the South Manchester Back Pain Survey. Spine 1995;20:1889–1894

11. Macfarlane GJ, Jones GT, McBeth J. Epidemiology of pain. In: McMahon SB, Klotzenburg M, eds. Wall and Melzack's textbook of pain, 5th edn, Chapter 76. Philadelphia: Elsevier; 2006

12. De Inocencio J. Epidemiology of musculoskeletal pain in primary care. Arch Dis Child 2004;89:431–434

13. Chitkara DK, Rawat DJ, Talley NJ. The epidemiology of childhood recurrent abdominal pain in Western countries: a systematic review. Am J Gastroenterol 2005;100:1868–1875

14. Ferrell BA. Pain management in elderly people. J Am Geriatr Soc 1991;39:64–73

15. Ferrell BA. Pain evaluation and management in the nursing home. Ann Intern Med 1995; 123:681–687

16. Schwartz BS, Stewart WF, Simon D, Lipton RB. Epidemiology of tension-type headache. JAMA 1998;279:381–383

17. Guinsburg R, de Araujo Peres C, Branco de Almeida MF, de Cassia Xavier Balda R, Cassia Berenguel R, Tonelotto J, Kopelman BI. Differences in pain expression between male and female newborn infants. Pain 2000;85:127–133

18. Edwards RR, Fillingham RB. Ethnic differences in thermal pain responses. Psychosom Med 1999;61:346–354

19. Videman T, Ojajarvi A, Riihimaki H, Troup JD. Low back pain among nurses: a follow-up beginning at entry to the nursing school. Spine 2005;30:2334–2341

20. Ernst E. Risk factors for back trouble. Lancet 1998;1:1305–1306

21. Ernst E. Jogging – for a healthy heart and worn-out hips? J Intern Med 1990;228:295–297

22. Jamison RN, Anderson KO, Slater MA. Weather changes and pain: perceived influence of local climate on pain complaint in chronic pain patients. Pain 1995;61:309–315

23. Linton SJ. A population-based study of the relationship between sexual abuse and back pain: establishing a link. Pain 1997;73:47–53

24. Croft P. The epidemiology of pain: the more you have, the more you get. Ann Rheum Dis 1996;55:859–860

25. Zimmermann M. Der chronische Schmerz. Orthopäde 2004;33:508–514

26. Potter RG, Jones JM, Boardman AP. A prospective study of primary care patients with musculoskeletal pain: the identification of predictive factors for chronicity. Br J Gen Pract 2000;50: 225–227

27. Andersson HI, Ejlertsson G, Leden I, Schersten B. Impact of chronic pain on health care seeking, self care, and medication. Results from a population-based Swedish study. J Epidemiol Community Health 1999;53:503–509

28. Johansson K, Oberg B, Adolfsson L, Foldevi M. A combination of systematic review and clinicians' beliefs in interventions for subacromial pain. Br J Gen Pract 2002;52: 145–152

29. Norrbrink Buddh C, Lundeberg T. Non-pharmacological pain-relieving therapies in individuals with spinal cord injury: a patient perspective. Complement Ther Med 2004; 12:189–197

30. Chrubasik S, Junck H, Zappe H, Stuzke O. A survey on pain complaints and health care utilization in a German population sample. Eur J Anaesthesiol 1998;15:408

31. Bassols A, Bosch F, Banos JE. How does the general population treat their pain? A survey in Catalonia, Spain. J Pain Symptom Manage 2002;23:318–328

32. Polkki T, Vehvilainen-Julkunen K, Pietila AM. Nonpharmacological methods in relieving children's postoperative pain: a survey on hospital nurses in Finland. J Adv Nurs 2001;34:492

33. Berman BM, Bausell RB. The use of non-pharmacological therapies by pain specialists. Pain 2000;85:313–315

MEASUREMENT OF PAIN   Luis F Buenaver, Robert R Edwards

Pain is a subjective, internal and personal experience that cannot be directly observed by others or exclusively understood in terms of tissue damage detected via physiological markers or bioassays. Thus, pain assessment almost exclusively relies upon the use of self-report measurements. While there are limitations to using self-report data, significant effort has been spent on testing and improving self-report methodology within the area of human pain research. The objective of this chapter is to give an overview of this research and to critically evaluate pain assessment tools to assist clinicians and researchers in selecting the pain assessment methods that most effectively serve their purposes.

CHALLENGES OF PAIN ASSESSMENT

The assessment of pain requires valid and reliable instruments in addition to the capability to communicate via language, movements, etc. Nevertheless, added difficulties persist even when these basic requirements are met. An example is the issue of the time period over which pain is to be measured, with various instruments querying current pain or pain during the previous week. However, longer time frames are also used in some cases, which may introduce important memory biases.[1] Pain is also a multidimensional experience that incorporates both sensory and affective components that, though correlated, can (and in some cases should) be separately assessed.[2] Overall, most of the self-report pain assessment instruments described in this chapter focus on pain intensity ratings (a quantitative estimate of the severity or magnitude of perceived pain) over a relatively brief and recent time period (e.g. the past week).

TYPES OF SELF-REPORT PAIN SCALES

The use of verbal rating scales, numeric rating scales and visual analogue scales to quantify the severity or magnitude of perceived patient pain are the three methods most commonly used to assess the pain experience.

VERBAL RATING SCALES

A verbal rating scale (VRS) is usually comprised of a group of adjectives or phrases that characterise different levels of pain intensity. The descriptors are arranged from least to most intense (or unpleasant). Ideally, the maximum possible range of the pain experience (e.g. from 'no pain' to 'extremely intense pain') should be spanned. Patients are generally asked to endorse the response (i.e. adjective or phrase) that best reflects their pain level. There are numerous examples of VRSs in the literature that have been described and validated; one of the most frequently used is presented in Table 2.8.[3]

Typically, VRSs are scored by arranging the descriptors in order of pain severity and assigning them a numerical value according to their rank (e.g. 0–4 in the example in Table 2.8). The advantages of the VRS lie in its simplicity along with the ease with which it can be administered and scored. Also, the VRS has face validity in that it appears to measure exactly what it claims (i.e. pain intensity), has demonstrated good reliability in various studies, and has frequently been positively correlated with other pain intensity self-report measures and with pain behaviours, thereby establishing its validity.[4] Additionally, compliance rates for the VRS

Table 2.8 **Verbal rating scale (VRS) for pain intensity**

5-point VRS scale
None
Mild
Moderate
Severe
Very severe

are generally better than those obtained with other scales because they are so easy to compre-hend, which can also be particularly useful with certain populations such as the elderly.[5]

Despite the strengths of the VRS, there are also some noteworthy weaknesses that should be addressed; these have led some pain researchers to hesitate in recommending it. One frequent criticism is that the scoring method of a VRS assumes equal intervals between adjectives, such that a change in pain from 'none' to 'mild' is quantified identically to the change from 'moder-ate' to 'severe'. This assumption is probably violated often and is rarely tested. VRSs can also be problematic if a patient is not familiar with all of the words on the scale and/or unable to find a descriptor that accurately describes their pain. A recent review of pain assessment procedures including self-report scales indicated that the VRS is being used less often than in the past.[6]

NUMERICAL RATING SCALES

One of the simplest and most direct ways of assessing pain is by asking the patient to rate their pain intensity on a numerical rating scale (NRS). Generally, NRSs consist of a range of numbers from 0 to 10 or 0 to 100, anchored with 0 indicating 'no pain' and 10 or 100 repre-senting 'the most intense pain imaginable' (see Figure 2.2 for an example). Similar to VRSs, there are various studies demonstrating that the NRS correlates positively with other pain measures and is sensitive to changes arising from the treatment of pain.[6–8] The NRS can be administered in different formats (i.e. verbally or written), is easy and practical to administer and score, is a non-intrusive method of measuring pain, and is easy to understand. The main weakness of the NRS is that, statistically, it does not have ratio qualities.[9]

VISUAL ANALOGUE SCALES

A visual analogue scale (VAS) is a variation of the NRS and typically consists of a 10-cm line with the ends anchored at 'no pain' on the left and 'the most intense pain imaginable' on the right. Unlike the NRS, a VAS does not contain marked intervals; patients indicate their pain intensity by marking a point on the line between 'no pain' and 'the most intense pain imaginable' and the results are essentially treated like ratio data. The patient's pain is meas-ured as the distance from 'no pain' to the point on the line representing their pain intensity. Though the VAS line may be depicted with a vertical orientation, it is usually represented horizontally (see Figure 2.3). Alternative versions of the VAS include a mechanical VAS, in which a sliding marker is superimposed on a horizontal VAS that is drawn on a ruler.[9] Scoring is easily carried out from the back, which includes numbers for each marker place-ment. Studies conducted in clinical settings support the reliability and validity of the VAS as well as its sensitivity to treatment effects.[10,11] Research generally indicates that there are

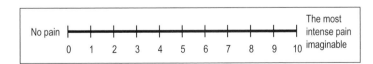

Figure 2.2 Sample numerical rating scale (NRS) for pain intensity.

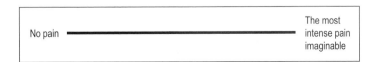

Figure 2.3 Sample visual analogue scale (VAS) for pain intensity.

minimal differences in sensitivity among the VAS, VRS and NRS; however, when significant differences are found they usually suggest that the VAS is more sensitive than the other two instruments. Further, VAS scores have been shown to correlate with pain behaviours and they also appear to possess ratio-level scoring properties.

However, the VAS also has some limitations. For example, scoring is more time-intensive and involves several steps (i.e. a VAS is scored using a ruler in which the score is the number of centimetres or millimetres from the end of the line), which consequently increases the likelihood of committing an error. A VAS can also be difficult to administer to patients with impaired motor function, a condition not uncommon when working with chronic pain populations. Lastly, research also indicates that compared to other pain intensity rating scales the VAS is difficult to understand, particularly for individuals with cognitive disabilities as well as for elderly populations (see below). This results in higher non-completion rates among these samples.

McGILL PAIN QUESTIONNAIRE

Unlike the unidimensional NRS or VAS, the McGill pain questionnaire (MPQ),[12] or its brief analogue the short-form MPQ,[13] is a widely used instrument for multidimensional pain assessment.[14–16] Though the MPQ was originally intended to be administered verbally, it is frequently given as a paper-and-pencil questionnaire. The MPQ was derived from the assumption that pain possesses three primary dimensions: sensory-discriminative, affective-motivational and cognitive-evaluative.[17] It is comprised of 20 sets of verbal descriptors, ranked in terms of pain severity from lowest to highest. The groups of descriptors are divided into those assessing the sensory (10 sets), affective (five sets), evaluative (one set) and miscellaneous (four sets) dimensions of pain. Respondents select the words that best capture their pain, which are then converted into a pain-rating index, based on the sum of all of the words after they are assigned a rank value, as well as the total number of words chosen. The full version of the MPQ also contains an outline of the human body for measuring pain location and a list of five adjectives to indicate overall intensity: a present pain intensity VRS (i.e. the PPI) that ranges from 'no pain' to 'excruciating.' Much research has yielded data supporting both the reliability and validity of the MPQ.[18–21]

The short form of the MPQ, which is more frequently used than the parent MPQ scale, is made up of 15 representative words from the sensory (11 items) and affective (four items) categories from the parent scale. The descriptors are ranked on a 0 ('none') to 3 ('severe') intensity scale. The PPI, along with a VAS, are also included (see Figure 2.4). The MPQ short form is highly correlated with the original scale, is able to discriminate among different pain conditions, and may be easier to use with geriatric patients than the original scale.[5]

PAIN RELIEF

In addition to measuring pain intensity, studies investigating pain management strategies usually measure the degree of perceived pain relief following treatment. The most common methods of assessing pain relief include VASs, generally anchored with 'no relief' and 'complete relief', and VRSs, measuring degrees of relief from 'none' to 'complete'.[1] Pain relief can also be evaluated using NRSs (i.e. assessing the percentage of relief). However, pain relief measures have been found to have validity difficulties. For example, despite an analysis of sequential pain ratings (i.e. baseline compared to post-treatment) revealing *increases* in reported pain intensity, a significant minority of patients were found to report at least moderate pain relief. In a recent clinical trial for the management of chronic myalgia of the jaw muscles, approximately 90% of patients reported some degree of pain relief on a VAS despite average pain ratings increasing by 28% early in the study.[22] This phenomenon (i.e. the over-reporting of relief) appears to be partly the result of a memory bias of past pain being considerably greater than the corresponding ratings would otherwise indicate.[1]

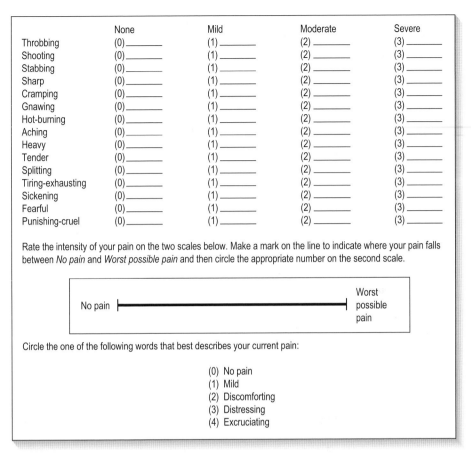

	None	Mild	Moderate	Severe
Throbbing	(0) _____	(1) _____	(2) _____	(3) _____
Shooting	(0) _____	(1) _____	(2) _____	(3) _____
Stabbing	(0) _____	(1) _____	(2) _____	(3) _____
Sharp	(0) _____	(1) _____	(2) _____	(3) _____
Cramping	(0) _____	(1) _____	(2) _____	(3) _____
Gnawing	(0) _____	(1) _____	(2) _____	(3) _____
Hot-burning	(0) _____	(1) _____	(2) _____	(3) _____
Aching	(0) _____	(1) _____	(2) _____	(3) _____
Heavy	(0) _____	(1) _____	(2) _____	(3) _____
Tender	(0) _____	(1) _____	(2) _____	(3) _____
Splitting	(0) _____	(1) _____	(2) _____	(3) _____
Tiring-exhausting	(0) _____	(1) _____	(2) _____	(3) _____
Sickening	(0) _____	(1) _____	(2) _____	(3) _____
Fearful	(0) _____	(1) _____	(2) _____	(3) _____
Punishing-cruel	(0) _____	(1) _____	(2) _____	(3) _____

Rate the intensity of your pain on the two scales below. Make a mark on the line to indicate where your pain falls between *No pain* and *Worst possible pain* and then circle the appropriate number on the second scale.

No pain ├───┤ Worst possible pain

Circle the one of the following words that best describes your current pain:

(0) No pain
(1) Mild
(2) Discomforting
(3) Distressing
(4) Excruciating

Figure 2.4 **Short-form McGill pain questionnaire (reprinted with permission from Melzack R. The short-form McGill Pain Questionnaire. Pain 1987;30:191–197).**

BEHAVIOURAL OBSERVATION

Though by definition pain is a subjective and private experience, its behavioural manifestations are often apparent to others. Individuals experiencing pain often convey their distress through facial expressions (e.g. grimacing), vocalisations (e.g. moaning), body postures (e.g. hunching over) and behaviours (e.g. rubbing/massaging the pain site). These verbal and non-verbal behaviours have come to be known as pain behaviours, and are an important component of behavioural models of pain. A multitude of methods exist to code pain behaviours, though a number of them are specific to particular pain conditions. One example includes the osteoarthritis pain behaviour coding system, which assesses the position, movement and particular pain behaviours observed in osteoarthritis patients during standardised tasks.[23] Assessing pain behaviours is important when determining a patient's level of physical function (e.g. how much activity they engage in), in understanding the factors that may reinforce pain behaviours (e.g. solicitous responses from others), or in evaluating pain in non-verbal individuals. Research indicates that although there is a moderate relation between self-reports of pain and pain behaviours, they are, in fact, not interchangeable.[24] Interestingly, the association between self-reports of pain intensity and pain behaviour was lower in the context of chronic pain relative to acute pain but, not surprisingly, was greatest when observations of pain behaviours and verbal reports of pain were recorded simultaneously.

EXPERIMENTAL PAIN ASSESSMENT

Administration of standardised aversive stimulation within a laboratory environment to examine the relationships of aversive stimuli to behavioural and sensory perceptions constitutes an important subdiscipline within the field of pain.[25] Within this field of study there are various forms of noxious stimulation that are employed to cause pain (e.g. thermal, mechanical, electrical, chemical, ischaemic, etc.). Outcome measures generally include pain threshold, pain tolerance and ratings of suprathreshold noxious stimuli using an NRS, a VAS or a VRS. The clinical relevance of experimental pain assessment is slowly being determined; quantitative sensory testing can be used to subtype patients afflicted with chronic pain conditions,[26] to identify mechanisms of chronic pain,[27] and to predict post-operative pain.[28]

PSYCHOPHYSIOLOGICAL ASSESSMENT

Psychophysiological data play an important adjunctive role in the assessment of acute and chronic pain. First, they are a necessary element for conducting biofeedback or similar procedures in which patients are taught to bring physiological processes under some degree of voluntary control. Second, psychophysiological data can help to clarify some of the accompanying phenomena of pain that are not easily measured by self-report (e.g. arousal, central processing of information related to noxious stimulation). However, it should be pointed out that none of the following measures constitute 'objective' measures of pain, because none can substitute for some type of patient rating of a patient's experience of pain.

Surface electromyography (EMG) is frequently used to record levels of local muscle tension in the context of musculoskeletal pain syndromes (e.g. low back pain, tension headache, etc.), in which elevated muscle tension is believed to contribute to the experience of pain.[29] Electroencephalography (EEG) has been used in various studies to measure cortical responses to noxious stimulation. Though the spatial resolution of EEG is somewhat limited, its temporal resolution is actually rather good; multiple studies have recently shown that brain responses to standardised noxious stimuli measured by EEG are enhanced in patients with chronic pain compared to healthy controls.[30] Heart rate and blood pressure are also often assessed in the context of laboratory pain testing. However, while pain responses and resting blood pressure are inversely related,[31] no consistent associations between cardiovascular reactivity and pain responses have yet been observed. Collectively, psychophysiological measures can provide unique information about pain responses, but they do not constitute an 'objective' measurement of an individual's pain experience.

SPECIAL POPULATIONS

CHILDREN

The assessment of pain in children presents numerous challenges. Often, treatment providers mistakenly assume that children are unable to provide accurate or reliable information about their pain experience. As a matter of fact, numerous pain assessment tools for use specifically in children have been developed and validated. Further, factors similar to those influencing pain in adults (e.g. degree of tissue damage, mood states, social responses, etc.) have also been shown to relate to children's pain in comparable ways.[32]

Various behavioural pain-rating scales for infants have been developed and validated. While establishing the validity of these instruments can frequently be difficult, several have consistently been shown to be reliable. One such example is the often used neonatal infant pain scale (NIPS),[33] which codes the presence and intensity of six pain-related behaviours: facial expressions, crying, breathing, arm movement, leg movement and arousal state. Even among older children who are better able to self-report sensory and affective experiences, researchers have

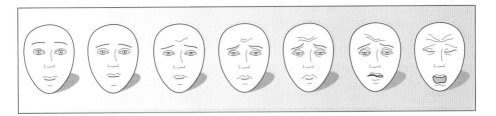

Figure 2.5 **The faces pain scale (reprinted with permission from Bieri D, Reeve RA, Champion GD, Addicot L, Ziegler JB. The faces pain scale for the self-assessment of the severity of pain experienced by children. Pain 1990;41:139–150).**

indicated that although direct questioning (e.g. 'How is your pain today?') can be clinically useful, it is particularly susceptible to bias and demand characteristics. Consequently, standardised pain assessment instruments for children of different ages have been developed, with some of the scales having been designed for use with particular ethnic groups. The faces scale and the Oucher scale[34] are two such examples that are intended for use with younger children who may be preverbal (see Figure 2.5). Other types of widely used pain measurement instruments designed for use with children include pain thermometers, comprised of a vertical NRS that is superimposed on a VAS shaped to resemble a thermometer, although a standard VAS is a valid and reliable pain measurement instrument for children older than 6 years of age.[35]

THE ELDERLY

In the last several years there has been a steady increase in research investigating pain in the elderly. The majority of pain assessment instruments validated in middle-aged adults have also been psychometrically evaluated in older subjects. Generally, research in this area has found that increasing age is associated with a higher frequency of incomplete or unusable responses on a VAS, though not on a VRS or NRS. Across different studies, rates of difficulty with the VAS (i.e. incomplete or unusable data) in cognitively intact samples of elderly subjects range from 7% to 30%, with the percentages substantially increasing (up to 73%) in cognitively impaired samples.[5] Studies examining elderly respondents' preferences of pain measurement instruments indicate that VRSs frequently receive the highest preference scores while VASs have been rated as one of the least preferred pain measures. Additionally, it has been suggested that the long form of the MPQ is not appropriate for use with elderly patients because of its level of complexity and time requirements. Indeed, multiple studies have now determined that older adults report less pain on the MPQ (i.e. choose fewer words) even when NRS-rated or VRS-rated pain does not differ.[36,37] These results may suggest that the MPQ differentially assesses the construct of pain as a function of age, suggesting that caution may be warranted when using this pain measurement instrument with older populations.

Collectively, recent findings suggest that the fewest 'failure' responses among samples of cognitively intact and cognitively impaired elderly subjects are produced with the VRS while the largest number is produced with a VAS. Consequently, it is recommended that studies investigating pain in elderly samples use, at minimum, a VRS to assess pain intensity.

BIASES IN PAIN MEASUREMENT

The consequences of inaccurate measurements of pain can be substantial with underestimation of pain potentially leading to improper management, unnecessary suffering and delays in recovery, while overestimation of pain can potentially lead to over-treatment and possible adverse iatrogenic consequences. Numerous studies have investigated the correspondence, or lack thereof, between patients' reports of pain and health-care providers' assessments of patients' pain. Generally, the results from this line of research indicate that substantial caution is warranted when health-care professionals attempt to estimate patients' pain levels.

Most studies investigating the level of agreement between health professional and patient ratings of pain have employed samples comprised of nurses. In one such study, 43% of nurses were found to underestimate the pain experienced by burn patients during a therapeutic procedure; nurses also overestimated the degree of pain relief subsequent to administration of analgesic medication.[38] Various other studies have reported similar results.[39] In one study,[40] there was virtually no agreement between nurses' and patients' ratings of post-surgical pain as agreement scores (i.e. κ statistics) ranged from 0.01 to 0.12, revealing no significant correlation. In a study examining congruence between cancer patients' VAS pain ratings and ratings of patient pain made by nurses, house officers or oncology fellows there were no significant correlations between patient ratings and provider ratings.[41] Lastly, in addition to findings associated with the inaccuracy or underestimation of patients' pain, there is little evidence supporting the validity of expert judgements regarding pain patients' prognoses. For example, there was no congruence between treatment providers' estimates of patients' rehabilitation potentials and actual rehabilitation outcomes among back pain patients who were followed longitudinally.[42]

SUMMARY AND RECOMMENDATIONS

A wide range of valid and reliable measurement instruments is available to assess pain despite the fact that pain is a private and subjective experience. Studies investigating pain should at the very minimum include one self-report measure, though it is often preferable to use either multiple measures or a multidimensional measure of pain (e.g. the short form of the MPQ comprised of both verbal descriptors and a VAS). A recent review investigating the validity and reliability of pain measures in adult cancer patients found that single-item VAS, VRS and NRS all showed good validity and reliability, and that all were generally comparable to one another.[4] However, the use of a VRS or NRS over a VAS is strongly recommended in studies using elderly or cognitively impaired subjects. It is preferable to measure pain relief using sequential ratings (i.e. changes from pre- to post-treatment) rather than retrospective impression. Behavioural observation, laboratory pain assessment and psychophysiological assessment are all useful and potentially informative adjunctive measures of pain responses; however, none can substitute for the patient's self-report of the pain experience. The assessment of pain in infants is the exception to this standard, where the coding of behavioural or facial expressions/responses is presently the gold standard for pain assessment. The faces or Oucher scales, which are pictorial scales, may be utilised for slightly older children, while in children aged 6 years and older a standard VAS may be preferable. Lastly, there is substantial research indicating that health-care providers, regardless of experience, are unreliable judges of patients' reports of pain. Treatment providers tend to frequently underestimate patients' experiences of pain.

Accurately assessing patients' pain is of vital importance to both clinicians and researchers. When selecting measures to assess pain, the decision should be based on as thorough a knowledge as possible of the properties, strengths and limitations of the various instruments.

REFERENCES

1. Haythornthwaite JA, Fauerbach JA. Assessment of acute pain, pain relief, and patient satisfaction. In: Turk DC, Melzack R, eds. Handbook of pain assessment, 2nd edn. New York: Guilford Press; 2001:417–430
2. Melzack R. Pain – an overview. Acta Anaesthesiol Scand 1999;43:880–884
3. Frank AJ, Moll JM, Hort JF. A comparison of three ways of measuring pain. Rheumatol Rehabil 1982;21:211–217

4. Jensen MP. The validity and reliability of pain measures in adults with cancer. J Pain 2003;4:2–21
5. Gagliese L, Melzack R. The assessment of pain in the elderly. In: Mostofsky DI, Lomranz J, eds. Handbook of pain and aging. New York: Plenum Press; 1997:69–96
6. Jensen MP, Karoly P. Self-report scales and procedures for assessing pain in adults. In: Turk DC, Melzack R, eds. Handbook of pain assessment, 2nd edn. New York: Guilford Press; 2001:15–34
7. Jensen MP, Karoly P, Braver S. The measurement of clinical pain intensity: a comparison of six methods. Pain 1986;27:117–126
8. Keefe FJ. EMG-assisted relaxation training in the management of chronic low back pain. Am J Clin Biofeedback 1981;4:93–103
9. Price DD, Bush FM, Long S, Harkins SW. A comparison of pain measurement characteristics of mechanical visual analogue and simple numerical rating scales. Pain 1994; 56:217–226
10. Price DD, McGrath PA, Rafi A, Buckingham B. The validation of visual analogue scales as ratio scale measures for chronic and experimental pain. Pain 1983;17:45–56
11. Scott J, Huskisson EC. Graphic representation of pain. Pain 1976;2:175–184
12. Melzack R. The McGill Pain Questionnaire: major properties and scoring methods. Pain 1975;1: 277–299
13. Melzack R. The short-form McGill Pain Questionnaire. Pain 1987;30:191–197
14. Melzack R, Katz J. The McGill Pain Questionnaire: appraisal and current status. In: Turk DC, Melzack R, eds. Handbook of pain assessment, 2nd edn. New York: Guilford Press; 2001: 35–52
15. Melzack R, Torgerson WS. On the language of pain. Anesthesiology 1971;34:50–59
16. Turk DC, Rudy TE, Salovey P. The McGill pain questionnaire reconsidered: confirming the factor structure and examining appropriate uses. Pain 1985;21:385–397
17. Melzack R, Casey KL. Sensory, motivational, and central control determinants of pain: a new conceptual model. In: Kenshalo DR, ed. The skin senses. Springfield, IL: Charles C. Thomas; 1968:423–443
18. Lowe N, Noble Walker S, MacCallum RC. Confirming the theoretical structure of the McGill pain questionnaire in acute clinical pain. Pain 1991;46:53–60
19. Pearce J, Morley S. An experimental investigation of the construct validity of the McGill Pain Questionnaire. Pain 1989;39:115–121
20. Reading AE, Everitt BS, Sledmere CM. The McGill Pain Questionnaire: a replication of its construction. Br J Clin Psychol 1982;21:339–349
21. Wilkie DJ, Savedra MC, Holzemer WL, Tesler MD. Use of the McGill Pain Questionnaire to measure pain: a meta-analysis. Nurs Res 1990;39:36–41
22. Feine JS, Lavigne GJ, Dao TT, Morin C, Lund JP. Memories of chronic pain and perceptions of relief. Pain 1998;77:137–141
23. Keefe FJ, Caldwell DS, Queen K, Gil KM. Osteoarthritic knee pain: a behavioral analysis. Pain 1987;28:309–321
24. Labus JS, Keefe FJ, Jensen MP. Self-reports of pain intensity and direct observations of pain behavior: when are they correlated? Pain 2003;102:109–124
25. Gracely R. Studies of pain in human subjects. In: Wall P, Melzack R, eds. Textbook of pain. Edinburgh: Churchill Livingstone; 1999:385–407
26. Pappagallo M, Oaklander AL, Quatrano-Piacentini AL, Clark MR, Raja SN. Heterogenous patterns of sensory dysfunction in postherpetic neuralgia suggest multiple pathophysiologic mechanisms. Anesthesiology 2000;92:691–698
27. Sarlani E, Greenspan JD. Evidence for generalized hyperalgesia in temporomandibular disorders patients. Pain 2003;102:221–226
28. Granot M, Lowenstein L, Yarnitsky D, Tamir A, Zimmer EZ. Postcesarean section pain prediction by preoperative experimental pain assessment. Anesthesiology 2003;98:1422–1426
29. Jensen R, Olesen J. Initiating mechanisms of experimentally induced tension-type headache. Cephalalgia 1996;16:175–182
30. Flor H. Cortical reorganisation and chronic pain: implications for rehabilitation. J Rehabil Med 2003;41 Suppl:66–72
31. Ghione S. Hypertension-associated hypalgesia: evidence in experimental animals and humans, pathophysiological mechanisms, and potential clinical consequences. Hypertension 1996;28: 494–504
32. McGrath PA. Pain in the pediatric patient: practical aspects of assessment. Pediatr Ann 1995;24: 126–128

33. Lawrence J, Alcock D, McGrath P, Kay J, MacMurray SB, Dulberg C. The development of a tool to assess neonatal pain. Neonatal Netw 1993;12:59–66
34. Luffy R, Grove SK. Examining the validity, reliability, and preference of three pediatric pain measurement tools in African-American children. Pediatric Nursing 2003;29:54
35. McGrath PA, Gillespie J. Pain assessment in children and adolescents. In: Turk DC, Melzack R, eds. Handbook of pain assessment, 2nd edn. New York: Guilford Press; 2001:97–118
36. Gagliese L, Melzack R. Age-related differences in the qualities but not the intensity of chronic pain. Pain 2003;104:597–608
37. Gagliese L, Katz J. Age differences in postoperative pain are scale dependent: a comparison of measures of pain intensity and quality in younger and older surgical patients. Pain 2003;103: 11–20
38. Choiniere M, Melzack R, Girard N, Rondeau J, Paquin MJ. Comparisons between patients' and nurses' assessment of pain and medication efficacy in severe burn injuries. Pain 1990;40:143–152
39. Stephenson NL. A comparison of nurse and patient: perceptions of postsurgical pain. J Intraven Nurs 1994;17:235–239
40. Thomas T, Robinson C, Champion D, McKell M, Pell M. Prediction and assessment of the severity of post-operative pain and of satisfaction with management. Pain 1998; 75:177–185
41. Grossman SA, Sheidler VR, Swedeen K, Mucenski J, Piantadosi S. Correlation of patient and caregiver ratings of cancer pain. J Pain Symptom Manage 1991;6:53–57
42. Jensen IB, Bodin L, Ljungqvist T, Gunnar BK, Nygren A. Assessing the needs of patients in pain: a matter of opinion? Spine 2000;25:2816–2823

CURRENT MEDICAL CONCEPTS OF PAIN   Anita Holdcroft

DEFINITIONS AND TAXONOMY OF PAIN

The symptom of pain is almost universally experienced by humans and epidemiological studies show that subjects report back, hip and shoulder pains at a frequency of one in four. There are a few individuals who are insensitive to pain, for example they may have a genetic disorder affecting nerve function. Pain is a common presentation of many different disorders but, because it is subjective, the interpretation of its behavioural and verbalised responses has changed over the years from labelling people as hysterical to an understanding that there may be no tissue damage to account for the sensation. The sensation may be induced by alterations in the dynamic activity of nerves and their supporting structures. Hence, definitions, taxonomy and pain classifications are a subject of scientific debate.

Pain is defined as an unpleasant sensory and emotional experience that is usually associated with actual or potential tissue damage or is described in terms of such damage. This approach acknowledges its unpleasant nature, which originates in brain regions (the reticular and limbic areas) that are slowly activated by spinal mechanisms. The sensation of pain originates in the nociceptive, rapidly conducting, protective, neural systems that extend from the periphery or deep body tissues to the cerebral cortex. Other dimensions of the pain experience include central nervous system processes, such as those generated by past experiences, and hormonal changes, as well as environmental influences.

Acute pain is of recent onset and limited duration. It frequently has an identified temporal and causal relationship to tissue injury or disease state. Conditions associated with acute pain include surgery or trauma, and acute exacerbations of disease such as pancreatitis, cholecystitis, sickle cell disease and angina (coronary artery disease). However, pain from trauma (accidental or surgical) may not subside so that pain progresses to a chronic stage. A feature of acute pain may be its recurrence, e.g. migraine, such that, between exacerbations, pain is absent.

Chronic pain persists beyond the point at which healing would be expected to occur or it accompanies a lack of healing. It may also be present without tissue damage. The symptom may be accompanied by alterations in behaviour, psychological functioning and social inter-actions. The precise time when acute pain becomes chronic is not readily defined and because some of the mechanisms of chronic pain relate to the long-term effects of acute pain the classification of pain into acute and chronic is questionable. What is considered clini-cally important is the alleviation of acute pain so that mechanisms that maintain pain are not established.

The purpose of taxonomy is to use definitions and classifications that are acceptable to the majority of health-care workers. Their evolving nature is dependent on current research and patient diagnoses. Their limitations are often visible where a group of patients have a cluster of symptoms and the diagnosis lacks the power to distinguish between those patients who will benefit from a treatment and those who will not. Over the years, diagnoses are refined to establish subgroups within a particular diagnostic category or to eliminate certain subgroups because it becomes clear that they do not have the newly identified causative pathophysiology. Once the characteristic features of a disorder are defined it then becomes easier to compare treatments and prognoses, leading the way to evidence-based manage-ment. There have been examples of this development in the diagnosis of angina pain in women (i.e. formerly misdiagnosed and treated) and in chronic regional pain syndrome (i.e. formerly called causalgia or reflex sympathetic dystrophy).

CLASSIFICATION OF PAIN

Pain can be classified for an individual patient according to:

- its temporal relations, e.g. acute, chronic, recurrent; neonatal, elderly, reproductive
- the underlying pathology, e.g. genetic, infection, immune reactions, toxic/metabolic, can-cer, trauma, vascular, mechanical/degenerative
- the organ/system affected, e.g. cutaneous, visceral, muscular
- the site of the pain, e.g. arm, leg, head
- the pain intensity, e.g. to enable pain management using the World Health Organization's pain 'ladder'.

Chronic pain as classified by the International Association for the Study of Pain is based on the premise that the majority of pain conditions have a specific body location. Their clas-sification describes a small general group and then the majority of conditions are identified according to site. This concept has led to many pain assessment tools including body images on which to record the site of the pain. The benefits of using pain classifications include accurate enumeration of cases and data capture for analyses and clinical trials.

There are a number of diagnostic features that are used to topographically classify pain:

1. *Pain quality* distinguishes cutaneous pain from deep tissue pain. Superficial pain is often sharp, pricking or burning whereas deep pain, e.g. from the viscera, may be aching in quality and dull. Pain from the skin is usually easily localised compared with pain from deeper structures; deep tissue pain is more diffuse and may be felt superficially in an area of the body that is remote from the affected organ, so called referred pain. The pat-tern of referral has a characteristic distribution. For example, scapular pain may indicate referral from the diaphragm or gall bladder.
2. A *radiculopathy* (or polyradiculopathy) describes pain arising in the distribution of a nerve root. It may be caused by any process that compresses, distorts or inflames nerve roots. The pain is neuropathic and any associated sensory or motor effects unresolved after 4 weeks should be managed urgently.
3. *Central pain* is defined as pain caused by a lesion or dysfunction in the central nervous system. It is commonly caused by long-term lesions, such as multiple sclerosis, traumatic

injuries and cerebrovascular disorders, especially for thalamic and brainstem lesions. Diagnostic features include sensory disturbances to temperature and pain. The pain from a stroke is commonly felt on one side of the body whereas in multiple sclerosis it is often in the legs. Trigeminal neuralgia, caused by a lesion in the brainstem, is one manifestation of central pain.

Other diagnostic features that are beginning to be used clinically for quantitative sensory testing are pain threshold and pain tolerance.

PHYSIOLOGY/PATHOLOGY OF PAIN

A nerve cell has a baseline negative electrical potential (generated by potassium ions) so that when the cell fires an action potential is generated. On firing, the cell is depolarised and becomes positively charged. The action potential travels faster in myelinated than non-myelinated nerves because myelin acts as an insulator. The cell returns to its resting state once the ions are redistributed across the nerve membrane. The cell body of the nerve that is in the dorsal root ganglion or brainstem (for the head and neck) does not play a direct role in this process but provides all the materials the cell needs to fire and interact with other cells, e.g. neurochemicals, ion channels and receptors.

Pain-sensing nerve cells are widely distributed in the body (e.g. skin, muscle, viscera, joints, meninges). They have afferent neural input into the central nervous system that coordinates a response to a noxious stimulus through effector systems that include protective motor and autonomic reflexes. The events that produce a cortical response begin by transduction at the peripheral terminal of the primary afferent nociceptor. It is here that chemicals induce electrical activity in the neurone that is transmitted into the central nervous system. Through a series of synapses in the dorsal horn of the spinal cord, electrical activity is converted to chemical energy and back again to electrical signals. The impulse is then transmitted by second-order neurones through parallel afferent spinal pathways (e.g. the spinothalamic and spinoparabrachial tracts) to reach the thalamus and areas of the brain concerned with affect and it then synapses with third-order neurones that relay to the cortex.

At all levels of this nociceptive response, modulation can increase or decrease the activity within the cells from the peripheral termination of the primary afferent neurone to the spinal cord and higher centres. For example, at the nerve ending in the peripheral tissues there are receptors that can excite the nerve [e.g. transient receptor potential vanilloid receptor (VR1)], receptors that can inhibit its activity (e.g. cannabinoid receptor) and those that can be switched on to sensitise the nerve (e.g. specific sodium channels) in particular situations. These functions are also occurring at the dorsal horn with opioid and γ-aminobutyric acid ($GABA_A$) receptors inhibiting central transmission of nociceptive impulses and α-amino-3-hydroxyl-5-methyl-4-isoxazole (AMPA) initiating onward transmission into the second-order neurones, which travel in the contralateral side of the spinal cord to the thalamus. After brief bursts of activity, the dorsal horn neurones become sensitised in a number of different ways:

- Wind up is the phenomenon whereby repeated stimulation of the second-order neurone by the primary afferent neurone increases its electrical response. The release of substance P and glutamate from the primary afferent neurone onto the neurokinin-1 receptor enhances electrical activity in the second-order neurone through slow depolarisations.
- Central sensitisation potentiates activity in both nociceptors and non-nociceptor nerves through calcium influx through the N-methyl-D-aspartate (NMDA) receptors. This sensitisation can last for many minutes.
- Long-term potentiation occurs through NMDA activation.
- Through gene transcription-enhancing excitatory chemicals, e.g. cytokines.

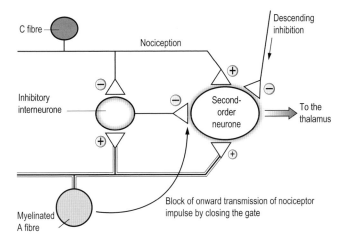

Figure 2.6 **Gate control theory of pain. A cartoon of the gate control theory of pain showing the inhibitory and second-order neurones in the dorsal horn of the spinal cord being activated and inhibited respectively by large fibre input from A fibres. The interneurone is tonically active and normally inhibits the second-order neurone unless it is itself inhibited by nociceptor C fibre activity. Further descending inhibition from higher centres in the brain is also shown acting on the second-order neurone.**

- Through a reduction in inhibition, e.g. from a reduction in activity in peripheral large nerve fibres thus opening the 'gate' (Figure 2.6).

The effect of these processes is to generate abnormal sensory responses such as allodynia and hyperalgesia.

BIOCHEMISTRY OF PAIN
PERIPHERAL NEUROCHEMICALS
The release of neurochemicals locally at the site of injury or inflammation is a general phenomenon in superficial and deep tissues. These include:

- kinins: bradykinin and kallidin act on bradykinin receptors
- serotonin: 5-hydroxytryptamine (5-HT) acts on several receptors
- adenosine triphosphate (ATP) acts on several receptors, importantly the P_2X_3 receptor on C-fibres
- protons: these act on acid-sensing ion channels
- prostaglandins: enhance the effect of other chemicals, e.g. bradykinin
- capsaicin: acts through VR1
- cannabinoids: act through peripheral cannabinoid receptors and VR1
- nerve growth factor mediates persistent pain.

DORSAL ROOT GANGLION NEUROCHEMICALS
In the dorsal root ganglion organisation there are two groups of cells: one synthesises peptides such as calcitonin gene-related peptide, substance P, galanin, somatostatin, brain-derived neurotrophic factor and vasoactive intestinal peptide and the other is non-peptidergic. Neurochemicals are released from the dorsal root ganglion and can travel in the axon to the peripheral or central nerve terminal.

SECTION TWO

DORSAL HORN NEUROCHEMICALS

The neurotransmitters on the ascending nociceptive pathways are GABA, an inhibitory neurotransmitter at the $GABA_A$ receptor, and excitatory amino acids. Glutamate is the major excitatory amino acid that acts on AMPA, NMDA and kainate receptors and is co-released with neuropeptides, e.g. substance P (a tachykinin) and calcitonin gene-related peptide.

The descending pathway neurotransmitters are excitatory (5-HT and acetylcholine) and inhibitory [opioids and noradrenaline (norepinephrine)]. Their release is controlled through mid-brain centres such as the periaqueductal grey and rostroventral medulla. The opioids act through pre- and post-synaptic modulation of nerve conduction. There are three opioid receptor subtypes with the following endogenous ligands: endorphins (MOR; μ opioid receptor), enkephalins (DOR; δ opioid receptor) and dynorphin (KOR; κ opioid receptor).

GLIAL NEUROCHEMICALS

Glial cells are now known to interact with neurones. Microglial cells have an immune function, releasing cytokines and enhancing sensitisation following nerve injury.

BRAIN NEUROCHEMICALS

Glutamate, GABA, 5-HT, acetylcholine, noradrenaline, opioids (including nociceptin) and cannabinoids all act supra-spinally (e.g. periaqueductal grey and rostroventral medulla).

GENERAL ASPECTS OF CHRONIC PAIN

The patient who attends a chronic pain clinic is characterised by a history of failed treatments such as analgesics, rest and time off work, a level of disability that is not commensurate with pathology and frequent psychosocial distress. These combine to alter affect (e.g. anxiety and depression), sleep patterns and social activities and to cause distraction and preoccupation with pain. The behavioural impact may reflect cognition, finances and compensation issues. There is evidence that multidisciplinary cognitive–behavioural therapy is effective for chronic back pain management compared with an active exercise programme with analgesic cover for acute back pain. In chronic severe cancer pain the World Health Organization recommends opioids but their safe use in non-cancer pain requires close control. However, a systematic review has shown them to be effective for neuropathic and musculoskeletal pain relief although with a high frequency of side effects.

Wherever possible, a diagnosis is sought and co-morbidities are recorded. An emerging characteristic of some forms of chronic pain is that some conditions co-exist, for example chronic cystitis and endometriosis, irritable bowel syndrome and fibromyalgia. A full pain history may reveal multiple episodes of pain, especially in women. Recognition of the potential disabling outcome for patients should generate a more robust approach to pain so that sensitisation becomes less frequent as patients are given pain relief through timely therapies that are designed to manage all the disabling aspects of pain.

GENERAL ASPECTS OF ACUTE PAIN

An acute pain team may be formed to effectively manage pain relief in hospitals. There is a wide range of structures from simple methods to enhance education, documentation, monitoring and guideline development to a multidisciplinary service for 'high-tec' forms of pain relief with multiprofessional input over 24 hours. Evidence for their effectiveness despite their organisational diversity has been found in the form of improved pain relief and reduced side effects, especially in post-operative patients. Other areas in hospitals where acute pain should be effectively managed include medical patients, e.g. those with sickle cell disease and human immunodeficiency virus infection, and obstetric patients, e.g. labouring women. A diagnosis is always required in case a readily remedied condition presents, e.g. acute urinary obstruction.

The mechanisms of nociception such as transduction, transmission, modulation, sensitisation and perception act as a framework to describe therapeutic approaches to acute pain management. Peripherally acting drugs such as cyclo-oxygenase 1 and 2 inhibitors and steroids may reduce inflammatory mediators. Opioids may act peripherally, at opioid receptors that become expressed in inflammatory states, or centrally to generate inhibitory activity. Local anaesthetics block the sodium channels of primary afferent neurones at different levels of the nociceptive pathway, e.g. regional nerve block. However, despite the apparent number of analgesics available, most work in <50% of patients and many have side effects through their pharmacology or route of administration that preclude their use, e.g. cyclooxygenase inhibitors. It is therefore standard practice to administer at least two of these drugs in combination so as to target different neurochemical activities. One of the best oral combinations is that of codeine (which is broken down to morphine) and paracetamol. Morphine remains the standard drug for comparison in clinical trials.

Effective management of acute pain is required not only for pain relief but also to modify the response to injury. There is a release of cytokines and neural, humoral, metabolic and immune physiological changes leading to catabolism, increased sympathetic nervous system activity, immunosuppression, inflammation and physical and mental deactivation. The psychological aspects of acute pain such as anxiety and loss of sleep and control interact adversely with these effects. There is clear evidence that effective analgesia modifies these responses and improves recovery.

FURTHER READING

Australian and New Zealand College of Anaesthetists and Faculty of Pain Medicine. Acute pain management: scientific evidence, 2nd edn. Australian Government National Health and Medical Research Council; 2005. Online. Available: http://www.nhmrc.gov.au/publications/synopses/_files/cp104.pdf 9 June 2005

Elliot AM, Smith BH, Hannaford PC, Smith WC, Chambers WA. The course of chronic pain in the community: results of a 4-year follow-up study. Pain 2002;99:299–307

Kalso E, Edwards JE, Moore RA, McQuay HJ. Opioids in chronic non-cancer pain: systematic review of efficacy and safety. Pain 2004;112:372–380

Royal College of General Practitioners. Clinical guidelines for the management of acute low back pain. London: Royal College of General Practitioners; 1996

Woolf CJ, Bennett GJ, Doherty M, Dubner R, Kidd B, Koltzenburg M, Lipton R, Loeser JD, Payne R, Torebjork E. Towards a mechanism-based classification of pain? Pain 1998; 77:227–229

World Health Organization. WHO's pain ladder. Online. Available: www.whi.int/cancer/palliative/painladder/en/January 2006

PSYCHOLOGICAL CONCEPTS OF PAIN — Stephen Morley

INTRODUCTION

> 'An unpleasant sensory and emotional experience associated with actual or potential tissue damage or described in such terms.'
>
> International Association for the Study of Pain (IASP)

The widely accepted definition of pain endorsed by the IASP clearly places pain as a psychological experience. The cardinal aspects of pain are its dual sensory and emotional components and its pervasive negative hedonic tone. The second half of the definition is concerned with presumed causal mechanisms (tissue damage). Current neurobiological research is concerned with elucidating the precise mechanisms that give rise to and modulate the experience of pain. Much of this work is conducted in animals and their experience can only be inferred through observation of their behaviour – a critical domain of psychology that is paradoxically missing from the IASP definition. There is no unified psychological conception of pain. The discipline of psychology recognises pain as a complex experience that can be approached from a range of psychological frameworks. The purpose of this article is briefly to elucidate strands of contemporary psychological constructs of pain.

PAIN AS SENSATION

In classical psychophysics, the oldest area of modern psychology, the primary aim is to scale the relationship between known properties of the pain-eliciting physical stimulus and the individual's subjective experience of pain. One practical outcome of these studies is the construction of reliable scales that facilitate the reporting of pain in a quantified manner.[1] The sensory experience of pain can be decomposed into several domains: the intensity of the sensation, its spatial location, temporal and sensory qualities, and its unpleasantness. A variety of scaling methodologies have successfully separated these domains and provide instruments that have appropriate scale properties. The McGill pain questionnaire captures the sensory quality of pain arranged on an underlying intensity continuum. Verbal descriptor scales (VDSs) and visual analogue scales (VASs) are able to represent the intensity and unpleasantness domains of pain as with properties of a ratio scale, i.e. having a true origin and a defined interval. Although judgement of intensity and unpleasantness are generally highly correlated, both experimental laboratory and clinical studies have demonstrated the separateness of the intensity and unpleasantness dimensions using a range of manipulations (pharmacological, hypnosis and induction psychological states such as expectation and anxiety).[2] For example, women who have undergone prepared childbirth classes report pain in the final phase of labour as being less unpleasant than women who have not been prepared, but both groups report pain as having a similar intensity. Studies that have explored the causal link between the experience of intensity and unpleasantness have demonstrated that intensity precedes the immediate experience of unpleasantness and is a significant cause of the degree of experienced unpleasantness.[3] Furthermore, emotional experience related to pain can modulate both intensity and unpleasantness.[3] For the most part, psychophysical studies study pain as a 'bottom–up' process, i.e. its experience as determined by the stimulus characteristics, but the influence of 'top–down' processes arising from the cognitive state or goal orientation of the individual have also been demonstrated.

PAIN AS ATTENTION

Pain is experienced as intrusive and interruptive of ongoing behaviour and cognitive activity: it enters consciousness and demands attention.[4] The analysis of the attentional processes underlying pain is grounded in the contemporary psychology of attention that considers an efficient attentional system as one that is sensitive to two competing needs. First, it must maintain attentional focus on the current behavioural goal, protecting it from less important demands that might interrupt its control and flow and, second, it must attend to important new information that may change the goal priority, e.g. threatening information that requires escape or avoidance activity. In this analysis, pain can demand attention because it is either relevant to ongoing behavioural goals, e.g. the goal to avoid pain or its exacerbation (as in the case for many people faced with chronic pain) or pain may interrupt because of its threat value. Pain is, par excellence, a signal of physical threat designed to interrupt attention in situations where the individual's current goal is not related to pain. The key features of pain that determine its interruptive capacity are its intensity, unpredictability, novelty and its threat value – the mere anticipation of a higher-intensity pain stimulus leads to greater interruption by a standard stimulus. In chronic pain, high-intensity pain retains its interruptive and attention-demanding capacity despite prolonged experience. It is associated with degradation of task performance

and subtle cognitive changes, e.g. memory impairment. In addition to the stimulus parameters of pain, individual differences in constructing the meaning and threat value of pain
determine its attention-demanding characteristics. Individuals reporting a high fear of pain
and high levels of catastrophising (see below) show the greatest decrement in task performance. Once a painful stimulus has captured the attention, it is a significant task to disengage
one's attention from it. Experimental analyses of brief pain again suggest that stimulus characteristics contribute to the ease of disengagement but little is known about processes influencing disengagement in chronic pain, although distraction is a common self-help strategy
used by sufferers.[5]

PAIN AS BEHAVIOUR

Painful stimulation gives rise to a wide range of behavioural expression ranging from involuntary flinching and withdrawal from an acute painful stimulus to verbal and para-verbal
utterances, postural adjustments such as guarding and bracing and the use of prostheses and
aids in the presence of chronic pain. From a psychological perspective, the essential issue is
that behaviour is susceptible to change by its consequences (reinforcers) and its future
occurrence can be shaped as a function of these consequences and the characteristics of the
antecedent conditions. Behavioural analysis offers a potentially valuable way of understanding the variation across individuals in response to pain, particularly chronic pain, and it has
been the cornerstone of contemporary treatment for chronic pain.[6]

There are three broad classes of reinforcers of which two, positive and negative reinforcement, act to increase and maintain the probability of particular behavioural sequences,
and one, punishment, decreases the probability of the behaviour that it follows. Extinction
occurs when the reinforcement no longer follows the behaviour: under this condition the
probability of the previously reinforced behaviour occurring will be reduced. It is well
established that it is not necessary for every occurrence of a given behaviour to be followed
by reinforcement for the probability of the occurrence of the behaviour to be changed.
Partial reinforcement is particularly effective in maintaining behavioural patterns and ren-
dering them resistant to extinction.

Positive reinforcement occurs when an event, often experienced as a pleasant event,
follows a behaviour. In the context of chronic pain, others in the person's environment
may express concern, suggest that the person rests and offer to help. Such complex social
reinforcing events may readily shape both expressions of distress and more frequent periods
of rest and recuperation. The presence of others and the environment in which positive
reinforcement occurs acquire the characteristics of a discriminative stimulus. This is a stimulus telling the individual that positive reinforcement is likely to occur and which signals
that the emission of the target behaviour is likely to be reinforced. An example of this in
medical settings is that the presence of medical and other health-care workers associated
with the delivery of help is often a discriminative stimulus for the expression of pain behaviour, ranging from verbal expressions of distress to exaggerated gait and movement. From a
behavioural perspective, treatment of behaviour that is controlled by positive reinforcement
is conceptually simple but often technically difficult. The essence of treatment is the withdrawal of the reinforcer, i.e. extinction, and the development of alternative behavioural
sequences.

Negative reinforcement also increases the frequency of behaviour but does so by the
removal of an aversive event. Pain is particularly susceptible to negative reinforcement. For
example, analgesics may be considered to be negative reinforcers because the act of taking
them results in the reduction of pain. The negative reinforcement inherent in taking analgesics is a powerful behavioural mechanism responsible for escalating ingestion of medication. A major aim of many chronic pain treatment programmes is to reduce medication
intake and transfer the control of medication ingestion to a time-contingent basis. Similarly,

avoidance of activity may result in the reduction of pain so it is possible to develop an extensive repertoire of avoidance behaviour. Understanding the role of negative reinforcement has been crucial to understanding avoidance behaviour and to developing treatment. When avoidance behaviour is established, it is, by definition, successful in avoiding the unwanted consequences. It is therefore difficult for extinction to occur because the individual cannot learn that the contingency between behaviour and reinforcement is changed. The major component of treatments for avoidance-motivated behaviour has been exposing the patient to the object of their fear and asking them not to avoid but to tolerate the experience of fear. Over time the fear reduces and the motivation to escape from or avoid the feared event is reduced. Recently, this paradigm has been extended to chronic pain where sufferers are afraid to engage in activity because of the fear that it will lead to further harm or injury.[7]

Finally, pain behaviour and its development, and particularly facial expression, have been considered in the context of the evolutionary advantages that its display might confer.[8] At a practical level this analysis provides a valuable tool for interpreting behaviour in neonates, infants and individuals whose cognitive capacity is impaired.[9]

PAIN AS COGNITION

It has long been observed that similar pain stimuli are associated with considerable variation in pain report and behaviour and that variation is not always easily explained by reinforcement histories. Beecher's classic observations of injured soldiers suggested that, paradoxically, severe injury could be accompanied by moderate pain.[10] He suggested that soldiers experienced a sense of relief on having escaped the battlefield. Similarly, anthropological observations of rituals that should be painful led many authorities to conclude that the context and the meaning of the pain were critically important.[11] These observations have, however, only recently been subjected to experimental test,[12] stimulated by the application of an explicit cognitive–behavioural theory to pain. The cognitive–behavioural account is now the dominant psychological model of pain. Its central precept is that individuals are active processors of information rather than passive responders to environmental contingencies.[13] From this perspective it is a person's cognitive representation of events and the contexts in which they occur that determine their subjective experience, behaviour and emotional responses. Studies of how people cognitively represent health and illness have identified cognitive domains relating to the cause, identity, timeline, consequences and personal control of illness. Particular patterns of attributions, expectations and appraisals are associated with a range of outcomes. An example of this is catastrophic appraisal.[14]

The appraisal of pain as potentially catastrophic has emerged as a critical cognitive component. Catastrophic appraisal comprises a complex of beliefs about pain, namely that it is difficult to control, that it will be unbearable and that it will lead to a range of unwanted negative outcomes; individuals who catastrophise tend to ruminate about catastrophic outcomes. Unsurprisingly, individuals who report catastrophic thinking report more severe pain intensity to standard pain stimuli, show greater behavioural expression of pain and report more fear and depression. Conversely, in psychological treatment programmes, good outcomes are associated with changes in catastrophising and there is some evidence that reduction of catastrophic thinking may be an important mechanism underpinning the effectiveness of such programmes.[15]

The combination of behavioural and cognitive concepts over the last three decades has resulted in cognitive–behavioural therapy, which is now the dominant psychological approach to treatment in pain. The fear avoidance model cited earlier[7] provides an excellent example of this, in which catastrophic appraisals of harm contribute to the development and maintenance of wider ranging, negatively reinforced, avoidance behaviour leading to a reduced behavioural repertoire associated with disuse, social withdrawal, increased analgesic intake and depression.

INDIVIDUAL DIFFERENCES – PERSONALITY

Early work (1940–50) focused on identifying the personality types associated with individual disorders and was characterised by two features: the use of selected samples of convenience from specialist clinics and psychological assessments based on the sapiential authority of the investigators' descriptive assessments of individuals. Subsequently, formal methods of assessment such as well-constructed, psychometrically robust, personality tests were introduced. However, these tests might be described as 'broadband', designed to capture many aspects of individual variation associated with a range of psychopathologies, e.g. the widely used Minnesota Multiphasic Personality Inventory (MMPI). A serious attempt was made to separate functional from organic pain, resulting in a diagnostic signature – the conversion V – named after the sequence of high–low–high scores on the three scales, hypochondriasis, depression and hysteria. The reliance on cross-sectional designs meant that separating the causal and consequential relationship between psychological state and pain was problematic. Furthermore, evidence accrued that personality profiles were not specific to pain disorders but were also present in other chronic illnesses[16] and that successful treatment of the pain was associated with a reduction in the extreme personality profile.[17,18] Extreme scoring on personality measures seems often to be caused by persistent pain rather than to be a cause of that pain.

A second strand to the research on individual differences has been the attempt to use measures of individual differences to predict the outcomes of interventions. This problem arises most frequently when high-cost invasive treatments, such as dorsal column stimulators and intrathecal pumps, are considered. Formal psychological testing, such as the MMPI, has been used in a number of studies but the use of highly selected clinic samples and relatively small numbers has made it difficult to reach any conclusions that could provide an actuarial basis for assessment. Nevertheless, most facilities offering these treatments do require a psychological assessment, which is often conducted around a thorough analysis of the patient's beliefs, attitudes and past behaviour and which incorporates a significant element of preparing the patient for the intervention.[19]

The study of individual differences in pain has persisted but has shifted emphasis to the development of typologies that reflect the ways in which individuals have adapted to chronic pain. These differ from earlier personality-based measures in that the focus of assessment has been specifically on pain-related behaviour. Turk has identified three profiles (adaptive copers, interpersonally distressed and dysfunctional) that are orthogonal to medical diagnostic categories and represent broad psychological responses to the experience of chronic pain.[20] Turk suggested that the profiles can be used to design interventions that match the treatment needs of individuals. There is some evidence that matching treatment to overt need is beneficial but this approach is challenged by analyses of chronic pain that explicitly model causal psychological processes in the development and maintenance of chronicity, i.e. take a functional approach such as the fear-avoidance model cited above.

REFERENCES

1. Gracely RH. Evaluation of pain sensations. In: Merskey H, Loeser JD, Dubner R, eds. The paths of pain 1975–2005. Seattle: IASP Press; 2005:271–283
2. Price DD, Riley JL 3rd, Wade JB. Psychophysical approaches to measurement of the dimensions and stages of pain. In: Turk DC, Melzack R, eds. Handbook of pain assessment, 2nd edn. New York: Guilford Press; 2001:53–75
3. Rainville P, Carrier B, Hofbauer RK, Bushnell MC, Duncan GH. Dissociation of sensory and affective dimensions of pain using hypnotic modulation. Pain 1999; 82:159–171
4. Eccleston C, Crombez G. Pain demands attention: a cognitive-affective model of the interruptive function of pain. Psychol Bull 1999;125:356–366
5. Van Damme S, Crombez G, Eccleston C, Roelofs J. The role of hypervigilance in the experience of pain. In: Asmundson GJ, Vlaeyen J, Crombez G, eds. Understanding and treating fear of pain. Oxford: Oxford University Press; 2004:71–90

6. Fordyce WE. Behavioral methods for chronic pain and illness. St Louis: Mosby; 1976

7. Vlaeyen JW, Linton SJ. Fear-avoidance and its consequences in chronic musculo-skeletal pain: a state of the art. Pain 2000;85:317–332

8. Williams AC. Facial expression of pain: an evolutionary account. Behav Brain Sci 2002; 25:439–455

9. Craig KD, Prkachin KM, Grunau RE. The facial expression of pain. In: Turk DC, Melzack R, eds. Handbook of pain assessment, 2nd edn. New York: Guilford Press; 2001:153–169

10. Beecher HK. The measurement of subjective responses. Oxford: Oxford University Press; 1959

11. Morris DB. Illness and culture in a postmodern age. Berkeley: University of California Press; 1998

12. Arntz A, Claassens L. The meaning of pain influences its experienced intensity. Pain 2004;109: 20–25

13. Turk DC. A cognitive–behavioral perspective on treatment of chronic pain patients. In: Gatchel RJ, Turk DC, eds. Psychosocial factors in pain, 2nd edn. New York: Guilford Press; 2002:138–158

14. Sullivan MJL, Thorn BE, Haythornthwaite JA, Keefe FJ, Martin M, Bradley LA, Lefebvre JC. Theoretical perspectives on the relationship between catastrophizing and pain. Clin J Pain 2001;17:52–64

15. Burns JW, Kubilus A, Bruehl S, Harden RN, Lofland K. Do changes in cognitive factors influence outcome following multidisciplinary treatment for chronic pain? A cross-lagged panel analysis. J Consult Clin Psychol 2003;71:81–91

16. Naliboff BD, Cohen MJ, Yellen AN. Does the MMPI differentiate chronic illness from chronic pain? Pain 1982;13:333–341

17. Naliboff BD, McCreary CP, McArthur DL, Cohen MJ, Gottlieb HJ. MMPI changes following behavioral treatment of chronic low back pain. Pain 1988;35:271–277

18. Sternbach RA, Timmermans G. Personality changes associated with the reduction of pain. Pain 1974;1:177–181

19. Doleys DM. Preparing pain patients for implantable technologies. In: Turk DC, Gatchel RJ, eds. Psychological approaches to pain management, 2nd edn. New York: Guilford Press; 2002: 334–348

20. Turk DC. The potential of treatment matching for subgroups of chronic pain patients: Lumping vs. splitting. Clin J Pain 2005;21:44–55

ALTERNATIVE CONCEPTS OF PAIN

Much of CAM is underpinned by a fundamentally different 'philosophy' to that of conventional medicine. This has implications for research as well as clinical practice. It seems important that conventional clinicians appreciate these differences. In the following chapters, we have invited leading experts from the most important branches of CAM* to present the concept of pain in their particular field. It is not our intention to present them as alternatives to the current scientific concepts of pain. We also abstain from judgements about their validity. However, we do feel that these short chapters are relevant. Patients who consult CAM practitioners will encounter these philosophies and conventional health-care providers might therefore want to be familiar with them. We hope that these chapters add greater depth to the descriptions of particular therapies as outlined in Section 3 on *Therapies*.

*We invited experts in anthroposophical medicine, Ayurveda, chiropractic, healing, homeopathy, naturopathy, osteopathy and traditional Chinese medicine. The chiropractic contribution was unfortunately withdrawn at a late stage.

ANTHROPOSOPHIC CONCEPTS OF PAIN   Peter Heusser

BACKGROUND: NATURAL SCIENCE AND SPIRITUAL SCIENCE IN ANTHROPOSOPHIC MEDICINE

While the natural sciences study the physical (material) phenomena related to pain, psychology examines the psychic phenomena involved. A holistic approach unites both and makes it possible to determine correlations between physical and psychic elements, thereby providing indirect evidence for the ongoing interaction between body and soul – just what today's psychosomatic medicine is striving for. Direct investigation of this interaction as such cannot, however, be undertaken because the action of such of our soul or mind on our physical body evades normal human consciousness. This is precisely the point from which the natural sciences and psychology give way to the approach of spiritual science as developed in anthroposophy. The origins of anthroposophy date back as far as the 19th century mid-European philosophers, physicians and anthropologists such as Ignaz Paul Vital Troxler (1780–1888) or Immanuel Hermann Fichte (1796–1879).[1,2] Anthroposophy was epistemologically and methodologically developed and implemented as a spiritual science by Rudolf Steiner (1861–1925), who had studied mathematics, natural sciences and philosophy, held a PhD in epistemology and was well known as the editor of Goethe's natural scientific work.

Anthroposophy as a science is based on an intricate method of systematic enhancement of human cognition, so that the actions of the soul or mind as such and their effect on the organism – which would otherwise remain unconscious – can be made fully conscious and thus directly accessible to empirical investigation.[3–6] The results of such research can provide a deeper understanding of human nature in general, with its interactions and interdependence of body, soul and spirit, and of a phenomenon such as pain in particular.[7] The practice of anthroposophic medicine consists of the complementary application of the results from both natural and spiritual science in an attempt to reach a truly holistic understanding and treatment of the human being.

THE FOUR-FOLD HUMAN BEING AS A BASIS FOR THE ANTHROPOSOPHIC CONCEPT OF PAIN

A human being is not merely made up of the material elements of the physical body that are the focus of the natural sciences today. If the forces of matter were the only ones exerting effects within the body, the body would deteriorate and disintegrate into the mineral kingdom, just as corpses actually do. But during the lifetime of an organism this does not happen. On the contrary, the organism is built to an astonishing degree of complexity and always at the expense of entropy, far off from the thermodynamic equilibrium. This can only happen if the otherwise inevitable decay is constantly prevented and if the material parts are forced into a higher order against their natural tendency to dissolve. According to anthroposophic research, this is the result of an immaterial organisation of life-giving forces – the so-called etheric body. The etheric body fully pervades the physical body as a living field of forces and organises its material processes so that the specific characteristics of life emerge in plants, animals and human beings: nutrition, metabolism, growth, reproduction, self-healing, etc. At death, the etheric forces separate from the physical body, which then inevitably decays.

If animals and human beings, however, only had a physical body and an etheric body, they would only have vital (living) properties, just as plants do, and would not develop consciousness. Animals and human beings, however, also have a soul in addition to their physical and etheric bodies. The soul (in anthroposophy often called the astral body) is a third organisation of forces, which pervades the physical and the etheric bodies. Based in the astral body are the emotions, sensations, feelings, drives, intentions, pleasure, sympathy and antipathy, lust and pain – in short, everything of which animals or human beings can be conscious. Large parts of the soul's contents and functions work in subconscious areas of the soul, but the soul is not active in isolation from the composition and the functions of the physical and etheric bodies but acts in interdependence with them. This is, of course, well known from the fields of psycho-neuroendocrinology and psychosomatic research. The difference between the prevailing conventional and anthroposophic explanations of consciousness is, however, that conventionally, the brain or other material structures or functions are considered to be the *cause* of consciousness, whereas in anthroposophic medicine these entities are just the necessary material *conditions* for the soul functions to become conscious.

Yet human beings are still different from animals in one respect. They do not only possess a physical body, an etheric body and a soul similar to those of animals, but they are also endowed with their own individual spirit. This spirit, which is essentially the core of the human soul, is its real 'I', which bestows human beings with reason, self-consciousness and self-determination.[6,8] The difference between soul and spirit can be seen in the different use of intelligence. Animals do show intelligent behaviour but this intelligence (lawfulness) is an intrinsic property of the functions of an animal's soul, i.e. instincts, etc., whereas humans, in contrast, can purposefully regulate their soul functions by intentions based on wilful reasoning (which is a function of the spirit), even against the intentions of the soul. In medicine, this fact plays an extremely important role in the phenomenon of coping: physical or emotional pain, for example, can be managed completely differently, depending on the way the individual is capable of consciously working on the sensation of pain or its emotional consequences by means of thought. Coping is a function of the human 'I' or spirit as opposed to the mere soul.

THE POLARITY OF CONSCIOUSNESS AND ORGANIC VITALITY AS AN EXPRESSION OF SOUL/SPIRIT–BODY INTERACTIONS

Just as the life of a plant is the opposite of death in the mineral kingdom, so the development of consciousness in human beings and animals is opposed to vitality: the more developed consciousness is in the evolutionary ladder of animals, the less potent vitality is as a regenerative force. For example, seemingly primitive worms like *Planaria*, which only have a set of nerve ganglia instead of a brain and which have a concomitant low-order form of consciousness, can regenerate a complete whole body from each of their parts if dissected in two, no matter where the dissection line is located in the body. Newts, which are of a higher evolutionary order and which already possess a simple brain with a correspondingly higher level of consciousness, can no longer regenerate whole bodies but can regenerate whole extremities if these are amputated. This ability is lost on the evolutionary path to the higher vertebrates with their even higher forms of consciousness. Additionally, the more an organ system serves consciousness in an individual animal or a human being, the weaker are its restorative powers. An instructive example of this fact can be seen in the tremendous difference between the regenerative capacities of nerve and liver tissues or, within the nerve system itself, between nerve tissues serving lower-order or higher-order forms of consciousness. Moreover, consciousness processes themselves are not related to the build-up of vitality in the corresponding nerve tissue, but rather to its use and subsequent deterioration if a new compensating build-up does not take place. In the eye, sensory processes are mediated through a corresponding decay, not build-up, of rhodopsin; repetitive action potentials exhaust the energetic potential of the nerve and necessitate a phase of recuperation before the nerve can exert its function to serve consciousness again; neurotransmitters, of which the release serves consciousness functions, are neurotoxic if not metabolised immediately after having accomplished their task. In other words, in many ways consciousness functions are only possible at the expense of build-up and vitality. The functions of soul and spirit (e.g. emotional and cognitive processes engendered by the astral body and the 'I') are in this sense opposed to the functions of the etheric body, with the result of a slight 'disease process' in *status nascendi*. This deterioration, however, as the result of the consciousness functions of the astral body and the 'I' is always balanced out, at least as long as the organism can maintain its status of health. Health, in this sense, is not the absence of decay, but is a harmonious equilibrium between the processes of build-up and decay. The latter are the inevitable corollary of our consciousness, which we owe to our soul and spirit functions. Disease results from a loss of that equilibrium. That is the reason why stress, a non-compensated overcharge with functions of consciousness, also results in organic disease. Sleep, on the other hand, regenerates the organs in charge of consciousness that deteriorate during the time the soul/spirit is awake. In sleep, the astral body and the 'I' detach themselves from the physical body and the etheric body to a certain degree. The etheric body can then release its regenerative and restorative powers in the physical body. From these perspectives the anthroposophic concept of pain can be understood.

THE ANTHROPOSOPHIC CONCEPT OF PAIN

Pain is clearly a phenomenon of consciousness. In pain, the affected part or region of the organism becomes conscious in a way that it normally does not. For example, the generally more or less comfortable yet barely noticeable feeling that normally accompanies a movement changes and becomes more noticeable to the point of discomfort or even pain: the astral body penetrates deeper than usual or in an abnormal way into the etheric and the physical bodies, resulting in pain and corresponding organic alterations. The reasons for pain can be manifold. The astral body itself may be the cause of the pain or illness, e.g. when it acts too strongly in relation to the other bodies, as in the case of various diseases with cramps of internal organs or external muscles. But also the 'I' may facilitate pain, e.g. if the 'I' is too weak to control strong yet disharmonious soul functions, as in the case of tiredness, nervousness or stress. On the other hand, the causes of pain can also lie in the etheric body or the physical body. In this case, the astral body, which may be normal in itself, encounters an already altered etheric and/or physical organisation when it interacts with them, with the consequence of an altered or sharpened state of consciousness, i.e. discomfort or pain. A weakened etheric body, as in chronic diseases or states of exhaustion, can result in too weak a regeneration; therefore, even normal deterioration as the result of the usual astral functions may not be properly balanced out and this may subsequently elicit pain. Physical injury as a reason for pain can be caused not only by external noxious factors, i.e. trauma, but also by dysfunctions of the etheric body. Cancerous tissue, for example, consists of a physical and etheric part of the organism which, when emancipated from the rest, results in deformation and destruction of normal tissue. In all of these cases, where the astral body cannot harmoniously penetrate the organisation because of the damage, pain is experienced. Pain is thus an expression of state in which the astral body (of the soul) interferes with the organism either too deeply or in an inappropriate manner.

CONSEQUENCES FOR THE THERAPY CONCEPT OF PAIN

Pain therapy means reversing the conditions described above either by curing or by remedying them. If the reason for organ damage lies in the physical body, it must be eliminated accordingly, e.g. by means of an operation in the case of a tumour, a gallstone or similar. On the other hand, if this cannot be done or if the pain is the result of a dominance of the astral body, the abnormal interaction between the astral body and the physical and etheric bodies must be influenced in such a way that the resulting phenomenon of consciousness, i.e. pain, is weakened or eliminated. In other words, the astral body must be freed from the too strong or irregular organic connection. In principle, any form of medication-based pain therapy works in this direction, although the effect may be mediated by a variety of different substances and physical and etheric pathways. The result is always that the astral body – and with it the 'I' – are loosened from the organism in one way or another. This can also be seen in the various side effects of painkillers, e.g. disturbed sensations, impaired consciousness, concentration or central breathing regulation (the astral body plays a major role in the regulation of respiration). Even the ultimate possibilities of pain management in desolate conditions, sedation and anaesthesia, and the dangers of going too far in this direction (death), show the basic principle of pain treatment: the detachment of soul and spirit from the affected organisation or its parts.

In anthroposophic medicine, both conventional as well as anthroposophic analgesics are used for the management of pain. In a Swiss National Foundation study (NFP 34) on quality of life in patients with advanced cancer receiving stationary palliative treatment in the anthroposophic Lukas Klinik in Arlesheim, Switzerland, we compared the use of analgesics for 4 months before and 4 months after hospitalisation with the 3 weeks of hospitalisation. The use of World Health Organization class III analgesics (strong opiates) was equivalent during all three phases of observation whereas the weaker analgesics (WHO classes I and II) were used less during and after the stay in the Lukas Klinik, and the average level of pain, measured with the EORTC QLQ-C30 (i.e. the European Organization for Research in Cancer Therapy, Quality of life questionnaire C30), decreased significantly during hospital-isation.[9] One of the reasons was that part of the weaker analgesic dose could be replaced by anthroposophic medication such as homeopathically potentised plants, including *Aconitum, Rhus toxicodendrum, Atropa belladonna, Colocynthis* and *Bryonia*.

Massage, baths or compresses, using calming oils like lavender, warming substances like rosemary, cooling ones like menthol, plant extracts with decongesting or anti-rheumatic effects like *Spiraea*, ointments with *Mandragora* or other analgesic plant preparations, and many other products, are used to calm, warm up, soothe, loosen and thus help to improve body–function and body–soul interactions, with positive consequences for pain control.

These processes, which are aimed at improving the way the astral body pervades the etheric body, can be enhanced from 'below' and from 'above'; from 'below', on the physical level by eliminating whatever obstacles can be eliminated with well-known medical procedures like sur-gery, radiotherapy, stents, etc. and on the etheric level by strengthening and improving the forces and functions of the etheric body. This can be achieved in various ways depending on the indi-vidual symptoms, necessities and possibilities. For example, liver function may be enhanced by oral or subcutaneously applied plant preparations from *Carduus marianus, Taraxacum* and oth-ers, thus engendering life processes that are related directly or indirectly to the liver. Substances with a general strengthening effect can be applied, like *Prunus spinosa* and Levico (an Italian mineral water with traces of iron, copper and arsenic used in small doses for its roborating effects), etc. A strengthened etheric body will more easily counterbalance the devitalising effects of the astral body and thus lift the threshold of pain.

The relationship of the astral body to the organism and thus pain can also be influenced 'from above'. This can be done, on the one hand, by influencing and harmonising soul func-tions through art therapies and curative eurythmy. The colours and forms in curative paint-ing and modelling, the rhythmic recitation in therapeutic speech, the harmonies and rhythms in music therapies, and the special body movements in curative eurythmy aimed at harmon-ising body, soul and spirit can all have harmonising effects on emotions and even on physi-ological processes, and in this way can influence the sensation of pain or the personal ability to manage pain. For example, the analgesic and relaxing effects of music therapy are well established.[10] With regard to therapeutic speech we recently succeeded in showing that the recitation of hexameters results in a harmonisation of respiration and circulation in a way that normally takes place at night during the regenerative phase of sleep.[11] This is the phase when the ether body exercises its main healing and regenerating activities. The physiology of healing can thus be understood.

On the other hand, to influence pain 'from above' also means to work on the soul from the spirit. An overly strong astral body or one that behaves in an irregular manner can be counter-balanced by means of a strong 'I'. It is well known that the effects of psychic events on illness or the intensity of pain experienced are determined not only by these psychic events or sensa-tions of pain themselves, but also by the way these events are dealt with consciously in the coping process. As explained above, coping is an achievement of the human 'I', and it is this 'I', the spiritual essence of the human soul, that is capable of searching for a deeper mean-ing in life, especially in the enigmas of disease and destiny. For this reason, meaningful physician–patient interaction, which includes regular counselling and, depending on individual patient needs, may also touch on questions of biography, destiny and spirituality, is an integral therapeutic element of anthroposophic medicine.

CONCLUSION

This means that according to the anthroposophic understanding of the human being, pain, which is a special phenomenon of consciousness indicating overly strong or irregular soul–body interactions in the affected part of the organism, can be caused and influenced by various internal and external factors acting on all levels of human organisation: the physical body, the etheric body, the astral body and the human 'I'. Accordingly, pain treatment can also encompass various – both conventional and unconventional – methods acting on these interacting levels. Extending natural science and psychology to include anthroposophically oriented spiritual science paves the way for a rational understanding of pain and pain therapy that integrates in a truly holistic way all four levels of the human being: body, life, soul and spirit.

REFERENCES

1. Troxler IPV. Naturlehre des menschlichen Erkennens oder Metaphysik, (1828); (edited by HR Schweizer). Hamburg: Felix Meiner; 1985
2. Fichte IH. Anthropologie, 3rd edn. Leipzig: Brockhaus, Leipzig; 1876
3. Steiner R. A theory of knowledge – implicit in Goethe's world conception, 3rd edn. Spring Valley, NY: Anthroposophic Press; 1988
4. Steiner R. Theosophy, 5th edn. London: Rudolf Steiner Press; 2005
5. Steiner R. Knowledge of the higher worlds, 6th edn. Bristol: Rudolf Steiner Press; 1993
6. Steiner R. Outline of esoteric science, 1st edn. Hudson, NY: Anthroposophic Press; 1997
7. Steiner R, Wegman I. Extending practical medicine, 2nd edn. London: Rudolf Steiner Press; 1996
8. Steiner R. Philosophy of freedom, 8th edn. London: Rudolf Steiner Press; 1999
9. Heusser P, Berger Braun S, Bertschy M, Burkhard R, Ziegler R, Helwig S, van Wegberg B, Cerny T. Palliative in-patient cancer treatment in an anthroposophical hospital II: quality of life during and after stationary treatment and subjective treatment benefits. Forsch Komplementärmed Klass Naturheilkd 2006;13:156–166
10. Aldridge D. Music therapy research and practice in medicine. London: Kingsley; 1996
11. Cysarz D, von Bonin D, Lackner H, Heusser P, Moser M, Bettermann H. Oscillations of heart rate and respiration synchronize during poetry recitation. Am J Physiol Heart Circ Physiol 2004; 287:H579–H587

AYURVEDIC CONCEPTS OF PAIN   Ram Harsh Singh

INTRODUCTION

Pain is a common manifestation of a wide range of pathologies. It is probably the most important symptom because of its greatly annoying nature and most unpleasant experience. This is why pain has been described prominently in all traditions of medicine since antiquity. Ayurveda is one of the most ancient systems of medicine in the world, its history going back to the *Vedas*. The science and art of Ayurvedic medicine has continued to be in uninterrupted practice for thousands of years and has survived in present times through the existence of two sets of ancient texts popularly known as *Brihattrayis* (three big books: Caraka-Samhita, 700 BCE, Susruta Samhita, 600 BCE, Samhitas of Vagbhatt, 300 CE) and *Laghuttrayis* (three small books: Madhava Nidan, 900 CE, Sharangdhara Samhita, 1300 CE and Bhavaprakasha, 1600 CE). All these texts describe the fundamental principles of Ayurveda besides the concept of disease, diagnostics and therapy including Ayurvedic materia medica. One can find descriptions of pain, its aetiopathogenesis, taxonomy and management. It is useful to look into the ancient concepts of pain management to advance an appropriate strategy to develop contemporary methods of pain management.[1–6]

DEFINITIONS AND TAXONOMY OF PAIN

Pain is the most important symptom of many diseases with a multi-faceted aetiology. Pain, being a most unpleasant experience and on many occasions turning into a pressing need for treatment, occupies the central place in clinical medicine and therapeutics. The nature and severity of pain widely varies with the nature and site of the tissues involved and the underlying mechanisms. Accordingly, pain is categorised in different forms and is given different nomenclatures. The Ayurvedic texts describe a wide range of pain, *Sula* (piercing pain), being the most prominent form. *Dank* (bursting), *Vedana* (unbearable sensation), *Dagdha* (burning pain) and *Cosa* (sucking pain) are some of the other expressions.[2]

CLASSIFICATION OF PAIN

Pain is classified in terms of the site or the organ and tissue involved or in terms of its mechanical, neurogenic, ischaemic, spasmodic or burning nature. The Ayurvedic texts mention most commonly the piercing pain termed *Sula*. The *Sula* could vary in its nature depending upon its site and tissue involvement, such as *Udarasula* (abdominal pain), *Parinama Sula* (dyspeptic pain), *Prista Sula* (backache), *Kati Sula* (lumbago), *Vasti Sula* (urinary pain), *Hicchula* (anginal pain) and so on. Classical Ayurveda describes eight kinds of *Sula* relevant to the *Tridosa* factor, most of which are visceral pain syndromes except *Vatika Sula*, which is again of five kinds and is related to extra-abdominal sites. A range of neurological and osteoarticular pains are described in the context of *Vata Vyadhi*.

PATHOPHYSIOLOGY OF PAIN

All considerations of health and disease in Ayurveda are based on the theory of *Tridosa*. The living body functions through three principal bio-factors namely *Vata, Pitta* and *Kapha*. It is difficult to correlate these three factors with contemporary medical language and understanding. For the purpose of a simplified approach it is understood that the *Kapha* component of the body represents the total solid substratum of the organism that is responsible for providing the body and body components with their shape and form through which the other two more vital *Dosa* factors operate. *Pitta* represents the entire range of the bio-fire system including its perceptible attributes like digestion of food and all metabolic activities including all the biochemical, enzymatic and hormonal moieties. *Pitta* is hot in nature and its excess produces fire-like actions and burning effects. *Vata* is essentially the energetic component and it encompasses all forms of energies and impulses including neural impulses that carry messages to the central nervous system and also carry the central impulses towards the periphery. Ordinarily it is presumed that the pain signal travels through the *Vata* system of the body. Ayurveda propounds that there can be no pain without involvement of the *Vata Dosa*. Hence, the *Vata Dosa* is the specific denominator of all kinds of pain. However, the nature of pain may change because of the mixture of the other two *Dosas*. The pain occurring as the result of the combination of *Kapha* with *Vata* transforms the nature of pain from sharp to dull. All dull aching pains are because of the *Kapha* factor associating with the *Vata* factor. Similarly, an association of the *Pitta Dosa* with the vitiated *Vata* may alter the pain from a simple sharp neurogenic pain to a burning pain.

Apart from the influence of *Tridosic* co-factors there are many other factors that may alter the nature of pain. The main ones are:

- tissue or *Dhatu* involved
- organ or *Kostha* and site involved
- specific functions of the tissue/organ involved

- the mental state of the victim
- environmental factors, both endogenous and exogenous.

For example, pain arising as a result of the pathology of *Vasti*, i.e. the urinary tract, will be different in nature and site from a pain arising as a result of the pathology of *Hridaya*, i.e. the cardiovascular system. The nature of the pain in the former case will be of a *Vataja* type while in the latter case it will be of *Paittic* type. The *Paittic* pain is usually ischaemic in nature while the pure *Vatic* pain is generally neurogenic and/or spasmodic in nature.

BIOCHEMISTRY OF PAIN

Pain is produced basically by mechanical causes. The stretching effect on tissues hurting the nerve endings has long been identified as the cause of pain but there are a range of intermediary factors that mediate the genesis and transmission of pain perception. Classical Ayurveda depicts the entire biochemical and metabolic functions in terms of its *Tridosa* theory where the entire function is presumed to take place in terms of three fundamental humors – *Vata, Pitta* and *Kapha*. These three factors are integrally in existence in each unit of the body, say each cell of the body, and they function together in a complementary manner in a tri-triangular fashion. These three *Dosas* have properties and functions that are opposed to each other. For example, *Vata* is light, cold and mobile, *Kapha* is heavy, solid and stable, while *Pitta* is liquid, hot and sharp. Because of these opposite attributes the three *Dosas* play complementary roles and control each other. These three bio-factors function in harmony with the three principal biospheric eco-factors, namely air, water and sun. In other words, the *Vata* system of the body represents the air component of the universe, the *Pitta* system of the body represents the sun and the *Kapha* system is the continuum of the water factor of the environment. Air, water and sun are the three angles of the ecological triangle while *Vata, Kapha* and *Pitta* are the three angles of the biological triangle. The *Vedic* traditions consider that the eco and bio triangles function as a continuum of the inner energetic triangle of the subtle body. The three angles of the subtle inner triangle are *Prana, Oja* and *Teja*. Thus, all considerations in Ayurvedic medicine are based respectively on the following tri-triangular eco-genomic model (Figure 2.7).

CHRONIC PAIN

Chronicity of a disease or a symptom in itself is an identifiable entity and it has its denominators, which are often multi-factorial. The most important factors are the virulence and

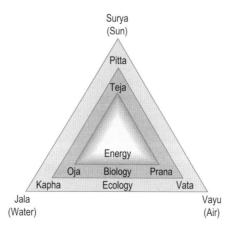

Figure 2.7 **Tri-triangular Ayurvedic model of eco-genomic holism**

SECTION TWO

perpetuation of the aetiological factor. The other denominators are the nature of local factors such as the tissue/organ involved, the mechanisms involved in the production of pain and their reversibility/irreversibility. The superimposed psycho-immune phenomena also play a significant role in determining the chronicity of the disease/symptom.

According to Ayurveda all pathologies are brought about through the phenomenon of *Dosa-Dusya Sammurchhana*, i.e. interaction of vitiated *Dosas* with the vitiable *Dhatus* or tissues. This morbid interaction is largely governed by two major biological factors:

- integrity of *Srotamsi* or the micro-channels of the body, i.e. the membrane system as known in western modern medicine, and
- integrity of *Oja Bala*, i.e. immune strength.

It is believed that the increasing degree of structural *Srotodistortion* and increasing humoral *Ojo-disorder* make the disease gradually chronic and after a stage of chronicity the disease becomes irreversible. This basic phenomenon, as conceived in Ayurveda, can be easily understood if one examines chronic pain conditions like rheumatoid arthritis, known as *Amavata* in Ayurveda, and other similar conditions. Management of such chronic pain/disease in Ayurveda involves bio-purification of channels of the body by *Panchkarma* therapy and immuno-correction by *Rasayana* therapy. This two-fold fundamental cure approach may be added with palliative symptomatic pain care whenever needed.

ACUTE PAIN

Acute pain in a new disease is usually the manifestation of acute or sudden stretching mechanisms in inflammatory conditions, non-inflammatory stretching and hyper-neural impulses. Such states may not be associated with the phenomenon of *Srotodistortion* and *Ojo-disorder* as mentioned above. Even if such disorders exist to some degree in acute pain, they are mostly reversible. Acute pain in Ayurveda is managed by tackling the *Vatic* angle of the *Tridosa* factor. Most of the painkillers are anti-*Vata* remedies.

MANOBALA AND PAIN

Apart from the *Tridosa* theory, Ayurveda also propounds the theory of *Triguna* factors, suggesting that the mind has three distinct properties: *Sattva, Raja* and *Tama. Rajas* represents activity while *Tamas* represents inertia. *Sattva* is essentially the balanced state. It is the balanced functioning of the *Trigunas* dominated by the *Sattva* state that determines the mental stamina or *Manobala* or *Sattva Bala* of an individual. Ayurveda describes three categories of *Sattva Bala*: *Pravara Sattva* (superior mental stamina), *Madhyam Sattva* (medium mental stamina) and *Avara Sattva* (weak mental stamina). A person of *Pravara Sattva* sustains and tolerates pain to a notable extent and does not require frequent doses of analgesics while a person of *Avara Sattva* fails to tolerate even a minor degree of pain and complains of pain disproportionate to the degree of actual pathology. Such persons have a tendency to consume large amounts of analgesic drugs. As a matter of fact, the *Avara Sattva* individuals need more psychotherapy and supportive counselling than chemical analgesics. Thus, according to Ayurveda, psychological management is an integral part of pain care.

CONCLUSION

The concept of pain in Ayurveda is based on the fundamental theories of *Tridosa, Triguna, Srotas* and *Ojas* and hence its management warrants a multifaceted approach. Pain management need not be merely a drug therapy. It can also involve bio-purification of body channels as well as immunostabilisation and management of the psyche.

REFERENCES

1. Charaka. Charaka Samhita. Translated and edited by Sharma PV. Varanasi, India: Choukhamba Orientalia; 2005
2. Madhava kara. Madhava Nidan. Translated and edited by Singhal GD. Varanasi, India: Choukhamba Surbharati; 2000
3. Singh RH. The holistic principles of Ayurvedic medicine. New Delhi, India: Choukhamba Surbharati Prakashan; 2003
4. Singh RH. Kayachikitsa, Vol. I, II. Varanasi, India: Choukhamba Surbharati Publications; 2003
5. Singh RH, Udupa KN, Ram Ji, Mamgain P, Rastogi S, Murthy KN. Advances in Ayurvedic medicine, Vol. 1–5. Varanasi, India: Choukhamba Visvabharati; 2005
6. Susruta. Susruta Samhita. Translated and edited by Singhal GD, et al. Varanasi, India: Choukhamba Surbharati; 2000

SECTION TWO

CONCEPTS OF PAIN IN SPIRITUAL HEALING   Daniel J Benor

INTRODUCTION

Spiritual healing (abbreviated here as *healing*) is arguably the oldest among all of the CAM modalities, found in one form or another in every culture. Shamans in traditional societies and healers in industrial societies are known for treating through the laying on of hands and through prayer/meditation/intent. This chapter reviews the common practices and concepts involved in the use of healing for treating pain.

METHODS

Healing through the laying on of hands is offered with a light touch (not involving manipulation of the body) or with the hands held near to but not touching the body. In shamanic and other healing traditions, the laying on of hands may be supplemented with prayers, meditations, imagery, healing rituals, chants and ceremonies. Prayers and the other methods may also be used alone, without the laying on of hands.

Various systems of healing have been developed and have grown in popularity in modern times,[1] including Therapeutic Touch,[2] Healing Touch,[3] Reiki[4] and many other, less well-known approaches. In the UK, *spiritual healing* is a generic term commonly used for any and all forms of healing. Each approach involves sets of rituals and recommendations of ways for healers to offer healing. Some healing traditions encourage healers to give themselves healing when in need, and some teach people to develop their own healing gifts for self-healing.

THEORIES EXPLAINING HEALING
BIOLOGICAL ENERGIES (BIOENERGIES) IN THE BODY

Healers and healees (those receiving healing) commonly report that during healings they sense heat, tingling, vibrations and other sensations between the hands of the healer and the parts of the body of the healee that are in need of treatment. This is often interpreted as a bioenergy exchange occurring between the healer and the healee. Healers claim to remove blocks to the flows of energies within the bodies of the healees; to release and/or remove excesses of energies; to harmonise energy imbalances; and to supplement missing energies. Bioenergies within the body can be addressed with spiritual healing, as well as by acupuncture, acupressure, reflexology, shiatsu, applied kinesiology and other CAM therapies.[5]

BIOLOGICAL ENERGY FIELDS

Healers and medical intuitives report that they perceive the bioenergy body as an energy field surrounding and interpenetrating the physical body, reflecting the health and illness of the body, emotions, mind, relationships and spirit. Healers report that the biofield is not only the product of physiological processes, it is also an informational template for guiding growth, maintaining integrity and promoting repair of body form and functions. Some sensitives can see changes in the biofield before the manifestation of these changes in the physical body, and can use these to predict the development of physical and psychological illnesses.[5]

Conventional science has confirmed Einstein's observation that matter and energy are interconvertible. The chair we sit on and the floor we stand on can be described as collections of particles; alternatively, they can be described as waves and energies. Conventional Newtonian medicine has been slow to absorb this lesson. Within the frameworks of modern physics, the body may be addressed as matter; it can equally be addressed as energies – which is what many healers believe.[5]

While thus far the definitive identification of biological energies related to healing has eluded measurement, preliminary research has indicated alterations in the infrared spectrum of water following treatment with spiritual healing.[6-8] Observational reports have indicated changes in the surface tension of water and in photographic film treated with healing.[9]

To some extent, all treatments of any sort involve self-healing. This applies to spiritual healing as well. It is speculated by healers that spiritual healing may be particularly effective in this regard because it adds bioenergy and intentional interventions to those present for all therapies through suggestion.

TRANSPERSONAL AGENTS FOR HEALING

Many healers report that they are not the agents for the healings but rather they are channels for healing from Christ, Mary, saints or other religious figures, from angelic or nature spirits, or directly from the Divine.

RELIGIOUS INTERPRETATIONS OF HEALING

Historically, healing has often been given within religious contexts, where it is sometimes claimed that faith in the teachings and tenets of the given religion is required for healing to occur – which has lent the name *faith healing* to this modality. People who are ill may respond better to a person who shares their religious beliefs. While faith may be helpful to members of a religion, the fact that animals, plants and other organisms respond to healing places this assumption in serious question. A further disadvantage to religious involvement in healing can be the engendering of guilt when people suffer blame for their inability to cure themselves or to respond to spiritual healing, interpreting their suffering as punishment for insufficient faith.[10]

SUGGESTION, PLACEBO AND OTHER SELF-HEALING RESPONSES

Suggestion, placebo and other self-healing responses have been documented with every known treatment. Thus, there is reason to believe that every treatment involves a measure of self-healing on the part of the healee, and spiritual healing is no exception.

SPIRITUAL SELF-HEALING

Spiritual self-healing is also possible. It is commonly held by healers that everyone has a measure of spiritual healing ability.[1] Much like playing the piano, some develop their healing gifts easily and spontaneously, some may become proficient with diligent practice and some are best off not engaging in healing lessons. Spiritual healing as taught by member groups of the UK Healers Organisation involves training and certification by peers. Some systems of healing are taught internationally, such as Therapeutic Touch and Healing Touch, and involve extensive training certification and ongoing professional development following certification.

Some systems, such as Reiki, involve inductions of healing abilities by the teacher (*master*) and may be learned in one to three weekends with no further supervision or certification. The UK Healers has a Code of Conduct that has been standardised for its various member organisations.

TOUCH, SKIN SENSITIVITY AND SPIRITUAL HEALING

One possible mechanism whereby laying on of hands healing may be effective is simply through the power of touch, unrelated to spiritual healing. Conversely, part of the potency of touch may reside in the effects of spiritual healing, which may occur even without the conscious knowledge or intention of the practitioner.[11]

RELAXATION, BREATHING AND A BROAD SPECTRUM OF OTHER SELF-HEALING CAPABILITIES

Relaxation, breathing and a broad spectrum of other self-healing capabilities could explain many of the effects of healing on pain. Most people notice a difference between their experiences of pain when they are rested and relaxed compared to when they are tired or anxious. When people are 'uptight' they have a lower tolerance for pain. Through mechanisms of suggestion and relaxation, healers could help to reduce pain.

CONTROLLED STUDIES

Rigorous controlled studies have indicated that there are probably factors related to spiritual healing beyond suggestion and self-healing that reduce pain. Some studies have suggested that spiritual healing is helpful in reducing headache,[12] back pain,[12] arthritis pain[12] and postoperative pain.[13–16] Other studies have explored healing for neck, menstrual and idiopathic pain, but these were not rigorous in either design or reporting or both.

POSSIBLE MECHANISMS FOR THE EXPERIENCE OF PAIN[5]

1. Pain perception is initiated by stimulation of nerve endings in the various organs of the body. Sources of stimulation can include:
   (a) *Mechanical factors* – trauma ranging from chronic external pressure to acute blows or cuts; internal trauma from heavy or chronic repetitive use of the musculoskeletal system beyond its natural capacities; and swelling or other deformity of organs and tissues from factors such as oedema (excessive body fluid), infection and direct trauma to nerves.
   (b) *Chemical or metabolic factors* – caustic external substances or toxins that damage tissues or cause muscle spasms; and accumulations of physiological toxins within the body.
   (c) *Thermal or electromagnetic stimulation* – reactions range from unpleasant sensations, through muscle spasms, to coagulation of tissues.
   (d) *Infections* – direct inflammation of nerves or indirect pain via swelling of tissues and organs.
   (e) *Neoplasms* – tumours with invasions of tissues and nerves, or indirect pain via swelling of, or encroachment upon, tissues and organs, especially nerves and bones.
   (f) *Degenerative factors* – wearing out of tissues and articulating surfaces, with pain felt as the body 'complains' about overuse.
   (g) *Immune system responses* – swelling or inflammation of tissues because of allergic reactions that produce inflammation (rheumatoid arthritis is included here because it is thought to be caused by autoimmune reactions).
   (h) *Neurophysiological factors* – malfunctions of the central and peripheral nervous systems leading to tension in muscles, which eventually tire or spasm producing pain, which in turn creates the vicious circle considered previously.

(i) *Psychological factors* – muscle spasms with tension or conditioned responses; metaphors for emotional problems that are expressed through muscle tensions; and *phantom limb* phenomena following amputations.

2. Pain perception is variable between different people. Pain is more than a simple chain of cause and effect of physical and psychological relationships. One person may have little reaction to a given painful stimulus, while another may writhe in agony under the (apparently) same stimulus or condition. Psychological factors influencing pain perception may involve:

   (a) *Innate differences in pain thresholds* – one person may have less sensitivity to certain stimuli than another.

   (b) *General state of the nervous system* (whether affected by tiredness, anxiety or other emotional factors) – this may relate to altered sensitivity thresholds or to the amount of energy a person has for coping with the added stress of pain.

   (c) *Specific psychological factors* – for example, people may tolerate post-surgical pain well if they know that the operation has resulted in a cure of their illness, or they may tolerate the same pain poorly if they hear that the surgery brought only a diagnosis of incurable disease.

   (d) *Cultural conditionings* – which teach a person to be stoic or vociferous in dealing with pain.

   (e) *Attention factors* – at the height of an emergency or exciting situation (accident, sports event), while engrossed in achieving some immediate objective, a person might not feel pain despite a severe injury. Only later, when attention is focused on the wound, is the pain perceived. People who have a goal to work toward may focus all their attention on this and even deliberately ignore their pain, subsequently finding that they also feel the pain less.

   (f) *Mood factors* – may influence responsivity to pain (anxiety and depression may increase pain, tranquillity and joy decrease it).

   (g) *Rewards associated with the expression of pain* – may influence the frequency of its occurrence and the severity of its expression. A person who unconsciously enjoys some benefit (secondary gain) from a pain, such as avoidance of unpleasant tasks or extra attention from family members, is likely to experience more pain. People who anticipate compensation following accidents are likely to relinquish their pains slowly, if at all.

   I enjoy convalescence. It is the part that makes illness worthwhile.

   George Bernard Shaw

   (h) *Phantom limb phenomena* – persistence of perceptions in a part of the body (limb, breast) that has been amputated, often associated with pains that are experienced as though the limb were still present. Paraplegics (paralysed from the waist down) may have phantom limb pains even when their spinal cords have been completely severed so that no ordinary sensations are felt from beyond the level of the nerves that were cut. Similarly, phantom limb sensations are reported in people with congenital absence of limbs.

   (i) *Fantasy pains* – sensations seemingly created by the mind, where no objective causes can be identified. These may be body metaphor equivalents for anxieties, emotions, traumatic experiences and psychotic misperceptions and misinterpretations of reality.

3. Transpersonal or spiritual awarenesses may contribute to how we experience and comprehend our pains:[10]

   (a) Pain may be experienced and interpreted as a stimulus for people to pray, or to question why they are suffering, and to ask God for help in understanding and dealing with their injury or illness. At the very least, pain may be the unconscious mind's way of forcing them to take a break from stresses or lifestyles that are in some way harmful. Many people who have serious health issues come to feel that their illness led them to re-examine their lives, and to make enormously enriching decisions for better relationships and more emotionally satisfying and rewarding careers, not to mention healthier lifestyles. This life-transforming process may come as a response to the physical challenges that force them to face their mortality and ask questions about the meaning of life.

(b) People may come to feel a spiritual causality that underlies and guides major life challenges, sensing that they might have been deliberately invited or pushed into such experiences by their higher self, by spirit or angelic guides, or by the Infinite Source – as a way of deepening their spiritual quest in life. Pain may be related to lessons chosen by their higher self or soul for their spiritual growth. When people are free of pain they tend to be complacent and coast along, enjoying life but not learning very much. When they are in pain they are challenged to find new solutions to their problems, to plumb the depths of their being, and to push beyond the limits of their ordinary capabilities and awarenesses.

> *We are not human beings having a spiritual experience, but spiritual beings having a human experience.*
>
> Pierre Teilhard de Chardin

(c) Pain may be a residual from a previous incarnation, which invites people to explore this dimension of their existence and to resolve ancient emotional scars.

MECHANISMS FOR HEALING TO RELIEVE PAIN

Any of the mechanisms of healing listed above can interact with the causal mechanisms for pain. The complexity of the human condition thus makes the study of pain a challenge.

PRACTICAL ISSUES

One of the major benefits of healing is that it is a safe intervention, in and of itself. There are no known detrimental effects of healing. It has occasionally been reported that pains may increase temporarily after initial healing treatments. This is viewed by healers as a positive sign, indicating that biological energies are being activated. With time and further healings, the pain levels return to baseline and below.

Where healing is misused as an alternative – rather than as a complement – to other therapies, there can be a danger that effective conventional or other therapies might be delayed to a point when they are no longer effective. In some cases, however, this could be a matter of patients' choices regarding the quality of life they prefer. They may decline to have chemotherapy, for instance, when this might offer limited hope but could seriously impair their enjoyment of life because of its major side effects.

IN SUMMARY

Pain is a multifactorial problem, extremely complex to understand, much less to treat. Spiritual healing is presumed to address many, if not all, of the factors through bioenergies and intent. Self-healing mechanisms present in organisms receiving healing may also be activated by the healing.

REFERENCES

1. Benor DJ. Healing research, volume I – spiritual healing: scientific validation of a healing revolution. Southfield, MI: Vision Publications; 2001

2. Krieger D. Living the therapeutic touch. New York: Dodd Mead; 1987
3. Hover-Kramer D. Healing touch: a guidebook for practitioners. Albany, NY: Thomson Delmar Learning; 2001
4. Barnett L, Chambers M, Davidson S. Reiki energy medicine: bringing healing touch into home, hospital, and hospice. Rochester, VT: Healing Arts; 1996
5. Benor DJ. Healing research, volume II (professional edition): consciousness, bioenergy and healing. Medford, NJ: Wholistic Healing Publications; 2004
6. Miller R. The relationship between the energy state of water and its physical properties. Research paper, Ernest Holmes Research Foundation; undated
7. Rein G, McCraty R. Structural changes in water and DNA associated with new physiologically measurable states. J Sci Explor 1995;8:438–439
8. Schwartz SA, De Mattei RJ, Brame EG Jr, Spottiswoode SJP. Infrared spectra alteration in water proximate to the palms of therapeutic practitioners. Subtle Energies 1990;1:43–72
9. Miller RN. Methods of detecting and measuring healing energies. In: White JW, Krippner S, eds. Future science: life energies and the physics of the paranormal. Garden City, NY: Anchor Press; 1997:431–444
10. Benor DJ. Healing research, volume III – personal spirituality: science, spirit and the eternal soul. Medford, NJ: Wholistic Healing Publications; 2006
11. Montagu A. Touching: the human significance of the skin. New York: Perennial Harper & Row; 1971
12. Redner R, Briner B, Snellman L. Effects of a bioenergy healing technique on chronic pain. Subtle Energies 1991;2:43–68
13. Green WM. The therapeutic effects of distant intercessory prayer and patients' enhanced positive expectations on recovery rates and anxiety levels of hospitalized neurosurgical pituitary patients: a double blind study. Doctoral dissertation. San Francisco: California Institute of Integral Studies; 1993
14. Meehan TC, Mersmann CA, Wisemann ME, Wolff BB, Malgady RG. The effect of therapeutic touch on postoperative pain. Pain 1990;41:S149
15. Silva C. The effects of relaxation touch on the recovery level of postanesthesia abdominal hysterectomy patients (abstract). Altern Ther Health Med 1996;2:94
16. Slater VE. The safety, elements, and effects of Healing Touch on chronic non-malignant abdominal pain. Doctoral dissertation. Knoxville: University of Tennessee, College of Nursing; 1996

CONCEPTS OF PAIN IN HOMEOPATHY — Martien Brands

THE ORIGINAL RECORDS OF PAIN: EXPERIMENTS AND CLINICAL CASES

Pain can be considered a symptom of disease and, as such, a noxious phenomenon, which needs to be eliminated. Pain can also be seen as a sign that requires a correct and precise interpretation; that interpretation depends on the cognitive framework of the observer, and, in a medical context, that knowledge is strongly influenced by emotions and personal experience.[1]

In a form of medicine such as homeopathy, which is based to a large extent on empirical data of experimental and clinical origin, this framework tries to link knowledge of pathophysiology with personal experience of pain. The units of diagnosis and remedy pictures reflect this connection between 'pathogenetic' effects of substances on certain 'target' organs and the sensations patients have experienced. The historical accounts are highly personalised and describe the agony of ill patients as well as the surprisingly strong effects that minute doses exerted on the healthy persons who participated in the 'provings', or experiments, which started around 1800.

These symptoms became connected with the substances that provoked them and were confirmed thereafter in clinical cases of cured patients in which patients received the same substance if their clinical symptom pattern (CSP) was similar to the experimental symptom pattern (ESP).

The ESP contained direct sensations of an acute disturbance of the balance of a healthy person, and the CSP also included pain symptoms, which had been engrained in ill patients already for a long time.

The application of a pattern arising from an acute state (the proving) to a match with the pattern of a chronic illness may in itself be problematic. However, apart from the pain sensations, the remedy pictures include many other symptoms that may assist in finding the remedy: mental, general and local features of those patients who reacted well to the remedy as a curative agent.

This richness of data in the homeopathic classification may seem confusing at first glance but upon closer observation it permits a very personalised diagnosis: peculiar sensations may be linked to specific remedies.

The relationship of the physiology and the patient's actual pain sensations is clarified by comparing Hughes's discussion of the pathogenic action of nux vomica: 'it is especially indicated when the muscular coat of the stomach is involved, making its churning movements irregular, inharmonious and painful'[2] with Boyd's description of the typical nux vomica pain: 'there is much retching with peristaltic movements and distension, usually 2–3 hours after food – vomiting tends to relieve the symptoms. It is a cramping or stitching pain.'[3]

So a specific sensation may become a 'sign' if it can refer to something. In other words, 'something is not there until you see it'; here, this something, this sensation, needs to be put into an experiential framework to be acknowledged. Hence, pain can be interpreted as a symptom of illness if we have the appropriate framework. If that framework is not available, pain unfortunately is often reasoned away or simply negated.

The illness is, however, the lived experience, in contrast to the disease, which reflects the classification system of the practitioners. This refers to the tension between *experienced* symptoms such as pain and *classifiable* symptoms. Hahnemann, the founder of homeopathy, saw this tension already when he asked to let the patient spontaneously tell – and finish – his or her story of illness.[4]

In the first general description of the homeopathic method, dated 1810, it was already advised to listen to this experience very carefully:[4]

> *'This individualising examination of a case of disease, for which I shall only give in this place general directions, of which the practitioner will bear in mind only what is applicable for each individual case, demands of the physician nothing but freedom from prejudice and sound senses, attention in observing and fidelity in tracing the picture of the disease.*
>
> *The patient details the history of his sufferings; those about him tell what they heard him complain of, how he has behaved and what they have noticed in him; the physician sees, hears, and remarks by his other senses what there is of an altered or unusual character about him. He writes down accurately all that the patient and his friends have told him in the very expressions used by them. Keeping silence himself he allows them to say all they have to say, and refrains from interrupting them unless they wander off to other matters. The physician advises them at the beginning of the examination to speak slowly, in order that he may take down in writing the important parts of what the speakers say.*
>
> *Every interruption breaks the train of thought of the narrators, and all they would have said at first does not again occur to them in precisely the same manner after that.'*

Key elements in homeopathic case taking therefore are:

- the spontaneous, uninterrupted flow of the patient's narrative
- the hetero-anamnesis of relatives and friends
- the almost literal recording of the patient's account.

The first brings about the associations that may guide the observer's insight into the inner world of the patient and the second may shed light on less emphasised features of the patient. The last may specify the sensations and link them to certain remedies as they are documented to liaise with specific expressions, either during the provings as provoked symptoms or from clinical cases which reacted well to the remedy.

Whether this careful method contributes to the so-called 'placebo effect' in homeopathy can only be clarified if, first, this *method* is compared with other consultations where the above techniques are not applied, through verbatim transcript and video recording (which may influence the context itself), and, second, the *outcome* of homeopathic consultations is compared with the outcome in similar illnesses treated in other medical specialties which pay comparable attention to the patient.[5] If the latter yielded similar results as homeopathy, one could argue that there would be little reason to continue prescribing analgesics as the consultation would lead to an 'effective healing context'. Psychogenic pain especially, or at least pain maintained by psychological factors, could then be treated with less analgesic medication.

Another important issue is that we need to distinguish between internal and external pain. Externally perceived pain, like chronic pain, presents in different forms such as headache, abdominal pain or musculoskeletal pain. These manifestations can be signs which refer to deeper layered, 'internal' pain requiring a multidisciplinary approach that clearly distinguishes between physical and psychological aspects. They may complement each other rather than be used as ammunition in an 'either/or' argument about the somatic or psychological aetiology of pain syndromes.

With regards to homeopathy, the hermeneutic or 'interpretational' approach of pain points to pain as part of a larger whole of lived experience. From this point of departure, if we consider acute pain as part of ESPs, and chronic pain as part of CSPs, we need to approach acute and chronic pain types from a different perspective, both diagnostically and therapeutically.

ACUTE PAIN

Especially for acute pain, its cause often shimmers through in its actual presentation. Acute pain is usually the result of a concrete impact of an external agent on the organism. The agent can be any sort of inflammation or trauma, and both causes demand quite specific homeopathic treatment. First of all, the target tissue, i.e. the tissue that is affected by the trauma, plays a major role in the choice of remedy. An example is the module from the training method of 'Homeopaths without Borders', where specific target organs are related to several remedies. The different remedies are indicated by very different types of pain (Table 2.9).

With inflammation, too, the pain is characterised by a specific sensation and often also by modalities (modifying circumstances which aggravate or improve the pain); together these form a very typical pattern. These types of pain are often 'key symptoms', i.e. their presence is highly predictive for the presence of other symptoms belonging to the same remedy picture.

Hughes described the pain quality with an example from his own practice, where someone had previously been treated with homeopathic remedies for gastric pain without result:

> 'He stated that he could compare it to nothing but a burning furnace within. I recollected that this was a leading symptom of arsenic and ... (administered) ... arsenic, a spoonful to be taken every 6 hours; the first dosis gave immediate relief; ... the next day the man was quite well, and required no further attendance.'[2]

The 'semantic marker' or key symptom 'burning furnace' guided the doctor to the choice of the effective remedy. This case is interesting because it highlights the relationship

Table 2.9 **Acute trauma: target tissues for remedies; example bruises**

Remedy	Target tissue	Indicative symptoms for choice*
Arnica	Soft tissue, blood vessel walls	Haematoma, extravasation S: Pain 'as if beaten', bruised M: worse and aversion to touch
Bellis perennis	Abdomen, pelvis	Deep wounds Sore, deep pain M: made worse by touch, cold, warm bed; better by motion, rubbing
Hypericum	Nerves, finger tips, coccyx, spinal cord	Sharp, 'electric' pain, shooting up the nerve M: made worse by cold, damp
Ledum	Sharp injury: bites, stitches	Long-lasting discoloration S: spots feel cold M: made worse by motion; better by cold
Ruta	Fibrous tissue, periosteum, tendons, ligaments	S: sore, bruised, aching M: made worse by rest, touch, cold; better by motion but aversion to motion

*S, sensations; M, 'modalities' (positive or negative influence on the sensation).

between a disease category and a clear individual sensation, but in general it is highly improbable that just one symptom will predict the right choice of a remedy; its 'referential power' increases only if it is *accompanied* by other symptoms. Then, the probability of finding the 'predicted' remedy increases rapidly.

CHRONIC PAIN

The other pain type is chronic pain encountered in syndromes such as osteoarthritis or migraine. Here, pain has become embedded in the patient's illness and has penetrated into his or her personality. The distinction in 'internal' and 'external' pain manifestations refers to the concept of blocking or discharging the original pain. 'Post-traumatic stress disorder' can serve as an example; the acute pain may indeed have been psychic pain, which has 'gone underground' in the course of time. It was pain such as this that trainers of organisations like 'Homeopaths without Borders' encountered in 2001 in an 'endemic' form in Bosnia after the war of 1992–1997. Almost everybody had experienced traumatic war situations; however, individuals suffered to a different degree from the aftermath. Roughly speaking, 'fight, fright and flight' are the three basic patterns of stress reaction and lead in post-traumatic stress disorder to three states, respectively aggression/acting out, anxiety and withdrawal. These reactive types are depicted in some homeopathic remedy pictures (Table 2.10).

However, in the course of time, the reactions become mixed with the patient's own personality, leading to the development of symptom patterns that bear the traces of several reaction patterns and that are also modulated by personal coping mechanisms. We can distinguish two approaches here: one focuses on the actual traumatic situation and the other addresses the modifications by biographical occurrences in the development of the personality.

Inadequate coping mechanisms fail to help the person to re-integrate the trauma into a newly organised, balanced personality; this implies that the 'root' of the disease, the original situation, seems to continue to exist, the 'root context' maintains the pathological process.[6] This is comparable with the cognitive psychological notion that a form of mental

Table 2.10 Different remedies for traumatic events

Aconite
Sudden shock
Terror of death
Anxiety, worse at night
Claustrophobia
Physical:
Chest palpitations
Great thirst
Urine retention
Pneumonia

Arnica
Physical and psychological trauma
Refuses help of doctor or nurse
Physical:
Haematoma and bruised feeling, pain on trauma sites
Everything feels too hard, even bed or pillow
Easy nosebleed
Brain concussion
Cough from weeping
Target action: on blood vessels: trauma plus bleeding or haematoma

Arsenicum
Anxiety and restlessness
Worried and tense
Fear of death, disease, robbers, being alone
Desire to be in control, precise
Generally worse around midnight
Physical:
Burning pains
Gastric ulcers
Frequent thirst for small sips
Offensive diarrhoea
Itching/burning eczema
Asthma worse between 00.00 h and 02.00 h
Cold extremities

Belladonna
Violence of sudden onset
Delirium, hallucination
Fear of dogs
Hot head, cold extremities
Physical:
Convulsions, twitches, jerks
Flushes of heat
Red, sweating face
Headache: relieved by pressure, worsened by noise, light, jarring
Any inflammation with heat, redness, swelling and pain

Opium
After fright
Stupor, dreaminess
Anaesthesia, painlessness of normally painful complaints
Alternation between stupor and restlessness
Physical:
Convulsions
Sleepiness
Dilated pupils
Constipation
Snoring in sleep
Heavy sleep

Stramonium
Violence, rage
Fears: violence, dark, death, water, mirrors
Mania, homicide

Nightmares,
Night terrors
Impulsive
Hyperactive children
Physical:
Convulsions
Jerking of the head
Strabismus
Violent sexual desire
Combined:
fears and convulsions;
tempers and fears or nightmares

Ignatia
Hypersensitive; contraction
Easily offended, touchy
Sighing; sobbing instead of crying
Physical:
Numbness, cramps
Convulsions
Lump in throat
Hiccough
Rectal spasms, prolapse
Trembling after coffee
Aversion to fruit and tobacco smoke
Exacerbated by sweets

Natrum muriaticum
Retention and inhibition
Silent grief
Withdrawal
Aversion to consolation
Retaining past grief
Physical:
Retention (salt and water):
Hypertension
Headache
Constipation
Low back pain, > pressure/hard bed
Craving for salty, sour foods
Aversion to sun and fatty, rich foods

Phosphoric acid
Exhaustion
Depressed, apathetic
Collapsed state
Answers slowly
Stupefied with grief
Physical:
Weakness after loss of body fluids (diarrhoea)
Bloody diarrhoea
Chilly
Hair loss from grief
Blue rings around eyes
Intolerance to fresh fruits, juices

Staphy-sagria
Sensitive to rudeness
Suppression of anger, outburst of anger
Wounded honour
Shy; sexual fantasies
Physical:
Styes/tumours on eyelids
Frequent cystitis, esp. after coitus
Complaints after suppressed anger
Sleepy by day, sleepless at night
Worse after surgery

conditioning has occurred that keeps the person in a stereotypical reaction form. Sankaran pleads for a search for the remedy that best fits the 'root situation', which in this context means the original 'painful situation'. Many case studies show that this can have positive effects if this origin is clearly identified.[6] However, the trauma may not only be covered by subsequent life experience but also it can have merged with the pre-existent personality. Vithoulkas introduced the concept of 'layers', an archaeological metaphor provoking associations with psycho-analytical concepts.[7] Often the ramifications do not manifest themselves as a clear single pattern referring back to the original trauma, so one single remedy cannot always resolve the psychic pain; several are needed in sequence to 'disclose' deeper layers.

In general, the potential diversity in pathological reactions requires the application of a much wider choice of remedies than can be given in a single table, although this table can indicate the accents that should be taken into account when approaching psychic pain. Many of these remedies have a wide range of application so may be applied to persons with more symptom patterns than are shown here.

INDIVIDUAL SENSITIVITY

One of the reasons for differences in pain experience is the different sensitivity to pain stimuli, be it physical or psychological. Pain thresholds have large inter-individual differences. This runs parallel to the homeopathic approach to pain, in terms of both diagnosis and treatment.

A contemporary representation of the homeopathic theory defines as the central concept: the *sensitivity* of the receiver and the receiver is a complex system. Moreover, the intervention is complex as well, as the aqueous structure of the solution is manipulated.

People are sensitive to a remedy if they have a specific reactive pattern, and part of this pattern is how they deal with pain. To get access to 'old' pain, that is to 'break open' certain pathways – we can consider them neuronal circuits in accordance with the well-known 'gate theory' of Melzack – neurones may be activated depending on the input of other neurones, so for reduction of pain the whole system needs to be influenced.[8] Therefore, it is essential that the substance 'matches' the receptor sensitivity. Receptors are empirically established entities and some of them are apparently sensitive to serially diluted and agitated (SDA) solutions, as used in homeopathic remedies.

Such a substance is histamine, which in its SDA form maintains its feedback mechanism in basophil degranulation, a key immune reaction.[8,9] As histamine has many connections to serotonin, receptors in the immune system are apparently linked to the nervous system, in which serotonin is a key neurotransmitter. Memory is established through the influence of serotonin on dendritic cells, which induce 'naive' T cells to proliferate to T memory cells.[10] There is therefore a close link between our immune and nervous systems in terms of the establishment of memory. Both are closely linked in pain management.

The following hypothesis is presented. If serotonin is neuro-immunologically so closely linked to histamine, then serotonin in SDA form may affect the serotonin receptors in a parallel mode to how SDA histamine influences histamine receptors. When this is empirically established, it will show that a main pathway of information distribution, the neuronal and immune systems, is sensitive to homeopathically prepared substances, substantiating the claim that self-healing processes are reinforced by homeopathic interventions.

PRINCIPLES UNDERLYING SENSITIVITY

In general, research into the homeopathic approach to pain can lead to a widening of the horizon of our understanding of receptor functioning. First of all, the measured physico-chemical changes in SDA aqueous solutions may redefine traditional linear pharmacological concepts in dose–effect relationships towards non-linearity – a feature of complexity.[11,12] Applied to specific receptors, this suggests that most probable receptors respond to signals rather than doses of certain medicines. These function as messengers, which has implications for pain syndrome treatment, both psychologically and physiologically: it is rather a matter of finding the right access to an unbalanced circuit than blocking entire nervous pathways with high doses.

The following summary can be made of the basic homeopathic concepts with regards to pain. First, the diagnostic principle is the matching of a sensitive person to a remedy intervention; this is the rule of similars. Homeopathic diagnosis is the description of a remedy picture or 'sensitivity profile', i.e. the pattern of features that someone needs to have to be sensitive to a certain remedy. These features belong to remedies as they come from patients who were sensitive to them. It is a case-based reasoning such as in law: jurisprudence compares the actual case to the rules established in law reference books.

The second principle is the intervention with a substance, which is prepared in such a way that it has become a 'non-linear dose–response agent'. That means that the response is not a linear function of the increase of dose. This is understandable if we consider the bipolarity of a biological agent. The same substance can, depending on the context – a healthy or ill person – suppress or stimulate the same reaction mechanism. For example, anti-epileptics, meant to suppress convulsions, can provoke convulsions in higher doses; similarly, digoxin has a similar bilateral relationship to arrhythmias and neuroleptics to hyperexcitation.[13]

Clinically, a sensitive person needs a small stimulus to achieve a measurable and often large clinical and biological effect on pain receptors. The small stimulus, however, can be small because of the special preparation which changes the original substance in a complex system, an aqueous solution of a biologically active agent. This solution is modified in its structure, although the chemical composition may finally not be different from distilled water.[14]

Therefore, the final pharmacodynamic concept is that of complexity, both on the level of medication processing and in the system into which the medication is introduced. This can form a bridge with more 'monocausal' approaches in medicine: one does not exclude the other, but complexity is a more comprehensive concept of reality in all its diversity and vicissitudes. Systems biology provides adequate models to test the interaction of multiple variables in complex systems, such as principal component analysis.[15]

Pain remains part of a larger whole and complexity analysis will support the clinical relevance of homeopathic case-taking for assessing the sensitivity of a specific person to pain treatment with this treatment modality.

REFERENCES

1. Brands M, Franck D, Leeuwen van E. Epistemology and semiotics of medical systems: a comparative analysis. Semiotica 2000;132:1–24
2. Hughes R. The principle and practice of homeopathy (repr). New Delhi: B Jain Publishers; 1985
3. Boyd H. Introduction to homeopathic medicine. Beaconsfield, UK: Beaconsfield Publishers; 1989
4. Hahnemann S. Organon of medicine. London: Victor Gollancz; 1983
5. Di Blasi Z, Harkness E, Ernst E, Georgiou A, Kleijnen J. Influence of context effects on health outcomes: a systematic review. Lancet 2001;357:757–762
6. Sankaran R. The system of homeopathy. Mumbai, India: Homeopathic Medical Publishers; 2000
7. Vithoulkas G. The science of homeopathy. New York: Grove Press; 1980
8. Kandel ER, Schwartz JH, Jessell TM. Principles of neural science, 4th edn. New York: McGraw-Hill; 2000:482–486
9. Belon P, Cumps J, Ennis M, Mannaioni PF, Roberfroid M, Sainte-Laudy J, Wiegant FA. Histamine dilutions modulate basophil activation. Inflamm Res 2004;53:181–188
10. Brown V, Ennis M. Flow-cytometric analysis of basophil activation: inhibition by histamine at conventional and homoeopathic concentrations. Inflamm Res 2001;50(Suppl. 2):S47–S48
11. O'Connell PJ, Wang X, Leon-Ponte M, Griffiths C, Pingle SC, Ahern GP. A novel form of immune signalling revealed by transmission of the inflammatory mediator serotonin between dendritic cells and T cells. Blood 2005;7:2903

12. Elia V, Napoli E, Niccoli M, Nonatelli L, Ramaglia A, Ventimiglia E. New physico-chemical properties of extremely diluted aqueous solutions: a calorimetric and conductivity study at 25°C. J Thermal Analysis Calorimetry 2004;78:331–342

13. Elia V, Marchese M, Montanino M, Napoli E, Niccoli M, Nonatelli L, Ramaglia A. Hydrohysteretic phenomena of "extremely diluted solutions" induced by mechanical treatments. A calorimetric and conductometric study at 25°C. J Solution Chem 2005;34: 947–960

14. Eskinazi D. Homeopathy re-revisited. Is homeopathy compatible with biomedical observations? Arch Intern Med 1999;159:1981–1987

15. Greef van der J, McBurney RN. Rescuing drug discovery: *in vivo* systems pathology and systems pharmacology. Nat Rev 2005;4:961–967

NATUROPATHIC CONCEPTS OF PAIN   Bernhard Uehleke

WHAT IS NATUROPATHY?

It is necessary to give a short definition of what can be understood by the term naturopathy because there are a number of different views on the subject. The idea that naturopathy, in its widest sense, is synonymous with CAM is not acceptable either historically or in its content. There is no unique definition of naturopathy but only divergent characteristics and descriptions. For this reason it makes sense to look at the history of naturopathy.

The term first appeared in the middle of the 19th century in Germany and had forerunners in the 18th century but they were not dogmatically opposed to mainstream medicine.[1] In its content the 19th century naturopathy based itself on the dogmatic and medicine-critical Hydropathic Movement. Step-by-step, the fanatic cold-water cures of the Hydropathic Movement were combined, at first at random but later systematically, with other natural healing methods such as sunlight, fresh air, physical training, healthy foods, herbs and *Ordnungstherapie* (see Table 2.11), which is a forerunner of psychosomatics and overlaps broadly with body and mind medicine.

Table 2.11 **Main naturopathic treatments**

Treatments	Description/functions
Hydropathy	Especially Kneipp treatments: effusions, partial baths, wraps, mostly cold, but also warm–hot and alternating
Exercise therapy	Natural movements patterns, sports (alone and with instruction, also in groups)
Massage, manual therapy	Classical massage and connective tissue massage according to Dicke; other manual therapies
Nutritional therapy	Diet of whole foods, calorie conscious, little meat, mostly vegetarian
Fasting	Restriction of food intake for detoxification, relief and rebalancing, according to the ideas of the pioneers Schroth, Buchinger and Mayr
Heliotherapy	Radiation with sunlight or with similar spectrum including ultraviolet B
Herbal therapy	Restricted to mildly active herbal plants with little risk
Ordnungstherapie	Stress-adapted healthy lifestyle, relaxation exercises like autogenic training, muscle relaxation, yoga, etc.

Up to this day, one of the characteristics of naturopathy is that it is based on natural remedies or on treatments based on natural sources but, for scientific theory, this is unsatisfactory because it comprises a relatively arbitrary listing of natural healing methods. For that reason a number of representatives consciously abstain from using a naturopathic nosology and diagnosis and do not talk of naturopathy or natural medicine but rather about natural healing methods.[2] These are the above-mentioned natural healing methods, which work with heat, cold, air, water, physical exercise including massage and manual therapy, diet and fasting, *Ordnungstherapie* and herbs. This list of natural healing methods has also been termed 'classical natural healing methods', because their use can also be found in the classical times of the ancient Greeks.

The other major characteristic relates to the supposed inherent mechanism of these therapies to stimulate the body's ability to heal itself. Apparently these self-regeneration forces are quite difficult to grasp and define, and therefore they are of little help in delineating the borders between naturopathy and other medical or complementary methods.[3] The strengthening of self-regeneration forces would be achieved by rather unspecific therapies instead of by modern specific ones. However, for a number of natural healing methods, particularly some herbal medicines, this cannot be upheld nowadays because of new discoveries of very specific modes of action.[4] A further problem is that the idea of stimulation of self-regeneration is put forward by many other complementary methods, especially by many discredited speculative therapies.

Both characteristics are often used in combination with each other or include other aspects, e.g. empowerment of self-competence, which considers natural instincts as part of the therapy.[5] In addition, it cannot be overlooked that many followers of naturopathy have their own religious or philosophical–evolutionary interpretation of life and that their motivation is therefore different from that of modern medical science. Just as the followers of naturopathy were trying to live a healthy life 150 years ago, so too are today's followers, not because there are new scientific medical studies but because man (be it through God as Kneipp, a water healer and priest and one of the best-known founders of naturopathy in the 19th century, and others believed, or through the evolutionary process according to Darwin) is best suited to a natural lifestyle and not to modern civilisation with its cars, TV and fast food.

All of these complex aspects of naturopathy allow little clarification of its characteristics and delineation of what is part of it and what is not. In this undefined free space, other treatment forms besides technical and mechanical methods have established themselves, such as reflex therapies, neural therapy, etc. Even many of the former academic medical practices like leeches, cupping and other drastic detoxification procedures, which were violently opposed by early naturopaths, have found their way into today's naturopathy after they were given up by academic medicine in the middle of the 20th century.[6]

Another possibility that might provide a concrete definition of naturopathy would be the restriction to only those methods that can be perceived through the human senses. That would mean that many of the naturally existing stimuli automatically become part of naturopathy – including acupuncture with its conscious use of pain stimuli. In this sense naturopathy could be found anywhere in the world, so this definition is not suitable to describe traditional European medical practices. Therefore, it might be better to speak of traditional European medicine, particularly because it is based on the knowledge that the classical naturopathic methods already played an important role in the writings of the Hippocratic School of ancient Greece, especially regarding maintenance of health and disease prevention. These classical naturopathic treatments are found throughout the medical history of Europe – in each period with their corresponding nosologies; the system of the four body fluids has especially been used predominantly and continuously in 'monastery medicine' up until the 20th century.[7] At the end of the 19th century, for example, Kneipp thought to encourage blood circulation through a cold-water stimulus and by this means to mobilise bad substances.[8] This is nothing but the old-fashioned *materia peccans* and he added mild medicinal herbs to eliminate them by natural excretion. Other naturopaths have developed more or less their own adaptations of the four body fluids system.

It is not surprising that naturopathy at the end of the 19th century became closer to academic medicine again. Academic medicine on the other hand was under political pressure to incorporate classical naturopathic treatments, although with a somewhat different emphasis on new specialties, e.g. physical medicine, sport medicine, dietetics and psychosomatics. For naturopathy on its own, the possibilities to develop its own scientific system were and still are quite limited because of the lack of a continual academic base, financial resources and experts.

PAIN – NOT AN INDEPENDENT TOPIC IN TRADITIONAL EUROPEAN MEDICINE AND NATUROPATHY

HISTORICAL PERSPECTIVE – PAIN AS A WARNING SIGNAL

Throughout the whole of European medical history, pain has been viewed as a warning signal that is precious in itself and gives rise to the treatment of the underlying cause. In as much as one will not find pain as an independent indication, pain relief is not in itself a goal. Of course, the various types of illnesses or conditions that are accompanied by pain or ache are known: toothache, headaches, abdominal pains, podagra (or gout), and treatment strategies were developed against them.

DIFFERENTIATION ACCORDING TO THE FOUR BODY FLUIDS SYSTEM OF TRADITIONAL EUROPEAN MEDICINE

The four body fluids system differentiates first of all between cramp-like pain and the pain accompanying inflammation. Deep constant pain of the musculoskeletal system is supposed to correspond more to the qualities of cold and dry and should benefit from a warming treatment. This treatment is not only made with application of warm water but also through hot foods and medicinal herbs with warming qualities.

Deposited harmful substances are supposed to be broken up or diluted and eliminated, for which outcome liquid has to be added to the body. Inflammation and fever are the efforts of the body to get rid of bad substances. The pain in an acute attack of gout is the prototype of an inflammatory pain, which is characterised by too much heat. When the patient can no longer bear this inflammation then the inflammation can be reduced by cooling.

Differences are made between attack-like pains (i.e. attacks of gout) and the time in between these attacks, which are always treated with warmth. Hardening using a short-duration cold stimulus to stimulate the inner heat was also known. All severe acute pain of the musculoskeletal system is cooled by cold-water treatments.[9]

On the other hand, forms of pain without inflammation (i.e. attack-like abdominal pains) are considered of a cold nature and therefore need to be treated with warmth. Stomach pains and the absence of digestive power are seen in connection with the inadequate fire of the stomach and are to be treated also with warming treatments and 'hot' foods or by drinking warm water.[10]

The advice for treatment of headaches is not always uniform. Some pour lukewarm water over the head,[11] others wash the head in cold water[12] or bath in cold water.[10] As a regulating measure to draw off the blood from the head down to the lower extremities, warm footbaths are advised for headaches.[13] From today's perspective the various forms of headaches, like migraines, tension headaches, etc., were not taken into account and this could be an explanation for the seemingly contradicting treatments. For earaches and toothaches both the cooling and warming treatments are recommended.

FURTHER CRITERIA FOR THE DIFFERENTIATION OF PAIN

The German forerunner of the dogmatic cold-water therapy, Johann Siegmund Hahn, differentiated in the middle of the 18th century between inner and outer pain and then treated these with either cold-water drinks or external cold-water applications. He had ideas about the fluidity of the blood; the blood of his patients had to be diluted with water, which then was supposed to relieve the pain.[14]

At the beginning of the 19th century, the English doctor John Currie dared to use cold water to lower fever with great success and he explained the effect by the subtraction of heat[15] while his opponent John Jackson already talked of an irritative stimulating reaction and anticipated the stress reaction.[16] According to John Hunter, the application of a stimulus is seen in connection with the idea that two functions cannot happen at the same time, which explains, for example, the effects of cold baths during epileptic fits.[17] Today's widely used idea in pain therapy about 'counter irritations' is a specific case of this much older and more general principle.

PAIN TREATMENT IN NATUROPATHY DURING THE 19TH CENTURY

The early naturopathy of the 19th century stayed with this idea but focused, in a one-sided dogmatic way, only on cold water. Painful processes of (from today's point of view) heroic cold-water cures were interpreted as a sign of an active healing crisis. Syphilis patients longed for the deep bone pain which showed the healing crisis and the break up of old deposits from previous medications (mercury salts) out of the bones. The cold-water treatments were used against all kinds of pain conditions. Oertel et al. also mentioned a forerunner of massages, namely brush massages, and suggested that pain can be 'spread but not eradicated' completely.[18] During the development of hydropathy, physical activity, staying in the fresh air ('air baths') and a vegetarian diet are also considered important for pain patients. For treatment of acute pain, ice and snow or a cooling salt mixture are sometimes used externally.[19] Ice water was also taken internally in acute cases of rheumatism, facial pain (*tic douloureux*) and hip pain.[20]

The first and very successful owner of a hydropathic–naturopathic spa Vincenz Prießnitz at first focused completely on drinking litres of cold water and taking cold baths or cold partial baths for all of his patients. Later he added, on the request of his patients, intensive sweating procedures, particularly against pain.[21]

Against stomach cramps, bloating and stomach pain his pupil Munde also recommended hot foot baths and, for a colic, either hot wraps or wraps with ice or snow.[22] Other naturopaths explained the effects of cold-water cures through the changing of a chronic illness into an acute phase[23] during which the bad substances are mobilised and eliminated.[24]

According to the idea of 'natural instinct' it is possible to go by one's own feelings, but if, through spoiling by civilisation or poisons, the natural instinct is lost, the naturopath has to intervene. If, nowadays, scholastic recommendations are no longer being made but the patient is involved in the choice of the treatment (i.e. cold or warm treatment) this should yield better results.

In 1856 Liébault from Nancy tried painless births with the help of hypnosis but this remains fragmentary and was not picked up by academic medicine or naturopathy before the beginning of the 20th century.

Kneipp, famous also for his use of medicinal herbs, used alternating warm and cold applications for pain and later introduced the steamed hot hay sack into naturopathic pain therapy. He also continued the ideas of traditional European medicine with treatments that were intended to dissolve congestions and to eliminate the 'bad matter'.[25]

In the course of the 20th century, pathophysiological ideas on the mode of action of natural healing methods changed in parallel with those of academic medicine.

At the beginning of the 21st century, evidence-based-medicine, even in naturopathy, focuses pragmatically on the clinical results of studies but neglects pathomechanisms, nosologies and explanations on mode of action. Hence, potentially more successful individualised naturopathic treatment of pain might be prevented.

TODAY'S VIEWPOINT ON THE NATUROPATHIC THERAPY OF PAIN
GENERAL VIEWPOINTS

As in the past, pain is viewed today as an alarm signal that develops its own unfavourable dynamic when it becomes chronic and needs intervention.

The forms of pain are still differentiated according to their phenomenological type, localisation and underlying disease, etc. Using this information, a plan for a differential therapy is drawn up. The old rule of 'cold against inflammatory pain and warmth against cramp-like pain' is not used as rigidly today as in the 19th century, and the instinct or feeling of the patient is taken into account. Furthermore, a patient-centred and holistic viewpoint including the patient's psyche, social surroundings, etc. is applied in today's naturopathy. Of course, one may question if this can be followed in everyday practice but it should at least be tried. Most importantly the strengthening of self-healing powers and resources on all levels is the aim of the therapeutic approach because they are formulated in the modern health model of Antonovsky.[26]

The idea of constitutional aspects, recently put forward by M. Bühring, seems more important for the tolerability of the treatments than for a differential diagnosis and therapy. All constitutional typologies have the disadvantage that most patients are of a mixed type and therefore cannot be easily categorised into the example types found in textbooks. Further research is needed to establish constitutional aspects in differential therapy.[28]

More interesting is the idea that specific malfunctions, such as a 'focus' or irritation centre, can have a triggering or promoting role in a completely different area of the body (see below). For an overview of important naturopathic principles of pain management see Table 2.12.

SPECIAL ACTIVE PRINCIPLES OF NATUROPATHY
Strengthening of the psyche/avoidance of stress/good sleep

At first it is important to obtain general psychological stabilisation and, if necessary, to improve mood and pain-disturbed sleep. After all, pain and stress reinforce each other so that sedation and stress reduction are sensible.

Even more fundamental is to increase resistance against the negative influence of too much psychic stress through serial use of somatic body stress factors, especially through the cold treatments according to Kneipp. Through psychotherapy or therapy with the herbal remedy St John's wort the depressive mood can also be improved.

Disturbed sleep as the result of pain is treated with simple naturopathic methods such as taking warm baths with the addition of citronella oil, long-term therapy with valerian root or hydropathic measures.

All in all the patient should not become dependent on the therapist but instead should develop self-reliance in handling the illness.

General strengthening and somatic resistance

Strengthening the body as well as the individual organ functions will indirectly help the self-healing of the pain syndrome. The basic idea of increasing the body's resistance is to stimulate the adaptation reactions through a series of stimuli to achieve better functioning of the immune system and have a better defence against harmful influences. Through such unspecific stimuli the adaptation processes and malfunctions are removed or improved. Through hydrotherapy an improvement of the circulation can also be achieved while physical exercise promotes muscular build-up, function, coordination, endurance, etc.

Foci/irritation centres/reflex zones

It is ancient medical knowledge that specific irritation centres or foci can trigger or promote a disease. Massage therapists are aware of trigger points, there are cutaneous–visceral

Table 2.12 **Important naturopathic principles of pain treatment**

Naturopathic principle	Naturopathic treatments	Explanation of mode of action
Hardening Unspecific strengthening	Hydrotherapy (cold stimuli); physical training (short maximal intensity); physiotherapy	Circulation; metabolism; resistance against stress; immune modulation; function
Influence to psyche	Herbals (sedativa, St John's wort); hydrotherapy; relaxation; psychotherapy	Sedative, antidepressive pharmacological effects; hardening against stress; stress reduction; sedation; perception of own body
Foci, reflex zones	Trigger point massages; reflexology; focal therapy	Influence the substrate of trigger points (gelosis); reflexive effects
Umstimmung	Fasting, nutritional therapy; Kneipp cure, *Klimakur* (rehabilitation programme at a health spa with emphasis on climatic stimuli)	Lowering of arachidonic acid, immune modulation; gut function
Dilution, deviation and mobilisation of *materia peccans*	Hydrotherapy, balneology, sauna, massage; herbs stimulating circulation	Circulation, metabolism
Elimination of *materia peccans*	Diuretic herbs, laxatives; immersion, leeches, cupping	Stimulation of excretion organs and excretion through the skin
Contra-stimulation	Cutaneous irritation (warm and cold), pain, cupping, massage	Counter-irritation, other feelings, mental distraction
Antiphlogistic effects	Cooling, nutrition, herbal remedies	Antiphlogenesis by lowering arachidonic acid and inhibition of cyclo-oxygenase; analgesia by capsaicin

connective tissue zones, pseudoradicular irritation and points of pain, and the neural therapists talk of a 'focus of disease'. Manipulations far away from the symptom are expected to help.

Rebalancing

The idea of rebalancing an out-of-balance organism is ancient and has persisted in naturopathy. Protective measures such as fasting are applied and, if necessary, are used in combination with eliminating measures or series of stimuli. Finally, a careful transition into normal life helps the 'newly programmed' body into healthy stability.

Dilution, deviation and elimination

There is the idea that a local accumulation of 'bad matter' or *materia peccans* can be the reason for disease or foci. Through warmth, dampness and a better circulation the bad matters are diluted and mobilised or deviated. For these detoxifying stimuli, wet cupping, artificially made wounds and leeches were previously used in traditional European medicine.

'Bad matter' is removed from the blood after mobilisation naturally by the excretory organs. Here one should not only think of the stimulation of the kidney and of laxation but also of the stimulation of the liver and gall bladder as well as of diaphoresis. The ancients in traditional European medicine used emmenagogues and blood letting and these were previously fought against by naturopathy but later partially incorporated.

Counter-irritation

Contra-stimulation and distractions are possibilities for influencing acute and chronic pain conditions. Deep-seated chronic pain is supposed to be covered up by peripheral and subcutaneous sensory stimuli, especially pain stimuli. The effects of leeches and wet cupping are explained today through irritation or contra-stimulation rather than through elimination.

CONCLUSION

Modern naturopathy has left its dogmatic isolation and offers pain therapy in conjunction with modern 'academic' treatments. Integrated concepts allow for new developments in modern pain therapy.

REFERENCES

1. Uehleke B. Zur Nennung des Begriffs Naturmedizin bei Daniel Fischer um 1745 als Vorgriff auf die ein Jahrhundert später entwickelte Naturheilkunde. Sudhoffs Archiv 1998;82:98–101
2. Hentschel HD. Naturheilverfahren – Grundlagen, Möglichkeiten, Grenzen. In: Hentschel HD, ed. Naturheilverfahren in der ärztlichen Praxis, 2nd edn. Köln: Deutscher Ärzteverlag; 1998
3. Uehleke B, Stange R. Re the editorial: 'Healing power—an art of natural healing of people or still only by natural therapy?' Forsch Komplementärmed Klass Naturheilkd 2005;12:47–48
4. Uehleke B. Phytotherapie: Schulmedizin oder Naturheilkunde? MMWR 2001;143:39–40
5. Stange R, ed. Naturheilkunde am Ende des 20. Jahrhunderts – Rückblick-Gegenwart-Perspektiven. Stuttgart: Hippokrates; 2000
6. Beer AM, Uehleke B. Geschichte stationärer Naturheilkunde. In: Beer A, ed. Stationäre Naturheilkunde – Handbuch für Klinik und Rehabilitation. München: Elsevier; 2005: 8–14
7. Mayer JG, Saum K. Handbuch der Klosterheilkunde. München: Zabert Sandmann; 2002
8. Kneipp S. Meine Wasserkur. Kempten: Kösel; 1887
9. Floyer J. An enquiry into the right use and abuses of the hot, cold and temperate baths in England. London: Smith & Walford; 1697
10. Smith J. The curiosities of common water, 6th edn. London: Clark; 1724
11. Alpinus P. De medicina methodica. Basel: C. Boutestein; 1719
12. Rolfinccius G. Ordo et methodus medicinae specialis. Jena: Goetz; 1671
13. Lucas C. An essay on waters. London: A. Miller; 1756
14. Hahn JS. Unterricht von Krafft und Würckung des frischen Wassers in die Leiber der Menschen besonders der Krancken bey dessen innerlichen und äusserlichen Gebrauch, 3rd edn. Breslau, Leipzig: Pietsch; 1749
15. Currie J. Medical reports on the effects of water, cold and warm, as a remedy in fever, and febrile diseases. Liverpool: M'Creen; 1797
16. Jackson R. An exposition of the practice of affusing cold water on the surface of the body, as a remedy for the cure of fever. London: J. Murray; 1808
17. Flittner CG. Gemeinfaßliche Anweisung über den Nutzen und den rechten Gebrauch der einfachen kalten und warmen Wasserbäder so wie der Dampfbäder. Berlin: Flittner'sche Buchhandlung; 1822
18. Oertel EFC, von Kolb AR, Kirchmayr AG. Anweisung zum heilsamen Wassergebrauche für Menschen und Vieh in den gangbarsten Krankheiten und Leibesgebrechen von A-Z. Ein Hülfsbuch für Aerzte, Chirurgen und Hebammen, Prediger, Schullehrer, Ortsvorsteher, Gutsbesitzer, 2nd edn. Nürnberg: Campe; 1835
19. Zoczek C. Triumph der Heilkunst mit kaltem Wasser. Leipzig: Hartleben; 1836
20. Weiß J. Handbuch der Wasserheilkunde für Aerzte und Laien. Leipzig: W. Einhorn; 1844
21. Selinger JEM. Vincenz Prießnitz – eine Lebensbeschreibung, 2nd edn. Wien: C. Gerold; 1851
22. Munde C. Hydrotherapie oder die Kunst, die Krankheiten des menschlichen Körpers, ohne Hilfe von Arzneien, durch Diät, Wasser, Schwitzen, Luft und Bewegung zu heilen und durch eine vernünftige Lebensweise zu verhüten. Ein Handbuch für Nichtärzte, besonders für Gichtkranke, 2nd edn. Dresden: Arnold; 1846:165–167

23. Rausse JH. Miscellen zur Gräfenberger Wasserkur, 3rd edn. Zeitz: Schieferdecker; 1846

24. Bleile J. Beiträge zur Kaltwasser-Heilkunde. Kempten: Dannheimer; 1852

25. Kneipp S. Meine Wasserkur. Kempten: Kösel; 1887

26. Bühring M. Naturheilkunde. Grundlagen – Ideen, Konzepte. Stuttgart: Beck; 1991

27. Uehleke B. Braucht die Naturheilkunde eine eigene Nosologie? Gedankensplitter. Würzburger medizinhistorische Mitteilungen 1998;17:535

OSTEOPATHIC CONCEPTS OF PAIN
CM Janine Leach

'Nature applies to you the switch of pain when her mandates are disregarded, and when you feel the smarting of the switch do not pour drugs into your stomachs, but let a skilful engineer adjust your human machine so that every part works in accordance with nature's requirements.'

Andrew Taylor Still[1]

INTRODUCTION

The aim of this chapter is to explore the concepts of pain that are specifically osteopathic, distinct from the current neurophysiological models, which are incorporated into osteopathic training and practice.[2]

Osteopathy is a system of medicine used for the diagnosis and treatment of physical pain, musculoskeletal dysfunction and a wide range of acute and chronic conditions. The unique contribution of osteopathy is its specialist use of manual methods of diagnosis and treatment.[3-6] It works with the soma, as a way to influence the function of the body–mind, the original biomechanical approaches having been expanded into subtler fields including cranial osteopathy.[7-9] The aim of treatment is to promote health through improved function of the musculoskeletal system, the circulation, the neuroendocrine system and, through somato-visceral effects, the organs including the brain.

Pain is the most common reason for patients to seek the help of an osteopath.[10,11] The most common sites of pain are the lower back, knee and neck, reflecting the epidemic of back pain in the western world.[12] Chronic pain represents a challenge to medicine and society and is therefore the focus of this chapter.

PAIN

There are few references in the osteopathic literature to the meaning and perception of pain. Andrew Taylor Still, who founded osteopathy in 1874 in Kirksville, US, rarely mentioned pain. His words quoted at the beginning of this chapter suggest that he viewed pain as a useful warning signal, and a sign that some part of the 'human machine' was not working in harmony with nature. Littlejohns viewed pain as 'a physiological condition arising from some disturbance of the vital economy; it is the voice of the vital force expressing itself through the body ... the body, represented by pain, is crying out for help'.[13]

However, there are specific osteopathic concepts associated with the biology of pain, central to which is the basic osteopathic principle that movement is fundamental to human life, to the expression of mind and spirit.[3,14] Everything that man does – running, playing, seeing, talking – requires movement. Even the activity of thinking is meaningless unless it results in external action or communication. The neuromusculoskeletal system is therefore seen as the 'primary machinery of life'. The other systems, including all the organs, exist to serve and maintain the primary machine by maintaining the correct supply of nutrients and disposal of wastes through the fine balance of homeostasis. Symptoms such as pain are viewed as the body's adaptive attempt to restore homeostasis. Our understanding of the precise mechanisms has been modified over time, notably by three neurophysiologists: Denslow and Korr who introduced the concept of segmental facilitation in the 1940s,[15] and Frank Willard who in the past few decades has interpreted osteopathic concepts in the light of current scientific knowledge.[16]

SOMATIC DYSFUNCTION

The early osteopathic pioneers based their concepts on decades of careful observation in practice. During physical examination of patients, they palpated areas of change in tissue texture which they called somatic dysfunctions (formerly 'osteopathic lesions'). In an area of somatic dysfunction there are changes in tissue texture, asymmetry of structure, restriction of motion and tenderness ('TART'). These may occur at local and distant body sites in relation to pain. Somatic dysfunction is formally defined as 'impaired or altered function of related components of the somatic (body framework) system: skeletal, arthrodial and myofascial structures, and related vascular, lymphatic and neural elements'. Somatic dysfunction is described by Frank Willard as a critical concept in osteopathy.[16]

Somatic dysfunction has been identified independently in all three manual therapy professions, being termed subluxation in chiropractic and joint fixation in physiotherapy; a reasonable rate of inter-examiner agreement can be achieved in the manual detection of areas of somatic dysfunction.[17]

The process which gives rise to the local findings of somatic dysfunction is very complex and involves the central sensitisation discussed in the next section. The local stimulus or injury which can initiate a somatic dysfunction includes trauma, possibly quite minor; sprain of joints such as the zygapophysial joints in the spine, resulting in capsule inflammation, pain and tenderness; joint effusion resulting in restricted motion; and periarticular inflammation resulting in tissue texture changes. The intervertebral discs are capable of producing reflex contraction in segmental muscles.[17] Finally, trigger points in muscles are thought to be one of the more common causes of regional musculoskeletal pain.[18,19]

SEGMENTAL FACILITATION

Following meticulous and innovative experimental work, Denslow and Korr proposed the concept of segmental facilitation, which they showed could give rise to the tissue changes observed in somatic dysfunction.[15,20]

Spinal facilitation is now well established and results in a 'gain' in output from the dorsal horn of the spinal cord to the higher centres and a magnified perception of pain. This occurs after excessive input, such as prolonged, severe or repeated injury to mechanical, chemical or temperature nociceptors in the peripheral tissues. Long-term and sometimes permanent change (plasticity) occurs in the dorsal horn neuronal circuitry. Facilitation may be induced by neuropeptide release within the dorsal horn, together with altered gene expression in the dorsal horn neurones. These are reversible changes. The dorsal horn neurones can also undergo irreversible cellular changes and enter a state of grossly enhanced output when they over-respond to minimal or even zero input.[16,21]

Of particular interest to osteopaths is the effect of spinal facilitation on the body tissues. In a facilitated segment, output to the body via efferent axons in the ventral roots is altered. Efferent fibres innervating skeletal muscle produce altered muscle tone in the associated spinal segments, which may then create distortions of the fascial connective tissue matrix, creating asymmetry. Altered sympathetic output to glands, vascular and organ wall smooth muscle associated with the spinal segments, causes changes in tissue texture and circulatory and functional changes. The osteopathic hypothesis that segmental facilitation can modify visceral activity via somato-visceral reflexes is not yet proven.[17]

HOMEOSTASIS AND ALLOSTATIC RESPONSE

The concept of the general adaptive response of the body to stresses was first described by Selye[22] and became part of osteopathic thinking.[5] Any kind of unexpected or unwanted stressor can trigger a state of arousal in the complex neural circuitry surrounding the medulla, pons and mid-brain.[16] The arousal system has descending tracts, which modulate spinal circuitry, and ascending connections to the forebrain, which influence behaviour. The arousal system is coupled to two important efferent pathways: the sympathetic nervous system and the hypothalamic–pituitary–adrenal axis. In a state of arousal, the three systems work together to shift neural, endocrine and immune function from a state of homeostasis to the protective state of allostasis. Allostasis is beneficial to 'fight and flight' – escape behaviour, wound repair, containment of infection. The body produces higher levels of noradrenaline, cortisol and cytokines for rapid defence of the body, to promote survival. Non-adaptive pathways such as digestion and reproduction will be suppressed. A prolonged compensatory state of persistent allostasis has serious adverse effects on the body, including chronic pain and chronic disease, because the organ systems are working in unnatural or compensated states.

Psychological stressors include cognitive and emotional events through the limbic system. Physical stressors can originate from somatic, mechanical or chemical stimuli or visceral dysfunction, acting through the spinoreticular and spinothalamic pathways. Stressful life experiences, especially those that appear inescapable, can dysregulate the neuroendocrine–immune axis. The lowered immunity and behavioural changes such as depression or anxiety observed in chronic pain can be explained in terms of allostasis. The various stressors can summate and augment the allostatic impact. The concept that the descent into chronicity starts when the body is unable to restore homeostatic mechanisms is now part of the scientific concepts of pain.[2] The osteopathic approach is to help to restore homeostasis by reducing the drives on the arousal system.

TISSUE MEMORY

The concept of tissue memory is the neuromusculoskeletal counterpart of allostasis. It is used in practice to explain why musculoskeletal symptoms tend to recur at the same body sites and with a pattern of sensation that the patient recognises. In the model, neural–myofascial retention of stressors in the body leads to barriers to function. Viewing the body as a tensegrity structure,[5] fascia is seen as the tissue that adapts to stress, adapting and integrating forces within the body to influence posture and movement.[23,24] Physiotherapists have proposed a similar stress–diathesis model.[25] The concept is also closely aligned to the 'neurosignatures' in the neuromatrix model, in which neural networks in many parts of the brain contribute to an image of self that incorporates genetic programmes and memories of past experiences.[2,26] The changes observed in repetitive strain injury add support to the concept. Neuroplasticity of the receptor fields in the somatosensory cortex widens the sensory fields and gives rise to inappropriate motor responses and altered function of the limb involved.

CONCEPTS IN PAIN MANAGEMENT

Patients usually come to an osteopath seeking physical treatment for a problem they perceive as musculoskeletal. Some come after a lengthy process of seeking orthodox treatment for chronic pain. Patients quickly perceive when a doctor is unable to make sense of the physical findings and test results. They lose confidence in the doctor, feeling that the doctor believes it is 'all in the mind'.[26] Patients become more distressed, feeling they are trapped in the system[27] with nowhere to turn for help, and this makes the symptoms worse. Osteopaths may provide support in a variety of ways.[28]

Attitudes to pain, the experience of pain and, hence, the needs of the patient differ according to race, gender, age and culture. The response of body tissues and the psychology of coping will also vary. For example, elderly chronic pain suffers have particular coping strategies including pacing, the use of prayer and looking good.[29]

Like other primary health-care physicians, an osteopath will take a detailed case history, conduct a physical examination and diagnostic tests, form a differential diagnosis and, if indicated, refer to an appropriate orthodox or complementary specialist.[6,30] Like other mainstream complementary therapies such as acupuncture, chiropractic, herbal medicine or homeopathy, osteopathy is holistic: time is taken to view the whole person in the context of their environment and lifestyle, to find the true underlying cause(s) of the symptoms and dysfunction. Patients are encouraged towards optimal health of body, mind and spirit through the osteopath listening and working in partnership with the patient to improve lifestyle, diet and exercise. The diagnosis is often non-specific in chronic conditions, and management aims to be constitutional rather than local, aiming to assist the body to restore homeostasis.[3,5]

The consultation and case history taking will initiate the therapeutic partnership with the patient, and will aim to understand the stressors that have caused allostasis. A lifelong perspective may be used, an approach termed 'evolutionary' in physiotherapy.[25] Biopsychosocial factors (yellow flags) will be assessed if the pain persists for more than a few weeks after onset.[26] The traditional distinction between acute (conventionally of less than 6 weeks duration) and chronic (more than 3 months duration) often does not reflect the true course of back pain, which is more typically an intermittent, fluctuating pattern of symptoms, with pain-free periods interspersed by acute episodes, exacerbations and recurrences.[12] There is good evidence that psychological distress, depressed mood and somatisation predict chronicity, at least in back pain.[31] Work stress may also play a role.[10,32] Informal methods for evaluating psychosocial factors appear sufficient[10,33] together with the use of narrative reasoning rather than empirico-analytic reasoning.[34] The depression, anxiety and positive outlook scale (DAPOS) questionnaire[35] may emerge as a useful tool in future.

The physical examination combines predominantly visual inspection and manual palpation. The clinical detection of somatic dysfunction has been shown to be reliable, specific and sensitive only if multiple criteria are combined, and the criteria must incorporate a pain provocation test.[17,36,37] The initiation of touch and non-verbal interaction is an important step in shaping the quality of the relationship and the healing response. Touch and narrative are powerful psychological tools, touch establishing 'the optimal bond between healer and healed.[38]' Treating the whole person rather than specific symptoms aims to resonate with the patient at spiritual and emotional as well as physical levels.[5]

The diagnosis for some patients may be specific, confirmed by pathology or imaging, such as rheumatoid arthritis or disc prolapse, or by specific items of clinical evidence, for example fibromyalgia or migraine. For many patients in osteopathic practice, however, the diagnosis is non-specific. A treatment plan is formed on the basis of the diagnosis and constitution of the person, and may be informed by guidelines in the case of back pain.[12]

MANUAL TREATMENT

The aim of manual treatment is to enhance the body's own healing capacity by removing barriers to physiological function,[6] using the bones as levers to relieve pressure on the nerves and blood vessels, producing metabolic, biochemical and circulatory changes. Manual therapy is believed to address many levels of a patient's life, not simply the musculoskeletal.[39] The adverse effects of sympathetic arousal make this a crucial area of influence for osteopathic practice.[14]

Osteopathic technique is far wider than spinal manipulation, including a wide variety of active and passive soft-tissue-release techniques and cranio-sacral techniques.[3] The choice of technique and dose depends on the purpose of the treatment. For example, postural or occupational strain may require an active approach aimed at influencing the mechanoreceptors and including exercises aimed at deconstructing and replacing the old movement patterns.[40,41] For distress, pain behaviour and emotional issues affecting body–mind, the choice may be education, advice, problem solving and manual therapies directed at somato-emotional release. For chronic allostasis, treatment may aim to modulate hyper-sympathetic activity, using breathing re-training, massage and rhythmic movement to mobilise oedema and lymphatic fluids.[40] For the treatment of trigger points, dry needling has been introduced[18] and neuroreflexotherapy is being evaluated in trials.[42]

Other modalities employed include cryotherapy, hydrotherapy, electrotherapy and pharmacological analgesia. As the risk of gastric bleeding when using non-steroidal anti-inflammatory drugs is rather high,[43] many osteopaths prefer to avoid drugs,[44] relying on natural remedies or the body's own pharmacy. Serotonin and dopamine levels increase, and endocannabinoids are thought to be produced during manual therapy.[45–47]

Education and advice on exercise and lifestyle aim to empower the patient. This may be informal or may be reinforced by authoritative home reading, e.g. *The back book*,[48,49] *The whiplash book*,[49] the wonderfully illustrated *Explain pain*,[50] or *Pain in later years*.[51]

The encounter with a practitioner is an encounter with a healing ritual,[52] the outcome of which depends powerfully on the patient's expectation.[53,54] Manual therapists are thought to enable the patients to re-configure their perception of the problem.[55]

SUMMARY AND CONCLUSIONS

The past 50 years or more has seen a growth in our understanding of the biomechanics and neurobiology of the body, of the value and limitations of the clinical trial,[56] and the important role of the placebo. We seem now to be entering a period in which there is growing recognition that treatment of the soma, the body, also treats the mind through the hypothalamic–pituitary–endocrine axis, and where the therapeutic relationship has become a therapeutic partnership. In this era, perhaps we will begin to understand the mechanisms behind the subtler forms of osteopathy, including cranial osteopathy, which bridge the 'mind in the body'.

While spinal facilitation and allostasis–homeostasis are now established scientifically and incorporated into the neurophysiological models of pain, the osteopathic concepts of somatic dysfunction and tissue memory are not yet fully understood. While more research is needed, the concepts remain useful as over-arching and unifying concepts linking body and mind. The advances in the science of pain of the past 50 years have informed the osteopath's choice of therapeutic technique. Outcomes research, to evaluate osteopathic management options, is also needed, perhaps using whole systems research methods rather than randomised trials alone.[56]

Pain continues to challenge orthodox and complementary practitioners at many levels. As science reveals the role of the mind in bodily pain, a major shift is occurring in the philosophy of medical science. The body and the mind are not separable, and the mind is as paradoxical to measurement as matter at the level of quantum physics: what is observed depends on the questions asked.[57] The nature of reality is that seemingly separate entities are entangled.[58]

ACKNOWLEDGEMENTS

I would like to thank the many osteopaths in practice and lecturers at the UK osteopathic colleges who have contributed to the development of this chapter, especially John Lewis and Dawn Carnes, Tim Oxbrow, Roderick MacDonald, Devan Rajandran, Jorges Esteves, Stephen Tyreman, Lawrence Butler and Martin Chorley; Nic Lucas, Editor of the *International Journal of Osteopathic Medicine*, and Professor Ann Moore and Carol Fawkes from the National Council for Osteopathic Research, University of Brighton, UK.

REFERENCES

1. Truhlar RE. Doctor A.T. Still in the living. Cleveland, Ohio: Privately published; 1950: p. 38. Reproduced with permission of the American Academy of Osteopathy
2. Loeser JD, Melzack R. Pain: an overview. Lancet 1999;353:1607–1609
3. Ward RC. Foundations for osteopathic medicine, 2nd edn. Philadelphia: Lippincott Williams and Wilkins; 2003
4. DiGiovanna EL, Schiowitz S. An osteopathic approach to diagnosis and treatment. Philadelphia: Lippincott-Raven; 1997
5. Stone C. Science in the art of osteopathy. Cheltenham: Stanley Thornes Ltd; 1999
6. Sammut EA, Searle-Barnes PJ. Osteopathic diagnosis. Cheltenham: Stanley Thornes Ltd; 1998
7. Magoun HI. Osteopathy in the cranial field. Kirksville, MO: The Journal Printing Co.; 1976
8. Upledger JE. Somatoemotional release and beyond. Upledger Institute, FL: UI Publishing; 1990
9. Sutherland WG, Wales AL (eds). Teachings in the science of osteopathy. Forth Worth, TX: Rudra; 1990
10. Lucas N. Psychosocial factors in osteopathic practice: to what extent should they be assessed? Int J Osteopath Med 2005;8:49–59
11. Pringle M, Tyreman S. Study of 500 patients attending an osteopathic practice. Br J Gen Pract 1993;43:15–18
12. Waddell G. The back pain revolution. Edinburgh: Elsevier; 2004
13. Wernham J. Notes on the principles of osteopathy by J M Littlejohns, centenary edn. London: Society of Osteopaths; 1974
14. Korr IM. The sympathetic nervous system as mediator between the somatic and supportive processes. In: Kugelmass IN, ed. The physiological basis of osteopathic medicine. New York: The Postgraduate Institute of Osteopathic Medicine and Surgery; 1982, pp. 21–38
15. Korr IM. The neural basis of the osteopathic lesion. J Am Ostopath Assoc 1947; 46:191–198
16. Willard FW. Nociception, the neuroendocrine system, and osteopathic medicine. In: Ward RC, ed. Foundations for osteopathic medicine. Philadephia: Lippincott, Williams and Wilkins; 2003, pp. 137–156
17. Fryer G. Intervertebral dysfunction: a discussion of the manipulable spinal lesion. J Osteopath Med 2003;6:62–73
18. Mense F, Simons DG. Muscle pain: understanding its nature, diagnosis and treatment. Baltimore: Lippincott Williams and Wilkins; 2001
19. McPartland JM. Travell trigger points – molecular and osteopathic perspectives. J Am Osteopath Assoc 2004;104:244–249
20. Korr IM, Wilkinson PN, Chornock FW. Axonal delivery of axonal components to muscle cells. Science 1967;155:342–345
21. Woolf CJ, Saler MW. Neuronal plasticity: increasing the gain in pain. Science 2000; 288:1765–1768
22. Selye H. The general adaptive syndrome and diseases of adaptation. J Clin Endocrinol Metab 1946;6:117–179
23. Oxbrow T. Ideas on tissue memory: informing osteopathic treatment and reflective practice. Presentation to Worcester Osteopaths Group, presented 19 February 2005 at Droitwich.
24. Barral JP, Croibier A. Trauma. Seattle: Eastland Press; 1997
25. Gifford L. An introduction to evolutionary reasoning: diets, fevers and the placebo. In: Gifford L, ed. Topical issues in pain 4. Physiotherapy Pain Association Yearbook. Falmouth, UK: CNS Press; 2004, pp. 119–146
26. Main CJ, Spanswick CC. Pain management: an interdisciplinary approach. Edinburgh: Churchill Livingstone; 2000
27. Walker J, Holloway I, Sofaer B. In the system: the lived experience of chronic back pain from the experience of those seeking help from pain clinics. Pain 1999;80:621–628
28. Pincus T, Vogel S, Breen A, Foster N, Underwood M. Persistent back pain – why do physical therapy clinicians continue treatment? A mixed methods study of chiropractors, osteopaths and physiotherapists. Eur J Pain 2006;10:67–76
29. Sofaer B, Moore AP, Holloway I, Lamberty JM, Thorp TAS, O'Dwyer J. Chronic pain as perceived by older people: a qualitative study. Age Ageing 2005;34:462–466
30. Goodman CC, Snyder TEK. Differential diagnosis in physical therapy. Philadelphia: WB Saunders; 1995

31. Pincus T, Burton AK, Vogel S, Field A. A systematic review of psychological factors as predictors of chronicity/disability in prospective cohorts of low back pain. Spine 2002;27:E109–E120

32. Jerome JJ. Pain management. In: Ward RC, ed. Foundations for osteopathic medicine. Philadelphia: Lippincott Williams and Wilkins; 2003, pp. 212–226

33. Watson P, Kendall N. Assessing psychosocial yellow flags. In: Gifford L, ed. Topical issues in pain 2. Physiotherapy Pain Association Yearbook. Falmouth, UK: CNS Press; 2000, pp. 111–139

34. Jones M, Edwards I, Gifford L. Conceptual models for integrating biopsychosocial theory in clinical practice. Manual Ther 2002;7:2–9

35. Pincus T, Williams AC, Vogel S, Field A. The development and testing of the depression, anxiety, and positive outlook scale (DAPOS). Pain 2004;109:181–188

36. Degenhart BF, Snider KO, Snider EJ, Johnson JC. Interobserver reliability of osteopathic palpatory diagnostic tests of the lumbar spine: improvements from consensus training. J Am Osteopath Assoc 2005;105:465–473

37. Seffinger MA, Najm WI, Mishra SI, Adams A, Dickerson VM, Murphy LS, Reinsch S. Reliability of spinal palpation for diagnosis of back and neck pain: a systematic review of the literature. Spine 2004;29:E413–E425

38. Kugelmass IN. The physiological basis of osteopathic medicine. New York: The Postgraduate Institute of Osteopathic Medicine and Surgery; 1982

39. Nash K, Tyreman S. An account of the development of the conceptual basis of osteopathy course at the British School of Osteopathy. Int J Osteopath Med 2005;8:29–37

40. Kuchera ML. Osteopathic manipulative considerations in patients with chronic pain. J Am Osteopath Assoc 2005;105:S29-S36

41. Edwards I, Jones M, Hillier S. The interpretation of experience and its relationship to body movement: a clinical reasoning perspective. Manual Ther 2006;11:2–10

42. Urrutia G, Burton K, Morral A, Bonfill X, Zanoli G. Neuroreflexotherapy for nonspecific low back pain: a systematic review. Spine 2005;30:E148–E153

43. Pirmohamed M, James S, Meakin S, Green C, Scott AK, Walley TJ, Farrar K, Park BK, Breckenridge AM. Adverse drug reactions as a cause of admission to hospital: prospective analysis of 18820 patients. Br Med J 2004;329:15–19

44. Grundy M, Vogel S. Attitudes towards prescribing rights: a qualitative focus group study with UK osteopaths. Int J Osteopath Med 2005;8:12–21

45. Lechin F, Pardey-Maldonado B, van der Dijs B, Benaim M, Baez S, Orozco B, Lechin AE. Circulating neurotransmitters during the different wake–sleep stages in normal subjects. Psychoneuroendocrinology 2004;29:669–685

46. Field T, Hernandez-Reif M, Diego M, Schanberg S, Kuhn C. Cortisol decreases and serotonin and dopamine increase following massage therapy. Int J Neurosci 2005;115:1397–1413

47. McPartland JM, Guiffrida A, King J, Skinner E, Scotter J, Musty RE. Cannabimetic effects of osteopathic manipulative treatment. J Am Osteopath Assoc 2005;105: 283–249

48. Burton K, Roland M, Waddell G, Klaber Moffat J, Main C. The back book. London: The Stationery Office; 2002

49. Burton K, McClune T, Waddell G. The whiplash book. London: The Stationery Office; 2002

50. Butler DS, Moseley GL. Explain pain. Adelaide: Niogroup Publications; 2003

51. Sofaer B. Pain in later years: practical ideas to help you cope. Brighton: Clinical Research Centre for Health Professions, University of Brighton; 2004

52. Kaptchuk TJ. The placebo effect in alternative medicine: can the performance of a healing ritual have clinical significance? Ann Intern Med 2002;136:817–825

53. Lucas N. To what should we attribute the effects of OMT? Int J Osteopath Med 2005;8: 121–123

54. de la Fuente-Fernandez R, Phillips AG, Zamburlini M, Sossi V, Calne DB, Ruth TJ, Stoessl AJ. Dopamine release in human ventral striatum and expectation of reward. Behav Brain Res. 2002; 15:359–363

55. Breen A, Breen R. Back pain and satisfaction with chiropractic treatment: what role does the physical outcome play? Clin J Pain 2003;19:263–268

56. Verhoef MJ, Lewith G, Ritenbaugh C, Boon H, Fleishman S, Leis A. Complementary and alternative medicine whole systems research: beyond identification of inadequacies of the RCT. Complement Ther Med 2005;13:206–212

57. Wallace AB. Choosing reality: a Buddhist view of physics and the mind. New York: Snow Lion Publications; 1996

58. Hyland ME. Does a form of 'entanglement' between people explain healing? An examination of hypotheses and methodology. Complement Ther Med 2004;12:198–208

CONCEPTS OF PAIN IN TRADITIONAL CHINESE MEDICINE

Ka-Kit Hui, Edward K Hui

Most clinicians and investigators are intrigued by the analgesic effect of inserting needles into various parts of the body, and acupuncture is becoming accepted as a useful and effective therapeutic tool in pain management with increasing validation by modern research. However, acupuncture is but one therapeutic modality of traditional Chinese medicine (TCM), whose theoretical framework guides its use in the diagnosis, prevention, treatment and rehabilitation of pain in clinical practice. It is important to appreciate that TCM's utility in the relief of pain goes beyond the release of endorphins and other neurotransmitters by acupuncture or different prescriptions of acupuncture points for specific pain conditions. TCM has much more to offer this complex clinical problem, whether acute or chronic in nature. As western-trained physicians who recognise the importance of the theoretical framework of TCM in pain beyond its frequently used therapeutic modalities of acupuncture and massage, we attempt to distill and highlight major principles and themes in this short chapter on TCM's conceptualisation of health and disease, with a particular focus on pain. We have avoided the use of TCM terminology in presenting the key concepts. Readers interested in a more comprehensive treatment of this topic should consult the references listed at the end of the chapter. Much of what we describe below has been put into practice in a busy clinical programme at a major academic medical centre in the US.

TCM'S CONCEPTUALISATION OF PAIN AND ILL HEALTH

According to TCM, the disruption of normal flow and balance leads to ill health, and depletion of the homeostatic reserve leads to chronicity. Abnormal flow and imbalance are the end result of the struggle between the body's endogenous resistance and pathogenic factors originating in either the external environment or within the human body. If the person's endogenous resistance is weak or pathogenic factors are particularly strong, ill health ensues. Pain is a common manifestation in this state of disharmony.

The body's endogenous resistance is dynamic in nature and is dependent on the person's constitution, emotional state, natural and social environment, diet and amount and types of physical and mental activity. A person's constitution is determined by prenatal and postnatal components. The constitutions of the parents and occurrences around the time of conception and during pregnancy will be a factor in the individual's genetic make-up. Postnatally, TCM recognises the contribution of age-related decline in various physiological systems and overall infrastructure decline to a decrease in the individual's endogenous resistance to ill health and disease. This may explain the increased prevalence of pain and its chronicity in older individuals.

TCM's emphasis on the importance of the prevailing emotional state and the social environment cannot be overstated. Extremes in emotions, particularly anger, anxiety and worry, in conjunction with poor coping style impact directly on the individual's ability to ward off pain and disease. According to TCM theory, certain emotions are linked with specific physiological functions, and imbalances that arise in these emotions will be reflected by pathological changes in the corresponding physiological functions. For example, excessive anger is extremely detrimental to the body's overall ability to ensure proper flow and will expectedly result in pain. It is not difficult to understand how the individual's interaction with his social environment and interpersonal relationships might affect the prevailing emotional state.

TCM also recognises extremes and rapid or unforeseen changes in weather and climate as potentially destabilising and pathogenic. If too much homeostatic reserve is needed to counteract these destabilising forces, there is a disruption of normal flow and pain ensues. The interaction of these exogenous forces with weakened defence systems results in characteristic clinical manifestations in the individual specific to that pathogen. According to TCM, cool temperatures may give rise to pain that is accompanied by a sense of contraction, limitation of range of motion and aversion to cold while excessive humidity may lead to pain characterised by heaviness and fullness and accompanied by a sense of lassitude and fatigue. Often, several exogenous factors may interact and lead to characteristic manifestations of pain. For instance, non-inflammatory pain commonly seen in rheumatological practice may occur in certain individuals influenced by a combination of windy, cold and damp weather conditions.

Likewise, poor dietary practices and overwork of mind and body can further insult the system and result in the genesis or perpetuation of pain. Trauma, whether accidental or iatrogenic, i.e. surgery, as expected results in short-term pain, but multiple and consecutive hits without timely intervention, particularly in an individual with compromised homeostatic reserve, can result in persistent pain. Again, TCM emphasises the adverse consequences of noxious stimuli that deplete the homeostatic reserve.

Both western physicians and TCM practitioners collect subjective and objective data to arrive at a diagnosis to guide appropriate treatment. After identifying anatomical, physiological and biochemical perturbations, the former arrive at a disease diagnosis that is separate from the individual in which it manifests. In contrast, TCM practitioners discern functional dysregulation and assess homeostatic reserve to arrive at a pathophysiological pattern that is unique to the patient and to that particular point in time. This pattern diagnosis describes the body's dynamic response to endogenous and exogenous forces. The TCM practitioner weaves this pattern diagnosis by eliciting the patient's emotional and somatic complaints, dietary and climatic preferences, genetic and postnatal contributions to constitution, as well as prevailing emotional expression and coping style. The history is complemented by information gleaned from tongue and pulse examination as well as palpation of acupuncture points. This pattern diagnosis reflects the location and stage of pathogenesis created by the interaction between pathogenic factors and the body's defence and regulatory systems. In short, pattern diagnosis allows for a whole-person identification of dysfunction, dysregulation and depletion manifesting in the individual, thereby guiding treatment and providing prognostic information.

Because of this preference for describing pathophysiological patterns as opposed to disease entities to guide therapeutics, clinicians place less emphasis on specific causal factors. This is particularly useful in situations where aetiology is ill-defined or multifactorial. The patient with multiple diseases can be characterised by a single or mixed pattern diagnosis, with specific treatment directed at such pathophysiological patterns. Restoration of normal balance and flow in the body, strengthening and enhancing the body's endogenous resistance to disease, and individualisation are central to the overall therapeutic approach to the sick individual.

TCM'S APPROACH TO PAIN

Acute pain is unavoidable and probably necessary for survival. According to TCM, the preservation and strengthening of endogenous resistance will allow the individual to best cope with pain if it does occur and to prevent its perpetuation into a state of chronicity. Any noxious insult to the system, whether it is an emotional stressor, an infection, physical trauma or physiological derangement, which results in disruption of normal flow and balance, must be dealt with in a timely manner. The importance of prevention is emphasised throughout the health and disease spectrum.

Accurate delineation of the pathophysiological patterns allows identification of the matching therapeutic principles to guide lifestyle counselling, dietary recommendations, exercise prescription and acupuncture point and herbal formula selection. Careful adjustment of the therapeutic principles and appropriate modalities according to the changing pattern as the condition evolves, with ultimate restoration of flow and balance and repletion of functional reserve, is central to the eradication of pain and better health.

A CASE STUDY

The following case illustrates some of the concepts discussed above and may serve as an introduction to TCM's approach to the management of a patient with pain.

A 24-year-old female medical student presented with a complaint of neck pain. She reported a 1-year history of pain in the neck, shoulders and upper back complicated by a decreased range of motion of the neck and periodic swelling overlying the area of the left trapezius muscle. She first noted her symptoms during a time of intense stress in her family. Around the same time, she ended her relationship with her boyfriend. The pain worsened, exacerbated by stress and temporarily relieved by professional massage, self-massage and application of local heat. She did not use medications for her symptoms.

She was involved in a skiing accident several years earlier which led to knee problems requiring surgery the following year. She was on oral contraceptive agents, took psyllium to regulate her gastrointestinal tract and also used ginseng (*Panax* sp.), *Gingko biloba* and chrysanthemum tea. She did not smoke or use recreational drugs but drank four alcoholic drinks a week and a cup of coffee every morning. Her diet consisted of frequent sweets and red meat with craving for chocolate around the time of menses. She had difficulty falling asleep but did not awake early or have disturbed sleep. She walked a treadmill for 30 minutes twice a week and lifted 8-lb (3.6-kg) weights overhead. Her review of systems was notable for fatigue in the late afternoon, cold intolerance with frequent cold extremities, chronic dry and red eyes, intermittent dyspepsia relieved with an antacid and abdominal bloating and cramping without use of psyllium and heavy bleeding with clots during her menstrual periods, which usually lasted 9 days.

Physical examination revealed a prominent left trapezius on inspection, bilateral cervical and thoracic muscle tenderness on palpation and decreased range of motion of the neck. There was no thyromegaly. TCM examination revealed a tongue with slightly puffy body with teeth marks, dusky colour with purple spots and thin white coating, as well as a wiry right radial pulse and slippery left radial pulse. The medical workup was otherwise unrevealing.

This patient's presentation of myofascial neck pain with concomitant symptoms of dyspepsia with bloating, cold intolerance, dry eyes and insomnia in the context of significant psychosocial stress and history of injury will be managed separately from a biomedical standpoint with the myofascial pain treated with muscle relaxants, trigger-point injection and myofascial release and her other problems managed symptomatically or left alone. In contrast, from the perspective of TCM, her constellation of symptoms, including pain, will be categorised as a mixed pattern diagnosis of stagnation and depletion. Various external social stressors, overloading of muscles via weight training and previous injuries in combination with internalised anger contribute to a system breakdown manifesting in this specific pattern. Management will utilise therapeutic principles and modalities to address stagnation by restoring balance and flow, prevent further depletion and replete the homeostatic reserve. Patient education includes instruction in avoiding muscle overloading and direct wind or draughts to the neck and stress and anger management techniques. For her particular pathophysiological pattern, specific acupuncture points can be selected for stimulation and classic herbal formulations can be used alone or in combination. For the neck pain, local points, which often overlap with trigger points, will be used, but distal points relevant to the

SECTION TWO

pathophysiological pattern will also be used. Acupuncture points can be stimulated in many different ways including dry needling, direct electrical current through the needle, injection with various substances, moxibustion and manual pressure, which the patient can self-administer. In terms of herbs, prescription of the formula will be dictated primarily by the prevailing pattern with major herbs used to address the underlying pathophysiology and minor herbs to address symptoms.

CONCLUSION

From the TCM perspective, optimal prevention, treatment and rehabilitation of persistent pain require an intimate understanding of the person including a comprehensive assessment of the individual's constitution, natural and social environment, diet, previous and ongoing injuries and concomitant diseases. Addressing the corresponding pathophysiological pattern(s) of stagnation and depletion in a most dynamic way is paramount.

FURTHER READING

Audette JF, Ryan AH. The role of acupuncture in pain management. Phys Med Rehabil Clin N Am 2004;15:748–772

Cassidy CM. Contemporary Chinese medicine and acupuncture. Edinburgh: Churchill Livingstone; 2002

Chen X. Chinese acupuncture and moxibustion. Beijing: Foreign Languages Press; 1997

Hui KK, Hui EK, Johnston MF. The potential of a person-centered approach in caring for patients with cancer: a perspective from the UCLA Center for East-West Medicine. Integr Cancer Ther 2006;5:56–62

Hui KK, Zylowska L, Hui EK, Yu JL, Li JJ. Introducing integrative East–West medicine to medical students and residents. J Altern Complement Med 2002;8:507–515

Macioca G. The practice of Chinese medicine = [*Chung yao chen chiu chih liao hsueh*]: the treatment of disease with acupuncture and Chinese herbs. Edinburgh: Churchill Livingstone; 1994

Macioca G. Diagnosis in Chinese medicine: a comprehensive guide: Edinburgh: Churchill Livingstone; 2004

Melzack R, Stillwell DM, Fox EJ. Trigger points and acupuncture points for pain: correlations and implications. Pain 1977;3:3–23

Rachlin E, Rachlin I. Myofascial pain and fibromyalgia: trigger point management. St Louis, MO: Mosby; 2002

Sun P. The treatment of pain with Chinese herbs and acupuncture. Edinburgh: Churchill Livingstone; 2002

Xie Z. Practical traditional Chinese medicine. Beijing: Foreign Languages Press; 2000

Therapies

ACUPUNCTURE

Synonyms

Reflexotherapy (in former USSR); sensory stimulation.

DEFINITION

Insertion of a needle into the skin and underlying tissues in special sites known as points for therapeutic or preventive purposes.

RELATED TECHNIQUES

Point stimulation by electricity (electroacupuncture), laser (laser-acupuncture, low-level laser therapy), heat (moxibustion), pressure (acupressure, shiatsu, tui na), ultrasound or shockwaves; electroacupuncture after Voll; Ryodoraku; neural therapy. In Korea, bee venom acupuncture seems to have gained popularity.[1]

BACKGROUND

Acupuncture originated in China and is part of traditional oriental medicine. Its precise origin is still the subject of scholarly debate. Some experts state that 'at some time in the first century BCE, acupuncture was already a signature therapy of Chinese medicine'.[2] Others insist that 'the earliest clear-cut references to human acupuncture can be reliably dated only to the fifth to eighth centuries CE'.[3] Some authors even speculated that tattoos on human remains may indicate the use of acupuncture in Europe from about 3300 BCE.

Although acupuncture has been used for years within immigrant communities in the West, interest among westerners has fluctuated. The most recent wave of interest dates from about 1970.

Acupuncture is commonly used in China, Taiwan, Japan, Korea, Singapore and other Far Eastern countries. In the West, its popularity has grown rapidly,[2] particularly as a treatment for pain.

TRADITIONAL CONCEPTS

The fundamental concept is 'qi'[2] (pronounced 'chee'), which is usually, though inadequately, translated as 'energy'. It is believed that one form of qi is inherited at birth and maintained during life by the intake of food and air. Qi is thought to circulate through all parts of the body via 12 'meridians'. More than 350 acupuncture points are located on these meridians. Other points lie outside the meridian pathways.

Several different approaches to diagnosis have been developed, but some concepts are basic to all. For example, health is a balance of two opposites, yin and yang. Diseases are associated with disturbances, disharmony or imbalance (typically 'blockage' or 'deficiency') of energy. The body is believed to correct its own energy flow and balance after stimulation of acupuncture points and ill health is thought to reflect a disturbance of energy. Therefore, every medical condition may be amenable to treatment with acupuncture. It is also claimed that disturbances may be detected before they develop into conditions; therefore, even healthy individuals might benefit from acupuncture.

SCIENTIFIC RATIONALE

No evidence has been found to confirm the existence of qi or meridians.[4] Some acupuncture points coincide with sites at which nerves can be stimulated. Acupuncture could thus be a method of affecting the nervous and muscular systems. Considerable differences have been noted between the historical location of points or meridians and current practice.[4] Acupuncture has been found to release various neurotransmitters, including opioid peptides and serotonin.[5,6] Acupuncture may also be used as a form of trigger-point therapy.[7]

PRACTITIONERS

In the US, the certificates of the National Certification Commission for Acupuncture and Oriental Medicine (NCCAOM) are accepted for licensing in many states. In some states non-medically qualified practitioners are allowed to see patients without medical referral. In the UK, there are currently no legal restrictions on the practice of acupuncture; statutory regulation has, however, been drafted. In other countries, the practice of acupuncture is officially restricted to medical practitioners but the restrictions may not be enforced. In Germany, it is practised both by doctors and by *Heilpraktiker* [non-medically trained complementary and alternative medicine (CAM) practitioners].

CONDITIONS FREQUENTLY TREATED

All types of pain, addictions, allergies, digestive disorders, ear, nose and throat conditions, infertility and menstrual problems, maintaining health and preventing illness, mental health problems and stress. Considerable differences exist among the conditions treated according to the 'school' and the origin of the practitioner.

TYPICAL SESSION

Traditional acupuncturists take a medical history and ask about predisposing or psychological factors. Examinations may include inspection of the tongue, palpation of the pulse and abdomen and a search for tender points. Medical acupuncturists will typically incorporate acupuncture into their usual diagnostic and treatment process.

When the diagnosis has been made, needles are usually inserted into several acupuncture points. The needles are typically about 30 mm long, thin (0.3 mm) and disposable. They may be placed just under the skin or deeper into muscle and may be stimulated either by repeated manual rotation, electrically or by heat. This may cause an aching sensation called 'deqi' (pronounced 'der chee'). The needles may be left in position for up to 20 minutes. Occasionally, special needles are left in place for up to 2 weeks. Points in the ear are used in auriculoacupuncture.

Points may also be stimulated by pressure (acupressure); in the Japanese form, shiatsu, pressure is applied by fingers, hands, elbows or other parts of the body. In the Chinese method, tui na, a variety of methods of physical stimulation are used such as pulling and rubbing. In moxibustion, points are heated by smoldering moxa, the leaves of *Artemisia vulgaris*. Points may also be stimulated by laser, ultrasound, shockwaves or injection of substances. Self-treatment versions of acupuncture use pressure pads or electrical apparatus.

COURSE OF TREATMENT

Consultations usually start at weekly intervals. When symptom relief occurs, the interval between treatments may be increased until a course of about six to eight sessions is completed. For chronic conditions many acupuncturists recommend maintenance treatments.

CLINICAL EVIDENCE

Numerous systematic reviews of acupuncture trials have been published. Table 3.1 is a summary of the most up-to-date systematic reviews by indications.[8–32] According to these data, acupuncture is of documented effectiveness for back pain,[8,9] dental pain[10] idiopathic headache,[12] pain relief after oocyte retrieval,[13] as well as osteoarthritis of the knee.[14,33] Since the publication of these systematic reviews new trial data have emerged. A randomised clinical trial (RCT) with 298 patients suffering from chronic low back pain showed

SECTION THREE

Table 3.1 Results of systematic reviews of acupuncture

Positive	Inconclusive	Negative
Chronic back pain [8,9]	Cancer pain[15]	Rheumatoid arthritis[31]
Dental pain[10]	Chronic pain[16]	Tension-type headache[32]
Fibromyalgia[11*]	Facial pain[17]	
Idiopathic headache[12]	Inflammatory rheumatic diseases[18]	
Oocyte retrieval[13]	Labour pain[19]	
Osteoarthritis of knee[14†]	Lateral elbow pain[20]	
	Myofascial pain syndrome[21‡]	
	Neck pain[22,23]	
	Osteoarthritis[24]	
	Primary dysmenorrhoea[25]	
	Sciatica[26]	
	Shoulder pain[27]	
	Surgical pain[28]	
	Temporomandibular joint dysfunction[29]	
	Xerostomia [30]	

*More recent studies have cast doubt on effectiveness.
†Confirmed in a recent, large RCT.[33]
‡Overall the data suggest beneficial effects.

no difference between real and sham acupuncture but both were better than no treatment at all.[34] For fibromyalgia a positive systematic review of three RCTs exists[11] but a recent, relatively large RCT concluded that 'acupuncture was no better than sham acupuncture at relieving pain in fibromyalgia'.[35] Another RCT suggested that the effect does not depend on correct needle stimulation or location.[36] A Chinese RCT ($n = 66$) implied that acupuncture plus cupping plus amitriptyline is superior to amitriptyline alone.[37] For tension-type headache, acupuncture is deemed to be less effective than physical therapy[38] and no difference was found in a recent large RCT[39] or in a systematic review comparing real with sham acupuncture.[32] An RCT of 74 patients with 'chronic daily headache' concluded that acupuncture plus medical care generated better pain relief than medical care alone.[40] As a treatment of migraine, two large RCTs showed that acupuncture was no more effective than sham acupuncture although both interventions were more effective than a waiting list control[41] or were similarly helpful to standard therapy.[42] This may indicate that, for this condition, acupuncture is a 'powerful placebo'. Several recent RCTs have suggested that acupuncture may be useful in controlling procedural pain.[43,44] Acupuncture is likely to be ineffective for rheumatoid arthritis.[31] For the vast majority of other conditions, the data are either contradictory (and therefore inconclusive), e.g. chronic pain in general,[16] shoulder pain,[27] analgesia during surgery,[28] osteoporotic pain,[45] experimental pain,[46] pelvic pain[47] and temporomandibular pain,[48] or non-existent. Because of numerous methodological and other problems, the current evidence allows ample room for interpretation. The recent RCTs using sham devices (and thus controlling adequately for potential placebo effects) tend to show no differences between real and sham acupuncture in a range of different conditions.

This, and other data,[49] seem to suggest that the clinical effects of acupuncture are to a large degree the result of a placebo response.[50]

RISKS
CONTRAINDICATIONS
Severe bleeding disorders. Pregnancy (first trimester, see p. 4) and epilepsy are often regarded as contraindications. Indwelling needles should not be used in patients at risk from bacteraemia.

PRECAUTIONS/WARNINGS
Asepsis is a precondition. Electroacupuncture should be used with caution for patients carrying a pacemaker. Patients should be treated lying down because acupuncture causes drowsiness in 3% of patients;[51] operating machinery or driving after treatment could be hazardous. Children should be treated with care, if at all. To avoid injury to internal organs, special care should be taken when needling points on the thorax. Close supervision is essential if indwelling needles are used.

ADVERSE EFFECTS
Mild, transient adverse events occur in about 7–11% of patients.[51–53] Drowsiness, bleeding, bruising, pain on needling and aggravation of symptoms are the most frequent adverse effects. Serious adverse events, such as pneumothorax or infections, appear to be rare although well-documented cases, including fatalities, are on record.[54]

INTERACTIONS
Electroacupuncture may interfere with cardiac pacemakers (see above).

RISK–BENEFIT ASSESSMENT
In cases where conventional medical diagnosis and advice on best management have previously been obtained, competent acupuncture is relatively safe. For some, but by no means all, conditions acupuncture appears to be effective (Table 3.1). For these conditions acupuncture is likely to do more good than harm.

REFERENCES
1. Lee JD, Park HJ, Chae Y, Lim S. An overview of bee venom acupuncture in the treatment of arthritis. Evid Based Complement Alternat Med 2005;2:79–84
2. Kaptchuk TJ. Acupuncture: theory, efficacy, and practice. Ann Intern Med 2002;136: 374–383
3. Imrie RH, Ramey DW, Buell PD, Ernst E, Basser S. Veterinary acupuncture and historical scholarship: claims for the antiquity of acupuncture. Sci Rev Altern Med 2001;5:133–139
4. Ramey DW. Acupuncture points and meridians do not exist. Sci Rev Altern Med 2001; 5:140–145
5. Han J, Terenius L. Neurochemical basis of acupuncture analgesia. Annu Rev Pharmacol Toxicol 1982;22:193–220
6. Andersson S, Lundeberg T. Acupuncture – from empiricism to science: functional background to acupuncture effects in pain and disease. Med Hypotheses 1995;45:271–281
7. Filshie J, Cummings TM. Western medical acupuncture. In: Ernst E, White A, eds. Acupuncture: a scientific appraisal. Oxford: Butterworth Heinemann; 1999:31–59
8. Manheimer E, White A, Berman B, Forys K, Ernst E. Meta-analysis: acupuncture for back pain. Ann Intern Med 2005;142:651–663
9. Furlan AD, van Tulder MW, Cherkin DC, Tsukayama H, Lao L, Koes BW, Berman BM. Acupuncture and dry-needling for low back pain. The Cochrane Database of Systematic Reviews 2005, Issue 1. Art No.: CD001351

SECTION THREE

10. Ernst E, Pittler MH. The effectiveness of acupuncture in treating acute dental pain: a systematic review. Br Dent J 1998;184:443–447

11. Berman BM, Swyers JP. Complementary medicine treatments for fibromyalgia syndrome. Baillières Best Pract Res Clin Rheumatol 1999;13:487–492

12. Melchart D, Linde K, Fischer P, Berman B, White A, Vickers A, Allais G. Acupuncture for idiopathic headache. The Cochrane Database of Systematic Reviews 2001, Issue 1. Art. No.: CD001218

13. Stener-Victorin E. The pain-relieving effect of electro-acupuncture and conventional medical analgesic methods during oocyte retrieval: a systematic review of randomized controlled trials. Hum Reprod 2005;20:339–349

14. Ezzo J, Hadhazy V, Birch S, Lao L, Kaplan G, Hochberg M, Berman B. Acupuncture for osteoarthritis of the knee: a systematic review. Arthritis Rheum 2001;44:819–825

15. Lee H, Schmidt K, Ernst E. Acupuncture for the relief of cancer-related pain – a systematic review. Eur J Pain 2005;9:437–444

16. Ezzo J, Berman B, Hadhazy VA, Jadad AR, Lao L, Sing BB. Is acupuncture effective for the treatment of chronic pain? A systematic review. Pain 2000;86:217–225

17. Myers CD, White BA, Heft MW. A review of complementary and alternative medicine use for treating chronic facial pain. Am Dent Assoc 2002;133:1189–1196

18. Lautenschläger J. Acupuncture in the treatment of inflammatory rheumatic disease. [In German.] Z Rheumatol 1997;56:8–20

19. Lee H, Ernst E. Acupuncture for labor pain management: a systematic review. Am J Obstet Gynecol 2004;191:1573–1579

20. Trinh KV, Phillips S-D, Ho E, Damsma K. Acupuncture for the alleviation of lateral epicondyle pain: a systematic review. Rheumatology (Oxford) 2004;43:1085–1090

21. Cummings TM, White AR. Needling therapies in the management of myofascial trigger point pain: a systematic review. Arch Phys Med Rehabil 2001;82:986–992

22. White AR, Ernst E. A systematic review of randomized controlled trials of acupuncture for neck pain. Rheumatology (Oxford) 1999;38:143–147

23. Irnich D. Acupuncture for neck pain – review of recent randomised controlled trials. Dtsch Z Akupunkt 2005;48:40–43

24. Ernst E. Acupuncture as a symptomatic treatment of osteoarthritis. Scand J Rheumatol 1997;26:444–447

25. Proctor ML, Smith CA, Farquhar CM, Stones RW. Transcutaneous electrical nerve stimulation and acupuncture for primary dysmenorrhoea. The Cochrane Database of Systematic Reviews 2002, Issue 1. Art. No.: CD002123

26. Longworth W, McCarthy PW. A review of research on acupuncture for the treatment of lumbar disc protrusions and associated neurological symptomatology. J Altern Complement Med 1997;3:55–76

27. Green S, Buchbinder R, Hetrick S. Acupuncture for shoulder pain. The Cochrane Database of Systematic Reviews 2005, Issue 2. Art. No.: CD005319

28. Lee H, Ernst E. Acupuncture analgesia during surgery: a systematic review. Pain 2005; 114:511–517

29. Ernst E, White A. Acupuncture as a treatment for temporomandibular joint dysfunction: a systematic review of randomized trials. Arch Otolaryngol Head Neck Surg 1999; 125:269–272

30. Jedel E. Acupuncture in xerostomia – a systematic review. J Oral Rehabil 2005;32:392–396

31. Casimiro L, Brosseau L, Milne S, Robinson V, Wells G, Tugwell P. Acupuncture and electroacupuncture for the treatment of RA. The Cochrane Database of Systematic Reviews 2002, Issue 3. Art. No.: CD003788

32. Li Y, Luo C. Acupuncture for tension-type headache: a systematic review. [In Chinese.] Chin J Evid Based Med 2005;5:117–124

33. Witt C, Brinkhaus B, Jena S, Linde K, Streng A, Wagenpfeil S, Hummelsberger J, Walther HU, Melchart D, Willich SN. Acupuncture in patients with osteoarthritis of the knee: a randomised trial. Lancet 2005;366:136–143

34. Brinkhaus B, Witt CM, Jena S, Linde K, Streng A, Wagenpfeil S, Irnich D, Walther HU, Melchart D, Willich SN. Acupuncture in patients with chronic low back pain: a randomized controlled trial. Arch Intern Med 2006;166:450–457

35. Assefi NP, Sherman KJ, Jacobsen C, Goldberg J, Smith WR, Buchwald D. A randomized clinical trial of acupuncture compared with sham acupuncture in fibromyalgia. Ann Intern Med 2005;143:10–19

36. Harris RE, Tian X, Williams DA, Tian TX, Cupps TR, Petzke F, Groner KH, Biswas P, Gracely RH, Clauw DJ. Treatment of fibromyalgia with formula acupuncture: investigation of needle placement, needle stimulation, and treatment frequency. J Altern Complement Med 2005;11: 663–671

37. Li CD, Fu XY, Jiang ZY, Yang XG, Huang SQ, Wang QF, Liu J, Chen Y. Clinical study on combination of acupuncture, cupping and medicine for treatment of fibromyalgia syndrome. [In Chinese.] Zhongguo Zhen Jiu 2006;26:8–10

38. Biondi DM. Physical treatments for headache: a structured review. Headache 2005; 45:738–746

39. Melchart D, Streng A, Hoppe A, Brinkhaus B, Witt C, Wagenpfeil S, Pfaffenrath V, Hammes M, Hummelsberger J, Irnich D, Weidenhammer W, Willich SN, Linde K. Acupuncture in patients with tension-type headache: randomised controlled trial. BMJ 2005;331:376–382

40. Coeytaux RR, Kaufman JS, Kaptchuk TJ, Chen W, Miller WC, Callahan LF, Mann JD. A randomized, controlled trial of acupuncture for chronic daily headache. Headache 2005;45:1113–1123

41. Linde K, Streng A, Jurgens S, Hoppe A, Brinkhaus B, Witt C, Wagenpfeil S, Pfaffenrath V, Hammes MG, Weidenhammer W, Willich SN, Melchart D. Acupuncture for patients with migraine: a randomized controlled trial. JAMA 2005;293:2118–2125

42. Diener HC, Kronfeld K, Boewing G, Lungenhausen M, Maier C, Molsberger A, Tegenthoff M, Trampisch HJ, Zenz M, Meinert R; GERAC Migraine Study Group. Efficacy of acupuncture for the prophylaxis of migraine: a multicentre randomised controlled clinical trial. Lancet Neurol 2006;5:310–316

43. Smith MJ, Tong HC. Manual acupuncture for analgesia during electromyography: a pilot study. Arch Phys Med Rehabil 2005;86:1741–1744

44. Resim S, Gumusalan Y, Ekerbicer HC, Sahin MA, Sahinkanat T. Effectiveness of electro-acupuncture compared to sedo-analgesics in relieving pain during shockwave lithotripsy. Urol Res 2005;33:285–290

45. Xu YL, Jin JJ, Xu DY, Zheng Y. Effects of acupuncture plus acupoint sticking on bone mass density and pain in the patient of primary osteoporosis. [In Chinese.] Zhongguo Zhen Jiu 2006;26:87–90

46. Barlas P, Ting SL, Chesterton LS, Jones PW, Sim J. Effects of intensity of electroacupuncture upon experimental pain in healthy human volunteers: a randomized, double-blind, placebo-controlled study. Pain 2006; (epub ahead of print)

47. Lund I, Lundeberg T, Lonnberg L, Svensson E. Decrease of pregnant women's pelvic pain after acupuncture: a randomized controlled single-blind study. Acta Obstet Gynecol Scand 2006;85:12–19

48. Schmid-Schwap M, Simma-Kletschka I, Stockner A, Sengstbratl M, Gleditsch J, Kundi M, Piehslinger E. Oral acupuncture in the therapy of craniomandibular dysfunction syndrome – a randomized controlled trial. Wien Klin Wochenschr 2006;118:36–42

49. Kaptchuk TJ, Stason WB, Davis RB, Legedza AR, Schnyer RN, Kerr CE, Stone DA, Nam BH, Kirsch I, Goldman RH. Sham device v inert pill: randomised controlled trial of two placebo treatments. BMJ 2006;332:391–397

50. Ernst E. Acupuncture, a critical analysis. J Int Med 2006;259:125–137

51. MacPherson H, Scullion A, Thomas KJ, Walters S. Patient reports of adverse events associated with acupuncture treatment: a prospective national survey. Qual Saf Health Care 2004;13: 349–355

52. White A, Hayhoe S, Hart A, Ernst E. Adverse events following acupuncture: prospective survey of 32000 consultations with doctors and physiotherapists. BMJ 2001;323:485–486

53. Melchart D, Weidenhammer W, Streng A, Reitmayr S, Hoppe A, Ernst E, Linde K. Prospective investigation of adverse effects of acupuncture in 97,733 patients. Arch Intern Med 2004;164:104–105

54. Ernst E, White A. Life-threatening adverse reactions after acupuncture? A systematic review. Pain 1997;71:123–126

SECTION THREE

ALEXANDER TECHNIQUE

DEFINITION
Process of psychophysical re-education to improve postural balance and coordination to enable movement with minimal strain and maximum ease.

RELATED TECHNIQUES
Feldenkrais method, Rolfing, Tragerwork, yoga.

BACKGROUND
The Alexander technique was developed around the turn of the last century by Frederick M. Alexander, an Australian actor, who suffered a recurring loss of voice. By observing himself in a mirror, he concluded that it was the result of the tense position in which he habitually held his head. By correcting the relationship between head, neck and spine during activity, he gradually solved the problem. This marked the beginning of the Alexander technique.

TRADITIONAL CONCEPTS
The Alexander technique is based on three principles:

● function is affected by use
● an organism functions as a whole
● the relationship of the head, neck and spine is vital to the organism's ability to function optimally.

Human movement is thought to be most fluent when the head leads and the spine follows. This is practised repeatedly in the hope of creating new motor pathways, improving proprioception and upright posture and leading to enhanced coordination and balance.

SCIENTIFIC RATIONALE
The notion that learning the Alexander technique allows a conscious change of habitual and detrimental physiological reactions receives some support from psychophysiology research, suggesting that the mind can modulate aspects of the autonomic nervous system. Specific investigations of the Alexander technique have demonstrated that it improves the efficiency of moving from the sitting to standing position.

PRACTITIONERS
There are several thousand Alexander teachers worldwide. They typically come from a background of performing arts, dance, theatre and music or, more recently, physical or occupational therapy and massage. Certified teachers undergo at least 3 years of education on an approved course involving 1600 hours of training.

CONDITIONS FREQUENTLY TREATED
Chronic pain, headaches, osteoarthritis, asthma, stress. Also frequently used by performing artists and sportspeople.

TYPICAL SESSION
Sessions last between 45 and 60 minutes and take place in an Alexander studio with the aid of a bodywork table and mirror. The client or student is encouraged to wear loose, comfortable clothing to facilitate movement. The Alexander process is taught using a gentle hands-on approach to guide movements with the head leading and the spine following. Within 5–10 lessons the student

is able to experience and recreate an expansive quality of movement known as poise. The skill can then be refined to specialist activities.

COURSE OF TREATMENT

Thirty lessons are recommended to learn the basic concepts. Serious students of the technique may undertake up to 100 lessons.

CLINICAL EVIDENCE

An uncontrolled trial of a multidisciplinary programme for 67 chronic back pain sufferers incorporating lessons in Alexander technique reported improvements in pain that persisted for 6 months.[1] Multiple cases of the successful application of the Alexander technique to people with craniomandibular disorders[2] have also been reported. A systematic review of all clinical trials concluded that the Alexander technique is under-researched but held considerable promise for a range of conditions.[3]

RISKS

CONTRAINDICATIONS

None known.

PRECAUTIONS/WARNINGS

None known.

ADVERSE EFFECTS

None known.

INTERACTIONS

None known.

RISK–BENEFIT ASSESSMENT

Whether learning the Alexander technique has a specific therapeutic effect is not clear, but because it is virtually risk-free and has been associated with positive outcomes in various conditions it may be worth considering as an adjunctive or palliative therapy for patients who express a strong interest.

REFERENCES

1. Elkayam O, Ben Itzhak S, Avrahami E, Meidan Y, Doron N, Eldar I, Keidar I, Liram N, Yaron M. Multidisciplinary approach to chronic back pain: prognostic elements of the outcome. Clin Exp Rheum 1996;14:281–288
2. Knebelman S. The Alexander technique in diagnosis and treatment of craniomandibular disorders. Basal Facts 1982;5:19–22
3. Ernst E, Canter PH. The Alexander technique: a systematic review of controlled clinical trials. Forsch Komplementärmed Klass Naturheilkd 2003;10:325–329

AROMATHERAPY

DEFINITION

The controlled use of plant essences for therapeutic purposes.

RELATED TECHNIQUES

Massage.

BACKGROUND

The medicinal use of plant oils has a long history in ancient Egypt, China and India. The development of modern aromatherapy is attributed to the French chemist René Gattefosse, who burned his hand while working in a perfume laboratory and immediately doused it in some nearby lavender oil. The burn healed quickly without scarring, leading him to study the potential curative powers of plant oils. He coined the term aromatherapy in 1937.

TRADITIONAL CONCEPTS

Essential oils can be applied directly to the skin through massage or a compress, added to baths, inhaled with steaming water or spread throughout a room with a diffuser. The oils are believed to have effects at the psychological, physiological and cellular levels. These effects are claimed to be relaxing or stimulating depending on the chemistry of the oil and the previous associations of the individual with a particular scent.

SCIENTIFIC RATIONALE

The scent from the oil activates the olfactory sense. This triggers the limbic system, which governs emotional responses and is involved with the formation and retrieval of learned memories. Essential oils are also absorbed through the skin. Laboratory studies suggest that molecules of the oil can affect organ function, although the clinical relevance of these findings is not clear.

PRACTITIONERS

In most countries aromatherapy is largely unregulated. In the UK it is currently in the process of becoming regulated. Various associations offer courses with the number of hours of training required ranging from 180 to 500. Many nurses and other health-care professionals seek aromatherapy qualifications.

CONDITIONS FREQUENTLY TREATED

Headaches, musculoskeletal pain, insomnia, anxiety and other conditions. Some therapists recommend regular aromatherapy as a means of maintaining general health and well-being. A US survey suggests that stress, musculoskeletal problems and pain are the most common conditions treated by aromatherapists.[1]

TYPICAL SESSION

During an initial session the aromatherapist takes the client's medical history and asks which aromas are liked or disliked. The therapist then selects essential oils deemed appropriate for the client. Treatment usually consists of an aromatherapy massage and advice may be given about home treatments involving the use of oils in baths or a diffuser. The initial session may last up to 2 hours. Subsequent sessions would typically last 1 hour.

COURSE OF TREATMENT

For chronic conditions, one weekly session would be recommended for several weeks, with fortnightly or monthly follow-ups.

CLINICAL EVIDENCE

A Cochrane review focused on aromatherapy and massage for symptom relief in patients with cancer. It included 10 RCTs and found that 'massage and aromatherapy confer short-term benefits on psychological well-being, with the effect on anxiety supported by limited evidence'.[2] A systematic review of CAM for labour pain found one RCT of aromatherapy; its results did not demonstrate that baths with essential oil of ginger or lemongrass reduced analgesic consumption.[3] Other RCTs fail to show benefit in terms of symptom control in cancer patients,[4] or pain control, anxiety or quality of life in hospice patients.[5] More recent controlled clinical trials (CCTs) or RCTs suggest that aromatherapy can reduce the pain of arthritis.[6] An RCT tested whether the mere olfactory absorption of lavender or rosemary essential oils affected pain sensitivity in healthy volunteers ($n = 26$); no such effect was demonstrated.[7]

RISKS
CONTRAINDICATIONS
Pregnancy (see p. 4), contagious diseases, epilepsy, local venous thrombosis, varicose veins, broken skin, recent surgery, circulatory disorders.

PRECAUTIONS/WARNINGS
Essential oils should not be taken orally or used undiluted on the skin. Some oils cause photosensitive reactions and some have carcinogenic potential. Allergic reactions are possible with all oils. Aromatherapy should generally be considered an adjunctive treatment, not an alternative to conventional care.

ADVERSE EFFECTS
Allergic reactions, phototoxic reactions, nausea, headache.

INTERACTIONS
Many essential oils are believed to have the potential to either enhance or reduce the effects of prescribed medications including antibiotics, tranquillisers, antihistamines, anticonvulsants, barbiturates, morphine, quinidine.

QUALITY ISSUES
Products marketed as 'aromatherapy oils' may be synthetic or adulterated rather than the pure essential oil.

RISK–BENEFIT ASSESSMENT
The trial evidence on aromatherapy is contradictory. Aromatherapy appears to have some benefits as a palliative or supportive treatment, particularly in reducing anxiety. In the hands of a responsible therapist there seem to be few risks. Aromatherapy may thus be worth considering as an adjunctive treatment for chronically ill patients or individuals with psychosomatic illness.

REFERENCES
1. Osborn CE, Barlas P, Baxter GD, Barlow JH. Aromatherapy: a survey of current practice in the management of rheumatic disease symptoms. Complement Ther Med 2001;9:62–67
2. Fellowes D, Barnes K, Wilkinson S. Aromatherapy and massage for symptom relief in patients with cancer. The Cochrane Database of Systematic Reviews 2004, Issue 3. Art. No.: CD002287
3. Huntley AL, Coon JT, Ernst E. Complementary and alternative medicine for labor pain: a systematic review. Am J Obstet Gynecol 2004;191:36–44
4. Wilcock A, Manderson C, Weller R, Walker G, Carr D, Carey AM, Broadhurst D, Mew J, Ernst E. Does aromatherapy massage benefit patients with cancer attending a specialist palliative care day centre? Palliat Med 2004;18:287–290
5. Soden K, Vincent K, Craske S, Lucas C, Ashley S. A randomized controlled trial of aromatherapy massage in a hospice setting. Palliat Med 2004;18:87–92
6. Kim MJ, Nam ES, Paik SI. The effects of aromatherapy on pain, depression, and life satisfaction of arthritis patients. [In Korean.] Taehan Kanho Hakhoe Chi 2005;35:186–194
7. Gedney JJ, Glover TL, Fillingim RB. Sensory and affective pain discrimination after inhalation of essential oils. Psychosom Med 2004;66:599–606

AUTOGENIC TRAINING

SYNONYMS

Autogenic therapy, autogenics.

DEFINITION

Autogenic training refers to a series of mental exercises involving relaxation and autosuggestion practised regularly. The aim is to teach individuals to switch off the 'fight/flight/fight' stress response at will. The resulting passive state is believed to allow the brain and body to tap into its own spontaneous self-regulatory mechanisms, which, in turn, can encourage an awareness of the origin of certain mental and physical disorders within. In the US, the term 'autogenic' often refers to any method that involves patients using their own resources to help themselves, usually involving relaxation, visualisation or autosuggestion.

RELATED TECHNIQUES

Relaxation, self-hypnosis.

BACKGROUND

Autogenic training developed in the last decade of the 19th century when it was noted that people who had previously undergone hypnotic sessions were able to put themselves readily into a state which appeared to be similar to hypnosis and that the regular use of this state reduced stress and improved efficiency. In the 1920s, the German physician Johannes Schultz explored these ideas and added autosuggestion, with the aim of developing a practice that avoided the therapist dependency of hypnosis and gave control to patients themselves. Heaviness and warmth were the two most common sensations during hypnosis, so Schultz taught patients to think about heaviness and warmth in the limbs. These constitute the first two exercises of autogenic training. Four other instructions, relating to heart rate, breathing, warmth in the abdomen and coolness of the forehead, were added to form the six standard exercises.

Later Schultz and Thomas developed the personal and motivational formulae (at first known as 'intentional formulae'), which are tailored to the individual experience, and involve repetition of therapeutic suggestions, designed, for example, to correct negative patterns of thought. A series of meditative exercises were added for those who have gained considerable experience.

In the 1970s, the chest physician Wolfgang Luthe developed the 'intentional off-loading exercises', whereby individuals are taught to off-load emotions. These exercises are thought to enhance the autogenic process by encouraging the release of stored and pent-up feelings that often manifest in psychosomatic 'stress' syndromes.

SCIENTIFIC RATIONALE

There is little neurophysiological research on autogenic training. It appears to combine the effects of profound relaxation, which probably involve the limbic system and the hypothalamo–pituitary axis, with psychotherapeutic aspects of autosuggestion.

PRACTITIONERS

Practitioners of autogenic training frequently have other health-care training and integrate autogenic training into their practice. There is no regulation or restriction on who may practice autogenic training. In some countries, associations exist which emphasise the classic method of Schultz and Luthe.

CONDITIONS FREQUENTLY TREATED

Pain, angina pectoris, anxiety, asthma, depression, dyspepsia, functional disorders of bladder and bowel, hypertension, phobia, premenstrual syndrome, sleep disorders, stress responses.

TYPICAL SESSION

Training is often carried out in groups in a quiet room, with patients first instructed in the three recommended postures. Then they learn to concentrate passively on the heaviness of the dominant arm and to generalise this sensation to the rest of the body. This is followed by instruction in the other standard exercises. These should be practised three times daily, for about 10 minutes each time. Students are asked to keep diaries of their experiences so that the process and reactions can be monitored by the tutor. When the standard exercises have been mastered, personal and motivational formulae are added, devised by the client with the help of the therapist. After gaining enough experience, advanced autogenic training can be learnt, which involves prolonging the autogenic state and performing meditative exercises on increasingly abstract concepts. A second advanced autogenic method, also prolonging the autogenic state and developed by Luthe, is 'autogenic neutralisation', a psychotherapeutic method of release or discharge (neutralisation) of the 'disturbing potency of neuronal record'.

COURSE OF TREATMENT

Typically between eight and 10 sessions are required to learn the standard exercises. There is no need for further attendance, unless advanced autogenic training is undertaken.

CLINICAL EVIDENCE

Recent RCTs or systematic reviews suggest that autogenic training can alleviate headaches in a variety of clinical situations.[1,2] A meta-analysis of all controlled trials reached positive conclusions for some conditions (hypertension, asthma, intestinal diseases, glaucoma and eczema) but made no assessment of the quality of the studies.[3] One RCT ($n = 18$) suggested that autogenic training may be a useful adjunctive therapy for complex regional pain syndrome.[4] A systematic review of CCTs suggested that autogenic training is equally effective in controlling chronic pain as hypnotherapy.[5]

RISKS

CONTRAINDICATIONS

Severe mental disorders. Latent psychosis and personality disorders, as these may become overt with introspection. Children under 5 years.

PRECAUTIONS/WARNINGS

For medical conditions, autogenic training should only be used as an adjunct to standard therapy. Some people have difficulty mastering the technique.

ADVERSE EFFECTS

Reactions to autogenic training may occur, such as unusual sensations in the body.

INTERACTIONS

Standard therapy (e.g. for hypertension) should be monitored more regularly while learning autogenic training in case alterations of medication are required.

RISK–BENEFIT ASSESSMENT

Autogenic training is likely to be effective and safe for a number of conditions including chronic pain. It can be recommended as an adjunctive treatment in suitable cases.

REFERENCES

1. Zsombok T, Juhasz G, Budavari A, Vitrai J, Bagdy G. Effect of autogenic training on drug consumption in patients with primary headache: an 8-month follow-up study. Headache 2003;43:251–257
2. Devineni T, Blanchard EB. A randomized controlled trial of an internet-based treatment for chronic headache. Behav Res Ther 2005;43:277–292
3. Stetter F, Kupper S. Autogenes Training – qualitative Meta-Analyse kontrollierter klinischer Studien und Beziehungen zur Naturheilkunde. Forsch Komplementärmed 1998;5:211–223
4. Fialka V, Korpan M, Saradeth T, Paternostro-Slugo T, Hexel O, Frischenschlager O, Ernst E. Autogenic training for reflex sympathetic dystrophy: a pilot study. Complement Ther Med 1996;4:103–105
5. Jensen M, Patterson DR. Hypnotic treatment of chronic pain. J Behav Med 2006;29: 95–124

AYURVEDA

SYNONYMS

Traditional Indian medicine.

DEFINITION

Ancient Indian philosophy that forms the basis of a traditional medical system.

RELATED TECHNIQUES

Meditation, yoga, herbal medicine, diet, massage.

BACKGROUND

The term 'Ayurveda' is derived from the Sanskrit words *ayur* (life) and *veda* (knowledge or science). Ayurveda evolved in India some 8000 years ago and is often quoted as the oldest medical system in the world. It was the dominant medical system in India for millennia. Today it is practised alongside modern medicine in India and Sri Lanka and has recently become popular in many other parts of the world.

TRADITIONAL CONCEPTS

Ayurvedic philosophy claims that all humans can be characterised by their unique mixture of three basic metabolic types or *Doshas* (or *Dosas*) known as *Vata, Pitta* and *Kapha* (concept of *Tridosha*). Illness occurs if the individual harmony between the three doshas is disturbed. The aim of Ayurvedic treatment therefore is to ensure a balance between the three doshas.

SCIENTIFIC RATIONALE

Ayurveda emphasises the need for harmony between body, mind and spirit, as well as the tridoshic equilibrium. Any disharmony can be addressed by cleaning, detoxification, palliation, rejuvenation or mental and spiritual hygiene. The principle of biological individuality is central. Many of the interventions thus employed have a scientific rationale. For instance, Ayurvedic herbal preparations include plants with well-documented pharmacological actions (e.g. *Rauwolfia*). Other Ayurvedic therapeutic principles, such as exercise or fasting, are equally well established in a scientific sense.

PRACTITIONERS

In India there are over 300,000 Ayurvedic practitioners, and about 100 Ayurvedic colleges exist. As the popularity of Ayurveda grows outside India, so does the number of practitioners. In most countries, the practice of Ayurveda is not strictly regulated.

SECTION THREE

CONDITIONS FREQUENTLY TREATED

Ayurveda is a 'whole system' of medicine that has survived for millennia. Most medical conditions are claimed to be treatable with it. Outside India, Ayurvedic practitioners tend to treat predominantly chronic benign conditions including many pain syndromes.

TYPICAL SESSION

During a first consultation, the therapist would take a medical history. A diagnosis might also rely on the palpation of the pulse and inspection of the tongue (not dissimilar to traditional Chinese medicine) as well as urine analysis and appearance of nails.

COURSE OF TREATMENT

Treatments are usually long-term and may include a variety of modalities: changes in lifestyle (e.g. diet), herbs, meditation, exercises, massage. Treatments are highly individualised and may follow a specially prescribed sequence.

CLINICAL EVIDENCE

There are no CCTs testing the effectiveness of the entirety of the Ayurvedic approach. Clinical trials invariably test one aspect of it, e.g. a herbal medicine. A systematic review of Ayurvedic medicines for rheumatoid arthritis found seven such studies. The totality of these data failed to convincingly demonstrate the effectiveness of these treatments.[1] Recent RCTs generated promising findings for Ayurvedic medicines as a treatment for osteoarthritis.[2,3]

RISKS

CONTRAINDICATIONS

Depends on specific modality.

PRECAUTIONS/WARNINGS

Depends on specific modality.

ADVERSE EFFECTS

Depends on specific modality. Herbal preparations have repeatedly been found to contain toxic levels of heavy metals.

INTERACTIONS

Depends on modality.

RISK–BENEFIT ASSESSMENT

Ayurveda is a whole system of medicine. Even though individual elements of this system have been tested for efficacy and safety (see elsewhere in this book), the whole system is insufficiently researched. Thus, its risk–benefit balance cannot be clearly defined at present.

REFERENCES

1. Park J, Ernst E. Ayurvedic medicine for rheumatoid arthritis: a systematic review. Semin Arthritis Rheum 2005;34:705–713
2. Chopra A, Lavin P, Patwardhan B, Chitre D. A 32-week randomized placebo-controlled clinical evaluation of RA-11, an Ayurvedic drug, on osteoarthritis of the knees. J Clin Rheumatol 2004;10:236–245
3. Singh BB, Mishra LC, Vinjamury SP, Aquilina N, Singh VJ, Shepard N. The effectiveness of Commiphora mukul for osteoarthritis of the knee: an outcomes study. Altern Ther Health Med 2003;9:74–79

SECTION THREE

BIOFEEDBACK

DEFINITION

The use of instrumentation to monitor, amplify and feed back information on physiological responses so that a patient can learn to regulate these responses.[1,2] Biofeedback is a form of psychophysiological self-regulation. When biofeedback is used to control brain activity, it is called neurofeedback or neurotherapy.[3]

RELATED TECHNIQUES

Biofeedback and neurofeedback are frequently used as adjuncts to relaxation, hypnosis, behaviour therapy and psychotherapy.

BACKGROUND

Biofeedback developed from several streams of research in the 1960s and 1970s: laboratory-based research on voluntary physiological controls, behavioural therapy efforts to identify reliable principles of behaviour change, and the search of humanistic psychology for the higher potentials of human beings.[4,5] Early research showed voluntary control of electroencephalographic (EEG) brainwave activity, internal visceral functioning and muscle activity. Biofeedback was shown to increase the human being's awareness and control of many bodily processes previously thought to be beyond voluntary control.

TRADITIONAL CONCEPTS

The process of becoming aware of physiological responses in the body offers the individual the opportunity to establish control over such processes. Any physiological response that can be monitored is suitable for biofeedback. The most common responses are electrical activity of the brain (EEG), skin temperature (thermal), muscle tension or surface electromyography (SEMG), galvanic skin response or electrodermal response, blood pressure, respiration, heart rate and heart rate variability and blood volume.[4,6] This information is presented to the patient through visual and/or auditory signals, often through a computer monitor display. The aim of the treatment is to establish the patient's control over the response independently of the biofeedback instrument. Biofeedback is also helpful in teaching the patient to recognise the link between mind and body, and more specifically to recognise the role of specific thoughts and emotions in the onset of physical symptoms. Biofeedback is frequently used as an adjunct to other therapies. Biofeedback-assisted relaxation training supports progress in cognitive–behavioural therapy and stress management. Biofeedback is also frequently used to monitor signs of affective arousal or disturbance in psychotherapy.

SCIENTIFIC RATIONALE

Biofeedback can modify physiological processes mediated by the central and peripheral nervous systems, impacting on both somatic and autonomic nervous pathways. The relaxation effects of biofeedback affect the limbic brain, the hypothalamic–pituitary–adrenal axis, autonomic control of a variety of internal organs and muscle function.[7]

PRACTITIONERS

Biofeedback is an interdisciplinary field. Clinical psychologists, health psychologists and behavioural therapists are among those who use the technique. Biofeedback procedures are also widely used by physicians, nurses, physical and occupational therapists, sports physiologists, social workers, counsellors, teachers and many others.

CONDITIONS FREQUENTLY TREATED

Conditions that can be alleviated by mental calming and/or affected more directly through the physiological changes achieved, such as pain, anxiety, asthma, attention deficit disorder, bruxism, encopresis, enuresis, epileptic seizures, essential tremor, hypertension, insomnia, irritable bowel syndrome, pelvic floor disorders including urinary and faecal incontinence, Raynaud's disease, substance abuse and tinnitus.

TYPICAL SESSION

An initial medical and psychosocial history provides evidence regarding relevant patterns and mechanisms active in the onset and maintenance of the patient's condition. The practitioner often conducts a psychophysiological profile, assessing the patient's baseline physiological patterns, reactivity under varied conditions such as stressors, and recovery ability and rate. The profile further identifies physiological systems though which this patient reacts that could be addressed and modified with biofeedback. The practitioner attaches sensors (SEMG, EEG, temperature, etc.) for measuring various physiological responses. The patient observes audiovisual displays and learns to reduce maladaptive responses, to correct abnormal physiological reactions and habits and to produce the desired physiological changes. The patient learns to recognise the maladaptive psychophysiological functioning such as the physiological responses and symptoms that are linked to thoughts, emotions, postures and breathing habits.

COURSE OF TREATMENT

Treatments with biofeedback vary, depending on a range of factors. Initial evaluations last typically about 60–90 minutes, and subsequent sessions vary from about 45 to 60 minutes. Therapists often recommend home practice such as varied relaxation procedures. Audiotapes or CDs are often used for training.

CLINICAL EVIDENCE

An overview provided a summary of all systematic reviews on biofeedback.[8] According to these data, various forms of biofeedback are effective as adjunctive treatments in a range of conditions such as paediatric migraine, rheumatoid arthritis and temporomandibular disorders. A recent RCT[9] and a systematic review[10] confirmed the value of biofeedback as a treatment for chronic headache. Another systematic review found encouraging but not conclusive evidence for biofeedback as an effective treatment for chronic pelvic pain.[11]

RISKS
CONTRAINDICATIONS

Patients with psychiatric conditions: examples include severe depression, acute agitation, acute or fragile schizophrenia, mania, paranoid disorders with delusions of influence, severe obsessive–compulsive disorder, delirium and dissociative reaction.

PRECAUTIONS/WARNINGS

As with other therapies that induce changes in mental state, biofeedback should be used only under medical supervision in cases of psychosis or personality disorder.

ADVERSE EFFECTS

There are occasional reports of biofeedback being associated with acute anxiety, dizziness, disorientation and floating sensations.

SECTION THREE

INTERACTIONS

In patients taking medication involved in homeostasis, such as insulin or antihypertensive therapies, the dose may need to be altered.

RISK–BENEFIT ASSESSMENT

Biofeedback is effective for a range of conditions, often as an adjunct to other interventions. The risks are small and adverse effects are rare. The risk–benefit balance is therefore positive for some conditions such as chronic headache.

REFERENCES

1. Schwartz M, Andrasik F, eds. Biofeedback: a practitioner's guide. New York: Guildford Press; 2003
2. Green JA, Shellenberger R. Biofeedback therapy. In: Jonas WB, Levin JS, eds. Essentials of complementary and alternative medicine. Baltimore, MD: Lippincott Williams & Wilkins; 1999: 410–425
3. Evans JR, Abarbanel A, eds. Introduction to quantitative EEG and neurofeedback. San Diego: Academic Press; 1999
4. Gilbert C, Moss D. Biofeedback. Biofeedback and biological monitoring. In: Moss D, Wickramesekera DI, McGrady A, Davies T, eds. Handbook of mind–body medicine in primary care: behavioral and physiological tools. Thousand Oaks, CA: Sage; 2003:109–122
5. Moss D. Biofeedback. In: Shannon S, ed. Handbook of complementary and alternative therapies in mental health. San Diego, CA: Academic Press; 2001:135–158
6. Lawlis GF. Biofeedback. In: Freeman LW, Lawlis GF. Mosby's complementary and alternative medicine: a research based approach. St Louis, MO: Mosby; 2001:196–224
7. Everly GS, Lating JM. A clinical guide to treatment of the human stress response. New York: Plenum; 2002
8. Ernst E. Systematic reviews of biofeedback. Phys Med Rehab Kuror 2003;13:321–324
9. Devineni T, Blanchard EB. A randomized controlled trial of an internet-based treatment for chronic headache. Behav Res Ther 2005;43:277–292
10. Biondi DM. Physical treatments for headache: a structured review. Headache 2005; 45:738–746
11. Capodice JL, Bemis DL, Buttyan R, Kaplan SA, Katz AE. Complementary and alternative medicine for chronic prostatitis/chronic pelvic pain syndrome. Evid Based Complement Altern Med 2005;2:495–501

CHIROPRACTIC

DEFINITION

According to the UK General Chiropractic Council, chiropractic is a health profession concerned with the diagnosis, treatment and prevention of mechanical disorders of the musculoskeletal system, and the effects of these disorders on the function of the nervous system and general health. There is an emphasis on manual treatments including spinal manipulation or adjustment.

RELATED TECHNIQUES

Osteopathy, manual therapy, spinal manipulation, spinal mobilisation.

BACKGROUND

Some therapeutic elements that chiropractors use, such as spinal manipulation, go back to antiquity and were used by bonesetters throughout the history of (folk) medicine. Chiropractic was developed in 1895 by the Canadian Daniel David Palmer (1845–1913). The term chiropractic is derived from the Greek *cheir* (hand) and *praxis* (action).

Chiropractic has a colourful history with tensions between various subsets of the chiropractic profession. The 'straights' adhered to Palmer's teaching as to a dogma, while the 'mixers' had a more liberal attitude. A fierce debate also raged between mainstream medicine and chiropractic. Today, chiropractors are accepted in many countries as health-care professionals and their treatments are now being tested according to the principles of evidence-based medicine.

TRADITIONAL CONCEPTS

Palmer reasoned that pressure on nerves, caused by misalignment or subluxation of the vertebral joints, produced disease. He surmised that correction of these misalignments was the only way of restoring health. The most important therapeutic method of chiropractors is spinal manipulation or adjustment. It often entails high-velocity, low-amplitude manual thrusts applied to spinal joints, which extend them just beyond their physiological range of motion. Spinal mobilisation, by contrast, is the application of manual force to such joints without thrust and within the normal passive range of motion.

SCIENTIFIC RATIONALE

The primary premise of Palmer and his followers that subluxation is the cause of all illness has no scientific rationale. Spinal mobilisation has been shown to have a number of physiological effects (such as reduction of muscle spasm, inhibition of nociceptive transmissions). Spinal manipulation and related techniques are thought to improve joint function and alleviate pain related to spinal abnormalities.

PRACTITIONERS

By definition, chiropractic is what chiropractors do. However, spinal manipulation and mobilisation are also used by osteopaths, naturopaths, physical therapists and doctors. Both in the US and the UK, chiropractors need a licence to practice. In the UK, chiropractors are regulated by statute.

CONDITIONS FREQUENTLY TREATED

Musculoskeletal pain and spinal pain syndromes, migraine, headache, asthma, cardiovascular problems, infantile colic, irritable bowel syndrome.

TYPICAL SESSION

A chiropractor takes a medical history and conducts a physical examination. In many cases, this is supplemented by spinal radiographs and possibly other diagnostic procedures. Subsequent treatments involve hands-on techniques, usually with the patient sitting or lying. These may last for 15 minutes or more and include reviews of patient progress, amendment of treatment plans and appropriate referral when clinically indicated.

COURSE OF TREATMENT

The number of sessions required is highly variable; on average it is about seven, ranging between four and 20. Repeat courses of treatments or continuing prophylactic or supportive sessions are often recommended.

CLINICAL EVIDENCE

Numerous reviews of spinal manipulation for back pain are available, many of which are overtly biased; thus its effectiveness is less certain than many reviewers suggest.[1] A systematic review of spinal manipulative therapies for back pain included 39 RCTs,[2] 29 of which assessed patients with acute pain, 29 studies evaluated patients with chronic pain, and 14 studies included patients with mixed or indeterminate durations of pain. For patients with acute low back pain, the only reported clinically significant improvement in short-term pain occurred among patients receiving spinal manipulation as compared with sham therapy. In comparisons with all other conventional therapies, spinal manipulative therapies showed no statistical or clinical difference among patients with acute low back pain. Similarly, among patients with chronic low back pain, the only clinically significant findings were in comparison with the sham therapy or, as the authors state, ineffective therapies groups. No differences were found for the outcomes of short-term or long-term function. More recent RCTs suggest that spinal manipulation in combination with individualised exercises is beneficial in reducing back pain[3] but not superior to a physiotherapeutic 'brief pain management programme'[4] nor to group exercises[5] nor to physician-led back care.[6]

As the above-mentioned review includes all types of manipulative therapies, it is pertinent to systematically review chiropractic spinal manipulation for back pain separately.[7] Twelve RCTs were found including all forms of back pain, many of which had considerable methodological shortcomings. Some degree of superiority of chiropractic spinal manipulation over control interventions was noted in five studies. More recent trials and those with adequate follow-up periods tended to be negative. It was concluded that the effectiveness of chiropractic spinal manipulation is not supported by compelling evidence. An RCT with 235 patients suffering from chronic back pain suggested that, compared to physiotherapeutic trunk exercise, chiropractic flexion distraction leads to greater pain relief.[8] An RCT with 681 back pain patients showed no 'clinically meaningful' differences between chiropractic and medical care.[9] Another RCT ($n = 252$) suggested that chiropractic care plus heat reduces osteoarthritic back pain more than heat alone.[10] It is conceivable that certain, as yet not clearly defined, subgroups of patients respond better to chiropractic treatment than others.[11,12] An RCT with 102 patients suffering from sciatica suggested that chiropractic spinal manipulation generates better pain control than sham manipulation.[13]

A Cochrane review of spinal manipulation and mobilisation for neck pain included 33 trials and found that, administered alone, these treatments were not beneficial.[14] Only four RCTs were located for a systematic review that were specifically on chiropractic spinal manipulation.[15] None of them convincingly demonstrated the superiority of manipulation over control interventions. Recent RCTs continue to generate contradictory results.[16–18]

Eight RCTs were included in a systematic review of spinal manipulation for headache disorders.[19] The results were inconclusive and no definitive conclusion about the effectiveness of this approach was drawn. Other reviewers stated that 'before any firm conclusions can be drawn, further testing should be done in rigorously designed … trials'[20] or concluded that there is 'no rigourous evidence that manual therapies have a positive effect in the evolution of tension-type headache'.[21]

Other systematic reviews generated no sound evidence for the effectiveness of spinal manipulation as a treatment for non-spinal pain,[22] infantile colic,[23] carpal tunnel syndrome[24] and secondary dysmenorrhoea.[25]

A systematic review of all sham-controlled RCTs of spinal manipulation (for any condition) concluded that 'the most rigorous of these studies suggest that spinal manipulation is not associated with clinically relevant specific therapeutic effects'.[26]

The above-named findings were also confirmed in a systematic review of systematic reviews of RCTs of spinal manipulation.[27]

RISKS

CONTRAINDICATIONS

High-velocity manipulations are contraindicated in advanced osteoporosis, bleeding abnormalities, malignant or inflammatory spinal disease, patients on anticoagulants, fractures, postoperative spinal instability, cervical spondylotic myelopathy and cauda equina syndrome.

PRECAUTIONS/WARNINGS

Elderly patients, people who feel uncomfortable with close contact. Overuse of X-ray diagnostics, advice of some chiropractors against immunisation, unreliability of diagnostic techniques used by chiropractors.

ADVERSE EFFECTS

Serious adverse effects include arterial dissection and stroke (upper spinal manipulation) and cauda equina syndrome (lower spinal manipulation).[28] Their incidence is probably low but reliable data are presently not available. Mild and transient adverse effects of high-velocity manipulations, such as local discomfort, are reported by about 50% of all patients.

INTERACTIONS

Patients on anticoagulants may be at a higher risk of cerebrovascular accidents after high-velocity manipulations of the upper spine.

RISK–BENEFIT ASSESSMENT

Chiropractic treatment might be helpful for acute low back pain but the evidence is not convincing. In view of the lack of convincingly effective conventional treatments for this indication, chiropractic might therefore be worth considering for such patients. For all other indications the evidence is even less compelling. Severe adverse events may be infrequent but mild transient complaints are common.

REFERENCES

1. Canter PH, Ernst E. Sources of bias in reviews of spinal manipulation for back pain. Wien Klin Wochenschr 2005;117:333–341
2. Assendelft WJJ, Morton SC, Yu EI, Suttorp MJ, Shekelle PG. Spinal manipulation therapy for low back pain. The Cochrane Database of Systematic Reviews 2004, Issue 1. Art. No.: CD000447
3. Geisser ME, Wiggert EA, Haig AJ, Colwell MO. A randomized, controlled trial of manual therapy and specific adjuvant exercise for chronic low back pain. Clin J Pain 2005;21:463–470
4. Hay EM, Mullis R, Lewis M, Vohora K, Main CJ, Watson P, Dziedzic KS, Sim J, Lowe CM, Croft PR. Comparison of physical treatments versus a brief pain-management programme for back pain in primary care: a randomised clinical trial in physiotherapy practice. Lancet 2005;365:2024–2030
5. Lewis JS, Hewitt JS, Billington L, Cole S, Byng J, Karayiannis S. A randomized clinical trial comparing two physiotherapy interventions for chronic low back pain. Spine 2005;30:711–721
6. Niemisto L, Rissanen P, Sarna S, Lahtinen-Suopanki T, Lindgren KA, Hurri H. Cost-effectiveness of combined manipulation, stabilizing exercises, and physician consultation compared to physician consultation alone for chronic low back pain: a prospective randomized trial with 2-year follow-up. Spine 2005;30:1109–1115
7. Ernst E, Canter PH. Chiropractic spinal manipulation for back pain? A systematic review of randomised controlled trials. Phys Ther Rev 2003;8:85–91
8. Gudavalli MR, Cambron JA, McGregor M, Jedlicka J, Keenum M, Ghanayem AJ, Patwardhan AG. A randomized clinical trial and subgroup analysis to compare flexion-distraction with active exercise for chronic low back pain. Eur Spine J 2006;15:1070–1082
9. Hurwitz EL, Morgenstern H, Kominski GF, Yu F, Chiang LM. A randomized trial of chiropractic and medical care for patients with low back pain: eighteen-month follow-up outcomes from the UCLA low back pain study. Spine 2006;31:611–621
10. Beyerman KL, Palmerino MB, Zohn LE, Kane GM, Foster KA. Efficacy of treating low back pain and dysfunction secondary to osteoarthritis: chiropractic care compared with moist heat alone. J Manipulative Physiol Ther 2006;29:107–114.
11. Axen I, Jones JJ, Rosenbaum A, Lovgren PW, Halasz L, Larsen K, Leboeuf-Yde C. The Nordic Back Pain Subpopulation Program: validation and improvement of a predictive model for treatment outcome in patients with low back pain receiving chiropractic treatment. J Manipulative Physiol Ther 2005;28:381–385

12. Fritz JM, Childs JD, Flynn TW. Pragmatic application of a clinical prediction rule in primary care to identify patients with low back pain with a good prognosis following a brief spinal manipulation intervention. BMC Fam Pract 2005;6:29

13. Santilli V, Beghi E, Finucci S. Chiropractic manipulation in the treatment of acute back pain and sciatica with disc protrusion: a randomized double-blind clinical trial of active and simulated spinal manipulations. Spine J 2006;6:131–137

14. Gross AR, Hoving JL, Haines TA, Goldsmith CH, Kay T, Aker P, Bronfort G. A Cochrane review of manipulation and mobilization for mechanical neck disorders. Spine 2004;29:1541–1548

15. Ernst E. Chiropractic spinal manipulation for neck pain: a systematic review. J Pain 2003; 4:417–421

16. Cleland JA, Childs JD, McRae M, Palmer JA, Stowell T. Immediate effects of thoracic manipulation in patients with neck pain: a randomized clinical trial. Man Ther 2006;10:127–135

17. Dziedzic K, Hill J, Lewis M, Sim J, Daniels J, Hay EM. Effectiveness of manual therapy or pulsed shortwave diathermy in addition to advice and exercise for neck disorders: a pragmatic randomized controlled trial in physical therapy clinics. Arthritis Rheum 2005;53:214–222

18. Palmgren PJ, Sandstrom PJ, Lundqvist FJ, Heikkila H. Improvement after chiropractic care in cervicocephalic kinesthetic sensibility and subjective pain intensity in patients with nontraumatic chronic neck pain. J Manipulative Physiol Ther 2006;29:100–106

19. Astin JA, Ernst E. The effectiveness of spinal manipulation for the treatment of headache disorders: a systematic review of randomized clinical trials. Cephalalgia 2002;22:617–623

20. Bronfort G, Assendelft WJJ, Evans R, Haas M, Bouter L. Efficacy of spinal manipulation for chronic headache: a systematic review. J Manip Physiol Ther 2001;24:457–466

21. Fernandez-de-Las-Penas C, Alonso-Blanco C, Cuadrado ML, Miangolarra JC, Barriga FJ, Pareja JA. Are manual therapies effective in reducing pain from tension-type headache?: a systematic review. Clin J Pain 2006;22:278–285

22. Ernst E. Chiropractic manipulation for non-spinal pain – a systematic review. NZ Med J 2003:116:1–9

23. Husereau D, Clifford T, Aker P, Leduc D, Mensinkai S. Spinal manipulation for infantile colic. Ottawa: Canadian Coordinating Office for Health Technology Assessment; 2003. Technology report no. 42

24. O'Connor D, Marshall S, Massy-Westropp N. Non-surgical treatment (other than steroid injection) for carpal tunnel syndrome. The Cochrane Database of Systematic Reviews 2003, Issue 1. Art. No.: CD003219

25. Proctor ML, Hing W, Johnson TC, Murphy PA. Spinal manipulation for primary and secondary dysmenorrhoea. The Cochrane Database of Systematic Reviews 2001, Issue 4. Art. No.: CD002119

26. Ernst E, Harkness E. Spinal manipulation: a systematic review of sham-controlled, double-blind, randomized clinical trials. J Pain Symptom Manage 2001;22:879–889

27. Ernst E, Canter PH. A systematic review of systematic reviews of spinal manipulation. J R Soc Med 2006;99:192–196

28. Stevinson C, Ernst E. Risks associated with spinal manipulation. Am J Med 2002;112: 566–571

CRANIOSACRAL THERAPY

SYNONYMS/SUBCATEGORIES

Cranial osteopathy, sacro-occipital technique.

DEFINITION

A subtle form of manual treatment which is tissue-, fluid-, membrane- and energy-oriented and very gentle in its application.

RELATED TECHNIQUES

Osteopathy.

BACKGROUND

The original concepts were first put forward in the 1930s by the American William G. Sutherland. Initially it was only practised by osteopaths but, in the 1970s, John E. Upledger made some refinements and was the first to teach it to non-osteopathic practitioners. Further refinements in both theory and practice continue to be made. Craniosacral therapy became popular first in the US and subsequently in Europe.

TRADITIONAL CONCEPTS

Craniosacral therapy is based on the premise that there are micro-rhythmic motions present in the body that play an important role in health. Emphasis is placed upon alleged rhythmic motion of tissues and fluids at the core of the body such as the cerebrospinal fluid, the central nervous system, the intracranial and intraspinal dural membranes, the cranial bones and the sacrum. The unrestricted motion of these subtle rhythms is believed to be fundamental to the self-healing capabilities of the body. According to Upledger,[1] the rhythmic motion of cerebrospinal fluid can be sensed in a similar way to the peripheral pulse. Treatment is based upon the palpation of any strains or restrictions that affect these subtle rhythms and the use of light touch to facilitate natural motion. Craniosacral therapy is thought to help alleviate a wide range of symptoms.

SCIENTIFIC RATIONALE

Subtle rhythmic motion at cranial bones and the sacrum not directly related to lung respiration or arterial pulse and motion of cerebrospinal fluid have been reported.[2–4] However, there is no published evidence that these movements affect health.

PRACTITIONERS

Craniosacral therapy is practised by chiropractors, osteopaths, naturopaths, physiotherapists, dentists, massage therapists, physicians and other regulated or unregulated health-care professionals.

CONDITIONS FREQUENTLY TREATED

According to Upledger the following conditions respond to craniosacral therapy: chronic pain, headaches, migraine, musculoskeletal problems, temporomandibular joint dysfunction, trigeminal neuralgia, birth trauma, cerebral dysfunction, cerebral palsy, colic, depression, dyslexia, ear infections, learning disabilities, Ménière's disease, sinusitis, strabismus, stroke. Young children are believed to respond particularly well.

TYPICAL SESSION

An initial diagnostic session is conducted to evaluate the nature of the problem. The patient may be lying down or seated. The procedure mainly involves lightly touching the skull and/or the sacrum or other locations depending on the physiological requirements of the patient. The first session may take about 1 hour. Subsequent therapeutic sessions are often shorter.

COURSE OF TREATMENT

The number of sessions required is extremely variable and depends on the nature and severity of the condition(s) treated. Upledger states that, if no effect is seen after about six sessions, craniosacral therapy may not be effective.

CLINICAL EVIDENCE

Upledger claims that craniosacral therapy 'is helpful in at least 90% of the patients'.[1] A systematic review of the evidence, however, concluded that there is 'insufficient evidence to support craniosacral therapy'[4] and an independent review supported these findings.[5] A systematic review of manual therapies for treating tension-type headache identified one trial of craniosacral therapy and concluded that there is presently no rigorous evidence of effectiveness.[6] An RCT compared osteopathic treatment employing parietal, visceral and craniosacral techniques with orthopaedic treatment using chiropractic techniques, antiphlogistics and cortisone in 53 patients with chronic epicondylopathia humeri radialis.[7] There was no difference between the treatments.

RISKS

CONTRAINDICATIONS

Intracranial aneurysm, cerebral haemorrhage, subdural or subarachnoid bleeding, increased intracranial pressure, recent skull fractures.

PRECAUTIONS/WARNINGS

None known.

ADVERSE EFFECTS

Some undesired effects were reported in patients with traumatic brain syndrome;[8] temporary worsening of symptoms and mild discomfort may occur.[1]

INTERACTIONS

May increase antidiabetic, antiepileptic or psychoactive treatments.[1]

RISK–BENEFIT ASSESSMENT

There is no convincing evidence for the effectiveness of craniosacral therapy for any disease or symptom. Several indirect and direct risks have been linked to craniosacral therapy. On balance, therefore, and until further more positive data emerge, craniosacral therapy cannot be recommended for any condition.

REFERENCES

1. Upledger JE. Craniosacral therapy. In: Novey DW, ed. The complete reference to complementary and alternative medicine. St Louis, MO: Mosby; 2000
2. Frymann VM. A study of the rhythmic motions of the living cranium. J Am Osteopath Assoc 1971;70:928–945
3. Tettambel M, Cicora A, Lay E. Recording of the cranial rhythmic impulse. J Am Osteopath Assoc 1978;78:149
4. Green C, Martin CW, Bassett K, Kazanjian A. A systematic review of craniosacral therapy: biological plausibility, assessment reliability and clinical effectiveness. Complement Ther Med 1999;7:201–207
5. Hartman SE, Norton JM. Interexaminer reliability and cranial osteopathy. Sci Review Altern Med 2002;6:23–34.
6. Fernandez-de-Las-Penas C, Alonso-Blanco C, Cuadrado ML, Miangolarra JC, Barriga FJ, Pareja JA. Are manual therapies effective in reducing pain from tension-type headache?: a systematic review. Clin J Pain 2006;22:278–285
7. Geldschlager S. Osteopathic versus orthopedic treatments for chronic epicondylopathia humeri radialis: a randomized controlled trial. [In German.] Forsch Komplementärmed Klass Naturheilkd 2004;11:93–97
8. Greenman PE, McPartland JM. Cranial findings and iatrogenesis from craniosacral manipulation in patients with traumatic brain syndrome. J Am Osteopath Assoc 1995;95: 182–188

FELDENKRAIS

SYNONYMS
Functional integration, awareness through movement.

DEFINITION
A technique of mind and body integration based on the assumption that correction of poor habitual movements improves self-image and health as well as providing symptomatic relief from some forms of pain.

RELATED TECHNIQUES
Alexander technique, physiotherapy.

BACKGROUND
Moshe Feldenkrais (1904–1984), a physicist, suffered from knee pain and developed this technique to overcome it. It gradually became popular in many countries of the world.

TRADITIONAL CONCEPTS
The method is based on the belief that guided exploration of movement promotes attention and awareness and improves the ability to detect information and perceptual discrimination. Feldenkrais stated that 'behaviour is acquired and has nothing permanent about it but our belief that it is so'.

SCIENTIFIC RATIONALE
The notion that re-education of wrong habitual movements can have health effects makes sense. However, attributing singular importance to such approaches does not seem rational.

PRACTITIONERS
Feldenkrais practitioners are usually not medically trained. Many come from other health-care professions such as physiotherapy and practise the technique as one of several therapeutic approaches, e.g. in rehabilitation.

CONDITIONS FREQUENTLY TREATED
Musculoskeletal pain, multiple sclerosis, psychosomatic problems and many other chronic conditions. Feldenkrais is also used in non-medical settings, e.g. education, performing arts.

TYPICAL SESSION
Initially, 'awareness through movement' is taught, often in groups, where attention is paid to the motion of specific body parts during simple everyday activities. This is followed by individual sessions of 'functional integration' aimed at developing more efficient movements through close supervision and manipulation by the therapeutist teacher. A session lasts around 1 hour.

COURSE OF TREATMENT
A series of group or individual sessions is required to learn the techniques. Patients, clients or students are taught exercises for regular home practice. Subsequently patients are requested to practise them regularly. Supervised refresher courses are recommended.

SECTION THREE

CLINICAL EVIDENCE

A systematic review included six RCTs.[1] All suffered from significant methodological flaws and all but one trial reported positive findings, e.g. decrease of neck, shoulder or back pain and improved balance in multiple sclerosis patients. More recent studies suggest that Feldenkrais improves quality of life in patients with non-specific musculoskeletal problems[2] but is not a promising approach for the treatment of fibromyalgia.[3]

RISKS

CONTRAINDICATIONS

Acute musculoskeletal injuries.

PRECAUTIONS/WARNINGS

Severe cardiovascular disease.

ADVERSE EFFECTS

None known.

INTERACTIONS

None known.

RISK–BENEFIT ASSESSMENT

The Feldenkrais technique is an under-researched rehabilitative approach that shows some promise for a range of muscoloskeletal pain syndromes. Its risks are small. It may be worth trying for appropriate patients who are interested in this technique and who show sufficient dedication to comply with the programme.

REFERENCES

1. Ernst E, Canter PH. The Feldenkrais method – a systematic review of randomised clinical trials. Phys Med Rehab Kuror 2005;15:151–156
2. Malmgren-Olsson EB, Branholm IB. A comparison between three physiotherapy approaches with regard to health-related factors in patients with non-specific musculoskeletal disorders. Disabil Rehabil 2002;24:308–317
3. Kendall SA, Ekselius L, Gerdle B, Sörén B, Bengtsson A. Feldenkrais intervention in fibromyalgia patients: a pilot study. J Musculoskelet Pain 2001;9:25–35

HERBALISM

SYNONYMS/SUBCATEGORIES

Ayurveda, botanical medicine, herbalism, traditional Chinese herbalism, Western herbalism, kampo, phytomedicine, phytotherapy.

DEFINITION

The medical use of preparations that contain exclusively plant material.

BACKGROUND

Plants form the origin of much of modern medicine (e.g. digoxin from *Digitalis purpurea* or aspirin from *Salix* spp.). Modern herbalism or phytomedicine as practised in many Western countries is integrated into conventional medicine with compulsory education and training for physicians and pharmacists. Other more traditional systems include Chinese herbal medicine, which is based on the concepts of yin and yang and qi energy. In Japan this system of traditional herbal medicine has evolved into kampo. Ayurveda, the traditional medical system of India, also frequently uses herbal mixtures. Characteristic of these systems is a high degree of individualisation of treatment, e.g. two patients with the same disease according to Western conventional diagnosis could receive two different herbal preparations. Contrary to modern phytomedicine, all traditional herbal medicine systems predominantly employ complex mixtures of different herbs.

TRADITIONAL CONCEPTS

The different constituents of a single plant or of herbal mixtures are claimed to work synergistically to produce a greater effect than the sum of the effects of the single constituents. It is also claimed that the combined actions of the various constituents reduce the toxicity of the extract compared with the single isolated constituent. These concepts of synergy and buffering extend to the use of different plant extracts in combination preparations. The diagnostic principles in traditional herbal medicine differ considerably from those in mainstream medicine with less emphasis on conventional disease categories and modern diagnostic techniques. Phytomedicine or botanical medicine as practised in most European countries and the US follows the diagnostic and therapeutic principles of conventional medicine.

SCIENTIFIC RATIONALE

Pharmacologically active constituents are contained within the herbal extracts. The active principle(s) of the extract, which is in many cases unknown, may exert its effects at the molecular level and may have, for instance, enzyme-inhibiting effects (e.g. escin). A single main constituent may be active or, more often, a complex mixture of compounds produces a combined effect. Known active constituents or marker substances may be used to standardise preparations.

PRACTITIONERS

Most traditional herbalists in the UK and the US are not medically qualified. In contrast to many European countries, there is little integration into the conventional health-care systems. In Germany and France much of herbalism, particularly Western phytomedicine, is practised by conventionally trained physicians and integrated into routine medical care.

CONDITIONS FREQUENTLY TREATED

A wide range of conditions are treated, for instance pain, intermittent claudication, menstrual problems, skin conditions, anxiety, depression, digestive complaints, respiratory conditions and benign prostatic hyperplasia.

TYPICAL SESSION

During an initial treatment session the practitioner will usually take the patient's medical history. Some herbalists will also seek information on the patient's personality and background, which may influence the selection of herbs. Individualised combinations of herbs are prescribed and may be taken as extracts, tinctures, infusions or decoctions. Follow-up appointments are arranged as necessary and the herbal preparations and regimen are reviewed and changed if appropriate. Practitioners may advise on lifestyle factors such as diet and exercise. Consultations and treatment as practised mainly on the European continent generally follow the principles of a conventional medical appointment.

COURSE OF TREATMENT

Depending largely on the nature and severity of the condition but generally one or two appointments per week for a treatment period of one to several weeks.

CLINICAL EVIDENCE

The clinical evidence has to be evaluated according to each individual herbal preparation (see Section 4 *Medicines*) or traditional approach. There is clinical evidence from Cochrane reviews and other systematic reviews for the effectiveness of a number of herbal preparations for treating various pain syndromes (see Table 3.2).[1–16] Safety has been assessed in systematic reviews in relation to individual herbs,[7,8] organ systems[18,19] or mechanism of action.[20,21]

RISKS

CONTRAINDICATIONS

Contraindications and precautions vary for each individual herbal preparation (see Section 4 *Medicines*) but usually include pregnancy and lactation (see p. 4).

PRECAUTIONS/WARNINGS

Precautions vary for each individual herbal preparation (see Section 4 *Medicines*).

ADVERSE EFFECTS

Plant extracts may have powerful pharmacological effects and therefore there is the risk of serious adverse events. The reader is referred to the information on the individual herbs in Section 4 *Medicines*.

Table 3.2 **Results of systematic reviews of herbal medicine**

Plant name	Evidence for effectiveness	Inconclusive evidence	Evidence for ineffectiveness
Avocado/soybean	Osteoarthritis (knee, hip)[1]		
Black cohosh		Menopausal symptoms[2]	
Chaste tree		Pre-menstrual syndrome[3]	
Devil's claw	Osteoarthritis[4,5] Low back pain[5]		
Evening primrose		Menopausal symptoms[6]	
Feverfew		Migraine prevention[7]	
Ginkgo	Intermittent claudication[8]		
Ginseng		Any condition[9]	
Green tea		Stomach, intestinal cancer[10] Breast cancer[11]	
Horse chestnut	Chronic venous insufficiency[12]		
Kava kava	Menopausal symptoms[6]		
Mistletoe		Cancer[13,14]	
Peppermint	Abdominal pain[15] Irritable bowel syndrome[16]		

INTERACTIONS

Interactions between different herbal preparations or with conventional drugs should generally be assumed and relevant patients should be closely monitored. Patients should be asked about self-prescribed drug use.

QUALITY ISSUES

The amount of active constituent may vary and depends on a variety of different factors such as time of harvest, type of soil or extraction method. Products may be contaminated with other plant material or adulterated or plants may be misidentified. The Register of Chinese Herbal Medicine in the UK operates an 'approved suppliers scheme' whereby suppliers of herbs and herbal products are assessed by independent auditors.

RISK–BENEFIT ASSESSMENT

Some of the most convincing evidence that exists in the area of complementary medicine relates to a number of herbal extracts, suggesting effectiveness for various pain syndromes. The possibility of adverse effects has to be considered and the risk–benefit ratio has to be assessed for each herbal preparation individually. A number of conditions exist for which conventional medical treatment is not satisfactory and herbalism may provide a possible option.

REFERENCES

1. Ernst E. Avocado–soybean unsaponifiables (ASU) for osteoarthritis – a systematic review. Clin Rheumatol 2003;22:285–288
2. Borrelli F, Ernst E. *Cimicifuga racemosa*: a systematic review of its clinical efficacy. Eur J Clin Pharmacol 2002;58:235–241
3. Fugh-Berman A, Kronenberg F. Complementary and alternative medicine (CAM) in reproductive-age women: a review of randomized controlled trials. Reprod Toxicol 2003;17:137–152
4. Soeken KL. Selected CAM therapies for arthritis-related pain: the evidence from systematic reviews. Clin J Pain 2004;20:13–18
5. Gagnier JJ, Chrubasik S, Manheimer E. *Harpagophytum procumbens* for osteoarthritis and low back pain: a systematic review. BMC Complement Altern Med 2004;4:13
6. Huntley AL, Ernst E. A systematic review of herbal medicinal products for the treatment of menopausal symptoms. Menopause 2003;10:465–476
7. Pittler MH, Ernst E. Feverfew for preventing migraine. Cochrane Database Systematic Reviews 2004, Issue 1. Art. No.: CD002286
8. Pittler MH, Ernst E. Ginkgo biloba extract for the treatment of intermittent claudication: a meta-analysis of randomized trials. Am J Med 2000;108:276–281
9. Vogler BK, Pittler MH, Ernst E. The efficacy of ginseng. A systematic review of randomised clinical trials. Eur J Clin Pharmacol 1999;55:567–575
10. Borrelli F, Capasso R, Russo A, Ernst E. Systematic review: green tea and gastrointestinal cancer risk. Aliment Pharmacol Ther 2004;19:497–510
11. Seely D, Mills EJ, Wu P, Verma S, Guyatt GH. The effects of green tea consumption on incidence of breast cancer and recurrence of breast cancer: a systematic review and meta-analysis. Integr Cancer Ther 2005;4:144–155
12. Pittler MH, Ernst E. Horse chestnut seed extract for chronic venous insufficiency. The Cochrane Database of Systematic Reviews 2006, Issue 1. Art. No.: CD003230
13. Kienle GS, Berrino F, Bussing A, Portalupi E, Rosenzweig S, Kiene H. Mistletoe in cancer – a systematic review on controlled clinical trials. Eur J Med Res 2003;8:109–119
14. Ernst E, Schmidt K, Steuer-Vogt MK. Mistletoe for cancer? A systematic review of randomised clinical trials. Int J Cancer 2003;107:262–267
15. Weydert JA, Ball TM, Davis MF. Systematic review of treatments for recurrent abdominal pain. Pediatrics 2003;111:e1–11
16. Koretz RL, Rotblatt M. Complementary and alternative medicine in gastroenterology: the good, the bad, and the ugly. Clin Gastroenterol Hepatol 2004;2:957–967

17. Coon JT, Ernst E. Panax ginseng: a systematic review of adverse effects and drug interactions. Drug Saf 2002;25:323–344
18. Pittler MH, Ernst E. Systematic review: hepatotoxic events associated with herbal medicinal products. Aliment Pharmacol Ther 2003;18:451–471
19. Ernst E. Serious psychiatric and neurological adverse effects of herbal medicines – a systematic review. Acta Psychiatr Scand 2003;108:83–91
20. Izzo AA. Drug interactions with St John's wort (*Hypericum perforatum*): a review of the clinical evidence. Int J Clin Pharmacol Ther 2004;42:139–148
21. Zhou S, Chan E, Pan SQ, Huang M, Lee EJ. Pharmacokinetic interactions of drugs with St John's wort. J Psychopharmacol 2004;18:262–276

HOMEOPATHY

DEFINITION

A therapeutic method, often using highly diluted preparations of substances whose effects when administered to healthy subjects correspond to the manifestations of the disorder (symptoms, clinical signs and pathological states) in the unwell patient.

RELATED TECHNIQUES

Autoisopathy, biochemic medicine, homotoxicology, isopathy, tautopathy.

BACKGROUND

Homeopathy was developed by the German physician Samuel Hahnemann (1755–1843) and became popular first in Europe and later in other parts of the world. With the success of pharmacology in the early part of the 20th century, its popularity decreased. Today, it is again becoming widely available as a result of the general trend towards CAM. Many different 'schools' of homeopathy exist.

TRADITIONAL CONCEPTS

Homeopathy is built mainly on two key principles. The law of similars or 'like cures like' principle states that a remedy which causes a certain symptom (e.g. a headache) in healthy volunteers can be used to treat a headache in patients who suffer from it. According to the second principle, homeopathic remedies become more rather than less powerful when submitted to 'potentisation'. Potentisation describes the stepwise dilution of the remedy combined with 'sucussion', i.e. vigorous shaking of the mixture. Thus, homeopathic remedies are believed to be clinically effective even if they are so dilute that they are unlikely to contain a single molecule of the original substance.

SCIENTIFIC RATIONALE

Examples can be found where the 'like cures like' principle does apply (e.g. digitalis), but it is not a universal principle or a natural law. There is no scientific rationale for understanding how remedies devoid of pharmacologically active molecules produce clinical effects. Homeopathic 'provings', which form the basis for the therapeutic selection of remedies, often yield negative results or lack scientific rigour.

PRACTITIONERS

Homeopathy is practised by both medically qualified and non-medically qualified practitioners. The latter therapists are often called 'professional homeopaths'.

CONDITIONS FREQUENTLY TREATED

Homeopaths do not usually use conventional disease categories. Their aim is to match a patient's individual symptoms and constitution with a 'drug picture' (i.e. a set of symptoms caused by a remedy in healthy volunteers). Homeopaths often see patients with benign chronic conditions, e.g. ear, nose and throat disorders, headaches, musculoskeletal and digestive problems, respiratory and skin complaints, stress and anxiety.[1-3] Many of them are associated with pain.

TYPICAL SESSION

A first consultation might take 90 minutes or longer. Homeopaths take a thorough history, exploring the patient's problems in much detail, with a view to finding the optimally matching homeopathic drug ('similimum'). They normally put much less emphasis on physical examination than conventional physicians.

COURSE OF TREATMENT

Homeopaths believe that long-standing problems necessarily require prolonged treatment. Thus, they would typically insist on several consultations during which their prescriptions can be altered according to the changes in symptomatology.

CLINICAL EVIDENCE

A meta-analysis[4] of all homeopathic, placebo-controlled or randomised trials suggested that the risk ratio for clinical improvement with homeopathy was 2.45 times that with placebo. This publication has attracted much criticism and six re-analyses of these data failed to demonstrate efficacy.[5] Similarly, 11 independent systematic reviews of homeopathy did not generate convincing evidence of efficacy.[5] A recent meta-analytic comparison of 110 homeopathy trials and 110 matched conventional-medicine trials concluded that the clinical effects of homeopathy were placebo effects.[6] Systematic reviews on specific diseases include conditions such as post-operative ileus, delayed-onset muscle soreness, migraine prophylaxis and osteoarthritis.[3] Only in two areas were the conclusions somewhat positive: influenza[7] and rheumatic conditions.[8] Since the publication of these systematic reviews, the results of RCTs have been mixed. Encouraging findings were reported for fibromyalgia[9] and low back pain[10] while negative results emerged for rheumatoid arthritis[11] and ankylosing spondylitis.[12] Many of the primary studies of homeopathy have serious methodological limitations.[13]

RISKS

CONTRAINDICATIONS

Life-threatening conditions, pregnancy and lactation (see p. 4).

PRECAUTIONS/WARNINGS

Homeopathic remedies should not be exposed to bright light or other radiation or pungent smells. Some homeopaths advise their clients against immunisation of children.[14,15]

ADVERSE EFFECTS

In about one-quarter of cases, homeopaths expect to observe an aggravation of symptoms (which is believed to be a positive sign indicating that the correct remedy has been given).[16] In low dilutions, homeopathic remedies can have adverse effects such as allergic reactions.

INTERACTIONS

Some medicines (e.g. corticosteroids, antibiotics) are thought to block the actions of homeopathic drugs.

RISK–BENEFIT ASSESSMENT

The totality of the available trial evidence does not demonstrate the effectiveness of homeopathic remedies. Although there are few risks associated with homeopathy the risk–benefit balance is not positive.

REFERENCES

1. Steinsbekk A, Fønnebø V. Users of homeopaths in Norway in 1998, compared to previous users and GP patients. Homeopathy 2003;92:3–10
2. Trichard M, Lamure E, Chaufferin G. Study of the practice of homeopathic general practitioners in France. Homeopathy 2003;92:135–139
3. Becker-Witt C, Lüdtke R, Weisshuhn TE, Willich SN. Diagnoses and treatment in homeopathic medical practice. Forsch Komplementärmed Klass Naturheilkd 2004;11:98–103
4. Linde K, Clausius N, Ramirez G, Melchart D, Eitel F, Hedges LV, Jonas W. Are the clinical effects of homeopathy placebo effects? A meta-analysis of placebo-controlled trials. Lancet 1997;350:834–843
5. Ernst E. A systematic review of systematic reviews of homeopathy. Br J Clin Pharmacol 2002;54:577–582
6. Shang A, Huwiler-Muntener K, Nartey L, Juni P, Dorig S, Sterne JA, Pewsner D, Egger M. Are the clinical effects of homoeopathy placebo effects? Comparative study of placebo-controlled trials of homoeopathy and allopathy. Lancet 2005;366:726–732
7. Vickers AJ, Smith C. Homeopathic oscillococcinum for preventing and treating influenza and influenza-like syndromes. The Cochrane Database of Systematic Reviews 2004, Issue 1. Art. No.: CD001957
8. Jonas WB, Linde K, Ramirez G. Homeopathy and rheumatic disease. Rheum Dis Clin North Am 2000;26:117–123
9. Bell IR, Lewis DA, Brooks AJ, Schwartz GE, Lewis SE, Walsh BT, Baldwin CM. Improved clinical status in fibromyalgia patients treated with individualized homeopathic remedies versus placebo. Rheumatology (Oxford) 2004;43:577–582
10. Gmünder R, Kissling R. The efficacy of homeopathy in the treatment of chronic low back pain compared to standardized physiotherapy [In German.] Z Orthop Ihre Grenzgeb 2002;140:503–508
11. Fisher P, Scott DL. A randomized controlled trial of homeopathy in rheumatoid arthritis. Rheumatology (Oxford) 2001;40:1052–1055
12. Schirmer KP, Fritz M, Jäckel WH. Wirksamkeit von Formica rufa und Eigenblut-Injektionen bei Patienten mit ankylosierender Spondylitis: eine doppelblinde, randomisierte Studie. Z Rheumatol 2000;59:321–329
13. Jonas WB, Anderson RL, Crawford CC, Lyons JS. A systematic review of the quality of homeopathic clinical trials. BMC Complement Altern Med 2001;1:12
14. Schmidt K, Ernst E. MMR vaccination advice over the internet. Vaccine 2003;21: 1044–1047
15. Lehrke P, Nübling M, Hofmann F, Stössel U. Impfverhalten und Impfeinstellung bei Ärzten mit und ohne Zusatzbezeichnung Homöopathie. Monatsschr Kinderheilkd 2004;152:752–757
16. Thompson E, Barron S, Spence D. A preliminary audit investigating remedy reactions including adverse events in routine homeopathic practice. Homeopathy 2004;93:203–209

HYDROTHERAPY AND BALNEOTHERAPY

DEFINITION

Hydrotherapy is defined as the external application of water in any form or temperature (hot, cold, steam, liquid, ice). A wide variety of water-related therapies are used, such as foot baths, wraps and rising temperature baths. In contrast to hydrotherapy, balneotherapy is defined as the use of baths with thermal mineral waters of at least 20°C and a mineral content of at least 1 g/l water from natural springs.

RELATED TECHNIQUES

Kneipp therapy, spa therapy, thalassotherapy.

BACKGROUND

Hydrotherapy and balneotherapy are used particularly in European countries where they are, at least in part, reimbursed by the health-insurance systems. They have traditionally been considered as part of the conventional medical system (e.g. in Germany). In countries such as the UK or the US these treatments are also used but are regarded as complementary. The use of natural means to cure ill health gained interest during the 18th and 19th centuries when the Germans Vinzenz Prießnietz (1799–1851) and particularly Sebastian Kneipp (1821–1897) established complex hydrotherapeutic interventions as a cure for many ailments. A disciple of Kneipp, Benedict Lust (1870–1945), introduced hydrotherapy to the US. Spa therapy employs additional treatments such as physiotherapy and diet at a spa resort.

TRADITIONAL CONCEPTS

Water has been used medicinally for thousands of years with traditions rooted in ancient Rome, Greece and Japan. In Germany, the ideas developed by Prießnietz include concepts rooted in humoral pathology, which were later refined by Kneipp.

SCIENTIFIC RATIONALE

Hydrotherapy and balneotherapy work mainly through physical (temperature, viscosity, pressure, buoyancy) and chemical (mineral content) stimuli and affect the whole body via the skin. This leads to adaptation processes on the level of the vascular, muscular and metabolic systems and includes the vegetative nervous system.

PRACTITIONERS

In many European countries hydrotherapy and balneotherapy are part of the conventional medical system. Many of those who practise it are conventionally trained medical doctors (*Arzt für Naturheilkunde*); in some cases patients are referred to other health professionals (*Medizinischer Bademeister*) after initial diagnosis by the doctor. In other countries (e.g. UK, US), these treatments are not regulated.

CONDITIONS FREQUENTLY TREATED

Low back pain, fibromyalgia, osteoarthritis, chronic venous insufficiency.

TYPICAL SESSION

During an initial consultation the practitioner or physician will usually take a medical history of the patient to obtain an overall impression of the medical status and screen for any serious conditions. The treatment plan will vary according to the diagnosed condition but may also include changes in lifestyle. The treatment of a particular condition may vary between practitioners. Follow-up appointments are arranged as necessary and medicines and regimen are reviewed and changed as appropriate.

COURSE OF TREATMENT

Depends largely on the nature and severity of the condition, but generally one or two appointments per week for a treatment period ranging from one to several weeks.

CLINICAL EVIDENCE

A systematic review assessing balneotherapeutic interventions identified evidence for a number of conditions including low back pain.[1] A meta-analysis of RCTs ($n = 230$) on low back pain found beneficial effects compared with controls.[2] A further RCT ($n = 60$) reported alleviation of local tenderness, enhanced rotation of the spine and improvements of the Schober's index in patients who bathed in mineral thermal water that did not occur in those who bathed in tap water.[3] Functional benefits were also shown in patients with chronic low back pain or back and leg pain after hydrotherapy compared with waiting list controls.[4] A Cochrane review of balneotherapy for osteoarthritis concluded that 'One cannot ignore the positive findings reported in most trials. However, the scientific evidence is weak … '.[5] Further RCTs of hydro- and balneotherapeutic interventions reported improvements of pain and function in patients with hip and knee osteoarthritis compared with baseline[6–8] and compared with waiting list controls.[9] For rheumatoid arthritis a Cochrane review of balneotherapy concluded that 'although one cannot ignore the positive findings reported in most trials, the scientific evidence is insufficient'.[10] Single trials report improvements for patients with psoriatic arthritis[11] and juvenile idiopathic arthritis.[12] A systematic review of non-pharmacological interventions for fibromyalgia identified evidence from RCTs for hydrotherapy but found it unconvincing.[13] Two RCTs of balneotherapy for patients with fibromyalgia reported beneficial effects[14,15] whereas, in a further study, improvements were found for balneotherapy with and without pool-based exercise but there were no intergroup differences.[16] For chronic heart failure, RCTs tested hydrotherapy and reported improvements in exercise capacity and heart failure-related symptoms.[17,18] For patients with varicose veins, hydrotherapy may improve symptoms and quality of life.[19,20] A systematic review of hydrotherapy for labour reported that there is some support for relief of pain and anxiety.[21] Single RCTs that require independent replication exist for psoriasis vulgaris, pressure ulcers and the common cold.[22–24]

RISKS
CONTRAINDICATIONS

Acute heart failure, decompensated heart failure, acute skin conditions, severe varicose veins.

PRECAUTIONS/WARNINGS

Non-swimmers should be carefully monitored during balneotherapy.

ADVERSE EFFECTS

Applications with water that is too hot or too cold may cause burns or hypothermia. May cause exacerbation of chronic venous insufficiency.

INTERACTIONS

None known.

RISK–BENEFIT ASSESSMENT

There is some evidence to suggest that balneotherapy is effective for chronic low back pain. It can be recommended for this condition considering the usually mild nature and low frequency of adverse events. For osteoarthritis, rheumatoid arthritis, varicose veins, fibromyalgia and chronic heart failure there is some encouraging evidence but no firm conclusions can be made. For all other conditions further evidence is required.

REFERENCES

1. Nasermoaddeli A, Kagamimori S. Balneotherapy in medicine: a review. Environ Health Prev Med 2005;10:171–179
2. Pittler MH, Karagülle MZ, Karagülle, M, Ernst E. Balneotherapy and spa therapy for treating chronic low back pain: meta-analysis of randomised controlled trials. Rheumatology (Oxford) 2006;45:880–884

3. Balogh Z, Ordogh J, Gasz A, Nemet L, Bender T. Effectiveness of balneotherapy in chronic low back pain – a randomized single-blind controlled follow-up study. Forsch Komplementärmed Klass Naturheilkd 2005;12:196–201

4. McIlveen B, Robertson VJ. A randomized controlled study of the outcome of hydrotherapy for subjects with low back or back and leg pain. Physiotherapy 1998;84:17–26

5. Verhagen AP, de Vet HC, de Bie RA, Kessels AG, Boers M, Knipschild PG. Balneotherapy for rheumatoid arthritis and osteoarthritis. The Cochrane Database of Systematic Reviews 2000, Issue 2. Art. No.: CD000518

6. Stener-Victorin E, Kruse-Smidje C, Jung K. Comparison between electro-acupuncture and hydrotherapy, both in combination with patient education and patient education alone, on the symptomatic treatment of osteoarthritis of the hip. Clin J Pain 2004;20:179–185

7. Sukenik S, Flusser D, Codish S, Abu-Shakra M. Balneotherapy at the Dead Sea area for knee osteoarthritis. Isr Med Assoc J 1999;1:83–85

8. Kovacs I, Bender T. The therapeutic effects of Cserkeszolo thermal water in osteoarthritis of the knee: a double blind, controlled, follow-up study. Rheumatol Int 2002;21:218–221

9. Foley A, Halbert J, Hewitt T, Crotty M. Does hydrotherapy improve strength and physical function in patients with osteoarthritis – a randomised controlled trial comparing a gym based and a hydrotherapy based strengthening programme. Ann Rheum Dis 2003;62:1162–1167

10. Verhagen AP, Bierma-Zeinstra SM, Cardoso JR, de Bie RA, Boers M, de Vet HC. Balneotherapy for rheumatoid arthritis. The Cochrane Database of Systematic Reviews 2003, Issue 4. Art. No.: CD000518

11. Elkayam O, Ophir J, Brener S, Paran D, Wigler I, Efron D, Even-Paz Z, Politi Y, Yaron M. Immediate and delayed effects of treatment at the Dead Sea in patients with psoriatic arthritis. Rheumatol Int 2000;19:77–82

12. Epps H, Ginnelly L, Utley M, Southwood T, Gallivan S, Sculpher M, Woo P. Is hydrotherapy cost-effective? A randomised controlled trial of combined hydrotherapy programmes compared with physiotherapy land techniques in children with juvenile idiopathic arthritis. Health Technol Assess 2005;9:1–59

13. Sim J, Adams N. Systematic review of randomized controlled trials of nonpharmacological interventions for fibromyalgia. Clin J Pain 2002;18:324–336

14. Evcik D, Kizilay B, Gokcen E. The effects of balneotherapy on fibromyalgia patients. Rheumatol Int 2002;22:56–59

15. Buskila D, Abu-Shakra M, Neumann L, Odes L, Shneider E, Flusser D, Sukenik S. Balneotherapy for fibromyalgia at the Dead Sea. Rheumatol Int 2001;20:105–108

16. Altan L, Bingol U, Aykac M, Koc Z, Yurtkuran M. Investigation of the effects of pool-based exercise on fibromyalgia syndrome. Rheumatol Int 2004;24:272–277

17. Michalsen A, Ludtke R, Buhring M, Spahn G, Langhorst J, Dobos GJ. Thermal hydrotherapy improves quality of life and hemodynamic function in patients with chronic heart failure. Am Heart J 2003;146:E11

18. Cider A, Schaufelberger M, Sunnerhagen KS, Andersson B. Hydrotherapy – a new approach to improve function in the older patient with chronic heart failure. Eur J Heart Fail 2003;5:527–535

19. Ernst E, Saradeth T, Resch KL. A single blind randomized, controlled trial of hydrotherapy for varicose veins. Vasa 1991;20:147–152

20. Mancini S Jr, Piccinetti A, Nappi G, Mancini S, Caniato A, Coccheri S. Clinical, functional and quality of life changes after balneokinesis with sulphurous water in patients with varicose veins. Vasa 2003;32:26–30

21. Benfield RD. Hydrotherapy in labor. J Nurs Scholarsh 2002;34:347–352

22. Gruber C, Riesberg A, Mansmann U, Knipschild P, Wahn U, Buhring M. The effect of hydrotherapy on the incidence of common cold episodes in children: a randomised clinical trial. Eur J Pediatr 2003;162:168–176

23. Burke DT, Ho CH, Saucier MA, Stewart G. Effects of hydrotherapy on pressure ulcer healing. Am J Phys Med Rehabil 1998;77:394–398

24. Delfino M, Russo N, Migliaccio G, Carraturo N. Experimental study on efficacy of thermal muds of Ischia Island combined with balneotherapy in the treatment of psoriasis vulgaris with plaques. Clin Ter 2003;154:167–171

SECTION THREE

HYPNOTHERAPY

DEFINITION

The induction of a trance-like state to facilitate relaxation. It makes use of enhanced suggestibility to treat psychological and medical conditions and effect behavioural changes.

RELATED TECHNIQUES

Self-hypnosis, imagery, autogenic training, meditation, relaxation.

BACKGROUND

Hypnotic practices can be traced back a long time, but the first therapeutic use has been attributed to charismatic Austrian physician Franz Anton Mesmer in 1778, hence the word mesmerism. He devised a treatment based on magnetism that was hugely successful until a Royal Commission investigated the method and concluded that the effects were entirely the result of the imagination. Mesmerism saw a revival in the 1800s when British surgeon James Esdaile used it as the sole anaesthetic when performing major operations in India. Another British physician, James Braid, is credited with making hypnosis respectable to the medical community and in the 1950s the British and American Medical Associations recognised hypnosis as a legitimate medical procedure.

TRADITIONAL CONCEPTS

The goal of hypnotherapy is to gain self-control over behaviour, emotions or physiological processes. This is achieved by inducing the hypnotic trance where the patients' focus of attention is directed inwards, thereby allowing easier access to the non-critical unconscious mind, which is more receptive to suggestion. A good rapport between the therapist and patient or client is important, but a fundamental principle of hypnotic phenomena is that the hypnotised individual is under his own control and not that of the hypnotist or anyone else. It is argued consequently that all hypnosis is really self-hypnosis and the therapist should actually be called a facilitator.

SCIENTIFIC RATIONALE

Hypnosis is usually associated with a deep state of relaxation. Whether this represents a specific altered state of consciousness has been the subject of fierce scientific debate. It has repeatedly been shown that analgesia and many other hypnotic phenomena can be achieved by means of suggestion alone without hypnotising individuals. However, in defence of the genuineness and importance of the hypnotic trance it has been argued that highly suggestible (or hypnotisable) individuals are easily able to enter a hypnotic state without requiring formal induction. The means by which hypnotic suggestion enables involuntary processes such as skin temperature, heart rate and gut secretions to be deliberately controlled is not fully understood. It may be that hypnosis is essentially just a specific type of relaxation technique.

PRACTITIONERS

The credentials and duration of training of hypnotherapists vary widely. The number of hours of training may range from 300 to 1600. Most therapists are not medically qualified. Some doctors, dentists or psychologists are trained as clinical hypnotherapists and make use of hypnosis during their practice.

CONDITIONS FREQUENTLY TREATED

Pain, psychosomatic conditions, post-traumatic stress disorder, addictions, anxiety and phobia.

TYPICAL SESSION

Sessions typically last between 30 and 90 minutes. The initial visit involves the gathering of the patient's medical history and discussion of hypnosis, suggestion and the client's expectations of the therapy. Tests for hypnotic suggestibility may also be conducted. Hypnotic induction may or may not be part of the first session. The hypnotic state is achieved by first relaxing the body, then shifting attention away from the external environment towards a narrow range of objects or ideas suggested by the therapist. Sometimes hypnotherapy is carried out in group settings.

COURSE OF TREATMENT

Varies according to the individual, but an average course is 6–12 weekly sessions.

CLINICAL EVIDENCE

For pain management, a meta-analysis[1] reported moderate to large hypnoanalgesic effects, which were supported by another meta-analysis[2] of controlled trials assessing surgical patients. RCTs suggested that hypnosis reduced chronic pain[3] and pain in patients with osteoarthritis compared with waiting list controls.[4] For burn patients, pain and anxiety caused by physiotherapy decreased compared with the no-hypnotherapy control group.[5] In an RCT of 30 severely burned patients both hypnosis and a stress-reducing strategy reduced pain and increased patient satisfaction compared with baseline.[6] For paediatric oncology patients, a systematic review aimed to assess the effectiveness of hypnosis for procedure-related pain and distress.[7] Seven RCTs and one CCT were found and the review concluded that hypnosis has potential as a clinically valuable intervention. For recurrent paediatric headache, a systematic review reported an approach of self-hypnosis, imagery and relaxation as an empirically supported therapy.[8] A review of 15 controlled trials of hypnosis in children found promising but not compelling evidence for relief of pain, enuresis and chemotherapy-related distress.[9] For pain relief in labour and childbirth, a meta-analysis including three RCTs reported beneficial effects compared with no-intervention control groups,[10] which is supported to some extent by another RCT.[11] Systematic reviews and Cochrane reviews found no convincing evidence of effectiveness for post-traumatic conditions[12] and terminally ill adult cancer patients.[13] Beneficial effects are reported in RCTs of hypnosis for treating irritable bowel syndrome.[14–17] An RCT failed to show that hypnotherapy accelerates the healing of bone tissue.[18]

RISKS
CONTRAINDICATIONS

Psychosis, personality disorders.

PRECAUTIONS/WARNINGS

Confabulation, epilepsy, very young children.

ADVERSE EFFECTS

Recovering repressed memories can be painful and psychological problems may be exacerbated. False memory syndrome has been reported. Studies investigating negative consequences of hypnosis have concluded that, when practised by a clinically trained professional, it is safe.

RISK–BENEFIT ASSESSMENT

There is evidence to suggest that hypnotherapy has analgesic effects. Encouraging data are also available for patients with irritable bowel syndrome. Some risks exist, but on balance it appears to be a valuable tool for pain management and conditions with a psychosomatic component, when performed by a qualified and responsible practitioner.

REFERENCES

1. Montgomery GH, DuHamel KN, Redd WH. A meta-analysis of hypnotically induced analgesia: how effective is hypnosis? Int J Clin Exp Hypn 2000;48:138–153
2. Montgomery GH, David D, Winkel G, Silverstein JH, Bovbjerg DH. The effectiveness of adjunctive hypnosis with surgical patients: a meta-analysis. Anesth Analg 2002;94: 1639–1645
3. Ray P, Page AC. A single session of hypnosis and eye movements desensitisation and reprocessing (EMDR) in the treatment of chronic pain. Aust J Clin Exp Hypn 2002;30: 170–178
4. Gay MC, Philippot P, Luminet O. Differential effectiveness of psychological interventions for reducing osteoarthritis pain: a comparison of Erikson [correction of Erickson] hypnosis and Jacobson relaxation. Eur J Pain 2002;6:1–16
5. Amini Harandi A, Esfandani A, Shakibaei F. The effect of hypnotherapy on procedural pain and state anxiety related to physiotherapy in women hospitalized in a burn unit. Contemp Hypn 2004;21:28–34
6. Frenay MC, Faymonville ME, Devlieger S, Albert A, Vanderkelen A. Psychological approaches during dressing changes of burned patients: a prospective randomised study comparing hypnosis against stress reducing strategy. Burns 2001;27:793–799
7. Richardson J, Smith JE, McCall G, Pilkington K. Hypnosis for procedure-related pain and distress in pediatric cancer patients: a systematic review of effectiveness and methodology related to hypnosis interventions. J Pain Symptom Manage 2006; 31:70–84
8. Tsao JC, Zeltzer LK. Complementary and alternative medicine approaches for pediatric pain: a review of the state-of-the-science. Evid Based Complement Altern Med 2005;2:149–159
9. Milling LS, Costantino CA. Clinical hypnosis with children: first steps toward empirical support. Int J Clin Exp Hypn 2000;48:113–137
10. Cyna AM, McAuliffe GL, Andrew MI. Hypnosis for pain relief in labour and childbirth: a systematic review. Br J Anaesth 2004;93:505–511
11. Mehl-Madrona LE. Hypnosis to facilitate uncomplicated birth. Am J Clin Hypn 2004;46:299–312
12. Cardeña E. Hypnosis in the treatment of trauma: a promising, but not fully supported, efficacious intervention. Int J Clin Exp Hypn 2000;48:125–138
13. Rajasekaran M, Edmonds PM, Higginson IL. Systematic review of hypnotherapy for treating symptoms in terminally ill adult cancer patients. Palliat Med 2005;19:418–426
14. Forbes A, MacAuley S, Chiotakakou-Faliakou E. Hypnotherapy and therapeutic audiotape: effective in previously unsuccessfully treated irritable bowel syndrome? Int J Colorectal Dis 2000;15:328–334
15. Simren M, Ringstrom G, Bjornsson ES, Abrahamsson H. Treatment with hypnotherapy reduces the sensory and motor component of the gastrocolonic response in irritable bowel syndrome. Psychosom Med 2004;66:233–238
16. Barabasz A, Barabasz M. Effects of tailored and manualized hypnotic inductions for complicated irritable bowel syndrome patients. Int J Clin Exp Hypn 2006;54:100–112
17. Roberts L, Wilson S, Singh S, Roalfe A, Greenfield S. Gut-directed hypnotherapy for irritable bowel syndrome: piloting a primary care-based randomised controlled trial. Br J Gen Pract 2006;56:115–121
18. Ginandes CS, Rosenthal DI. Using hypnosis to accelerate the healing of bone fractures: a randomized controlled pilot study. Altern Ther Health Med 1999;5:67–75

IMAGERY

SYNONYMS

Visualisation.

DEFINITION

A mind–body technique that involves using the imagination and mental images to encourage physical healing, promote relaxation and bring about a change in attitude or behaviour.

RELATED TECHNIQUES

Meditation, hypnosis.

BACKGROUND

Mind–body interventions constitute a major portion of the overall use of CAM by the public. In 2002, relaxation techniques, imagery, biofeedback and hypnosis combined were used by more than 30% of the adult US population.[1] Some techniques employed are based on psychological theory.

TRADITIONAL CONCEPTS

Imagery is a visualisation technique that is based on the idea that the mind can affect the functions of the body.

SCIENTIFIC RATIONALE

Stimulating the brain through visualisation has been suggested to have direct effects on the endocrine and nervous systems. This may lead to changes in immune function and other bodily functions.

PRACTITIONERS

Some psychologists practise imagery, as do many other professional groups such as nurses and social workers. There are no central licensing or certification procedures in place.

CONDITIONS FREQUENTLY TREATED

Chronic pain, headaches, patients undergoing conventional cancer therapy or surgery, stress and anxiety.

TYPICAL SESSION

Imagery is usually taught in small classes. Patients will be asked to wear comfortable clothing, and will either sit on a chair or lie on a treatment table or a floor mat. Sessions usually begin with general relaxation exercises and then move on to more specific visualisation techniques, introduced by the practitioner. Patients will be led to build a detailed image in their mind. If they have a specific medical condition, the practitioner may ask them to picture their body free of the problem. Patients may be encouraged to picture their pain, for instance, as tumours shrinking in a local area or their body freeing itself of cancer. Athletes or performers may picture themselves moving well and competing or performing perfectly.

COURSE OF TREATMENT

Sessions are usually 20–30 minutes, or longer if needed, once or twice weekly for several weeks.

CLINICAL EVIDENCE

A systematic review evaluating the evidence for imagery as a sole treatment for cancer patients concluded that it may be psycho-supportive and increase comfort.[2] Another systematic review reported that, in patients near the end of life, relaxation/imagery can improve pain from oral mucositis.[3] It has been suggested that the meaning of pain as a theme in patients' lives changes with the use of imagery.[4] Post-operatively, less pain and lower analgesic requirements compared with standard care are reported in patients after elective colorectal surgery[5] and gynaecological laparoscopic surgery,[6] whereas no differences are reported in proctological patients[7] or in cancer patients undergoing colorectal resection compared with progressive muscle relaxation.[8] In burn patients during debridement, there was a reduction in the self-reporting of pain in those who received music-based imagery compared to patients who did not.[9] In children, beneficial effects on post-operative pain and analgesic consumption are reported[10,11] as well as less distress during cardiac catheterisation.[12] Patients in rehabilitation for anterior cruciate ligament reconstruction reported less pain in those who received imagery compared with attention control.[13] Fibromyalgia patients ($n = 58$) who received imagery experienced a reduction in current pain and anxiety compared with a patient education programme.[14] These findings were confirmed when standard treatment was compared to imagery in patients with fibromyalgia.[15,16] Single trials reporting positive results are also available for chronic low back pain,[17] osteoarthritis[18] and sympathetic dystrophy.[19]

RISKS
CONTRAINDICATIONS
Severe mental illness. Latent psychosis and personality disorders, as these may become overt with introspection.

PRECAUTIONS/WARNINGS
Should only be used as an adjunct to standard therapy.

ADVERSE EFFECTS
None.

INTERACTIONS
None.

RISK–BENEFIT ASSESSMENT
Imagery may be helpful for patients with pain of different origins. Only a few studies have been conducted on a number of pain syndromes, but considering the few risks involved, imagery is worth trying.

REFERENCES
1. Wolsko PM, Eisenberg DM, Davis RB, Phillips RS. Use of mind-body medical therapies. J Gen Intern Med 2004;19:43–50
2. Roffe L, Schmidt K, Ernst E. A systematic review of guided imagery as an adjuvant cancer therapy. Psychooncology 2005;14:607–617
3. Pan CX, Morrison RS, Ness J, Fugh-Berman A, Leipzig RM. Complementary and alternative medicine in the management of pain, dyspnea, and nausea and vomiting near the end of life. A systematic review. J Pain Symptom Manage 2000;20:374–387
4. Lewandowski W, Good M, Draucker CB. Changes in the meaning of pain with the use of guided imagery. Pain Manag Nurs 2005;6:58–67
5. Tusek DL, Church JM, Strong SA, Grass JA, Fazio VW. Guided imagery: a significant advance in the care of patients undergoing elective colorectal surgery. Dis Colon Rectum 1997;40:172–178
6. Laurion S, Fetzer SJ. The effect of two nursing interventions on the postoperative outcomes of gynaecologic laparoscopic patients. J Perianesth Nurs 2003;18:254–261
7. Renzi C, Peticca L, Pescatori M. The use of relaxation techniques in the perioperative management of proctological patients: preliminary results. Int J Colorectal Dis 2000;15: 313–316
8. Haase O, Schwenk W, Hermann C, Muller JM. Guided imagery and relaxation in conventional colorectal resections: a randomized, controlled, partially blinded trial. Dis Colon Rectum 2005;48:1955–1963
9. Fratianne RB, Prensner JD, Huston MJ, Super DM, Yowler CJ, Standley JM. The effect of music-based imagery and musical alternate engagement on the burn debridement process. J Burn Care Rehabil 2001;22:47–53
10. Huth MM, Broome ME, Good M. Imagery reduces children's post-operative pain. Pain 2004;110:439–448

11. Lambert SA. The effects of hypnosis/guided imagery on the postoperative course of children. J Dev Behav Pediatr 1996;17:307–310

12. Pederson C. Effect of imagery on children's pain and anxiety during cardiac catheterization. J Pediatr Nurs 1995;10:365–374

13. Cupal DD, Brewer BW. Effects of relaxation and guided imagery on knee strength, reinjury anxiety, and pain following anterior cruciate ligament reconstruction. Rehabil Psychol 2001;46:28–43

14. Fors EA, Götestam KG. Patient education, guided imagery and pain related talk in fibromyalgia coping. Eur J Psychiatry 2000;14:233–240

15. Fors EA, Sexton H, Gotestam KG. The effect of guided imagery and amitriptyline on daily fibromyalgia pain: a prospective, randomized, controlled trial. J Psychiatr Res 2002;36:179–187

16. Menzies V, Taylor AG, Bourguignon C. Effects of guided imagery on outcomes of pain, functional status, and self-efficacy in persons diagnosed with fibromyalgia. J Altern Complement Med 2006;12:23–30.

17. Basler HD, Jakle C, Kroner-Herwig B. Incorporation of cognitive-behavioral treatment into the medical care of chronic low back patients: a controlled randomized study in German pain treatment centers. Patient Educ Couns 1997;31:113–124

18. Baird CL, Sands L. A pilot study of the effectiveness of guided imagery with progressive muscle relaxation to reduce chronic pain and mobility difficulties of osteoarthritis. Pain Manag Nurs 2004;5:97–104

19. Moseley GL. Graded motor imagery is effective for long-standing complex regional pain syndrome: a randomised controlled trial. Pain 2004;108:192–198

KINESIOLOGY

SYNONYMS

Applied kinesiology; the term 'kinesiology' is sometimes also used for physiotherapeutic exercise therapy, which is entirely different from applied kinesiology and considered a conventional approach.

DEFINITION

A method using muscle-strength monitoring to diagnose and treat illness.

RELATED TECHNIQUES

Other methods for testing muscular function.

BACKGROUND

This is a relatively recent method used for diagnosing and treating human illness. It was developed by the American chiropractor George Goodheart in the 1960s.

TRADITIONAL CONCEPTS

Practitioners of kinesiology believe that health problems are associated with weakness of certain muscle groups. By determining the muscular strength with simple manual tests, they diagnose predisposition to certain medical conditions or the adequacy of certain oral medications.

SCIENTIFIC RATIONALE

This method is not based on a scientific rationale.

PRACTITIONERS

Practitioners of kinesiology often practise another form of CAM in parallel, e.g. chiropractic. In most countries there is no regulation of kinesiology.

CONDITIONS FREQUENTLY TREATED

Most human conditions or predispositions to ill health, particularly allergies and intolerances.

TYPICAL SESSION

A kinesiologist would normally take a medical history. This is typically followed by muscle testing and often by various types of CAM treatment, e.g. chiropractic.

COURSE OF TREATMENT

A course of 6–10 treatments would be characteristic in the first instance. Practitioners often advise repeat courses as well.

CLINICAL EVIDENCE

A review evaluated 20 research projects on kinesiology, and the authors found them to be of such a low methodological standard that no firm conclusions about the validity of the technique could be drawn.[1] More recently, several controlled studies have become available.[2–7] They relate to a range of conditions, mostly allergies and intolerances. The results fail to demonstrate that kinesiology is a valid diagnostic technique. There are no trials of kinesiology as a therapy.

RISKS

CONTRAINDICATIONS

None.

PRECAUTIONS/WARNINGS

None.

ADVERSE EFFECTS

False-positive or false-negative test results.

INTERACTIONS

None.

RISK–BENEFIT ASSESSMENT

There is no good evidence that kinesiology is a valid diagnostic or therapeutic technique. Its risks are only minor. A risk–benefit analysis fails to arrive at positive conclusions.

REFERENCES

1. Klinkoski B, Leboeuf C. A review of the research papers published by the international College of Applied Kinesiology from 1981 to 1987. J Manipulative Physiol Ther 1990;13:190–194
2. Friedman MH, Weisberg J. Applied kinesiology – double-blind pilot study. J Prosthet Dent 1981;45:321–323
3. Garrow JS. Kinesiology and food allergy. Br Med J (Clin Res Ed) 1988;296:1573–1574
4. Haas M, Peterson D, Hoyer D, Ross G. Muscle testing response to provocative vertebral challenge and spinal manipulation: a randomized controlled trial of construct validity. J Manipulative Physiol Ther 1994;17:141–148
5. Lüdtke R, Kunz B, Seeber N, Ring J. Test–retest reliability and validity of the Kinesiology muscle test. Complement Ther Med 2001;9:141–145
6. Pothmann R, von Frankenberg S, Hoicke C, Weingarten H, Ludtke R. Evaluation of applied kinesiology in nutritional intolerance of childhood. [In German.] Forsch Komplementärmed Klass Naturheilkd 2001;8:336–344
7. Staehle HJ, Koch MJ, Pioch T. Double-blind study on materials testing with applied kinesiology. J Dent Res 2005;84:1066–1069

MASSAGE

DEFINITION

A method of manipulating the soft tissue of body areas using pressure and traction (with primary focus on 'Swedish massage').

RELATED TECHNIQUES

Aromatherapy, reflexology, shiatsu.

BACKGROUND

Massage is one of the oldest forms of treatment. The development of modern massage is attributed to the Swede Per Henrik Ling, who developed an integrated system consisting of massage and exercises, which was later termed 'Swedish massage'. In the middle of the 19th century it was introduced in the US and was practised predominantly by physicians until the early 20th century. The interest in massage therapy gradually declined but increased again in the 1970s. Today massage is considered a complementary therapy in many countries and gentler techniques than the vigorous treatment recommended by Ling are often used. In some European countries (e.g. Germany), however, massage continues to be part of the conventional medical system.

TRADITIONAL CONCEPTS

Various manual techniques are used in massage to apply pressure and traction to manipulate the soft tissues of the body. Massage therapy also allows the therapist to locate areas of muscle tension, which can then be treated using touch with the optimal amount of pressure.

SCIENTIFIC RATIONALE

Mechanical pressure and friction of the hands, which are exerted on cutaneous and subcutaneous structures, affect the body. The circulation of blood and lymph is generally enhanced, resulting in increased arterial and venous perfusion. Direct mechanical pressure and effects mediated by the nervous system beneficially affect areas of increased muscular tension.

PRACTITIONERS

In the US, massage is often practised by nurses and a variety of training courses are available. The number of hours of training required varies greatly and examinations by the International Therapy Examinations Council are the most widely accepted. In other countries such as Germany, massage is fully registered and a recognised profession.

CONDITIONS FREQUENTLY TREATED

Back pain, musculoskeletal conditions, constipation, depression, anxiety, stress and many other conditions.

TYPICAL SESSION

During an initial treatment session the therapist will usually take the patient's medical history to obtain an overall impression of the medical status and screen for contraindications. The duration of individual treatment sessions varies depending on the condition, but will typically be about 30 minutes. Patients are normally treated unclothed with a sheet or towel provided. Usually, the massage is performed on a specially designed massage couch. Therapists often use oil to facilitate movement of the hands over the patient's body. The five fundamental techniques used in massage are effleurage, pétrissage, friction, tapotement and vibration. Sometimes sessions are followed by other treatments such as hot packs, which essentially apply external heat. Most patients are advised to rest for about 20 minutes after a treatment session.

COURSE OF TREATMENT

Usually, one or two sessions per week for a treatment period of 4–8 weeks would be recommended initially.

CLINICAL EVIDENCE

For treating low back pain, a systematic review[1] conducted within the framework of the Cochrane Collaboration Back Review Group extended the findings of an earlier review[2] and concluded cautiously that massage might be beneficial for patients with subacute and chronic non-specific low back pain, especially when combined with exercises and education. This is supported by trials on back and neck pain.[3-6] Cochrane reviews of treating upper extremity work-related disorders[7] and tendinitis with deep transverse friction massage[8] found insufficient evidence for any firm conclusions. A systematic review[9] of massage for treating cervicogenic headache concluded that massage appears to be less effective than spinal manipulative therapy. Another systematic review found no clear evidence regarding the role of physical treatments such as chiropractic, osteopathy or massage in the management of patients with headache,[10] which is supported by another independent systematic review.[11] In stroke patients, an RCT reported reduced levels of pain and anxiety.[12] It has also been concluded in a systematic review that vibratory massage might be of benefit for musculoskeletal pain.[13] Massage did not affect the level or duration of pain or the loss of strength or function following exercise.[14] A further small RCT ($n = 22$), however, found that massage is effective compared with rest for decreasing delayed-onset muscle soreness.[15] In patients with fibromyalgia, massage alone and as part of a multidisciplinary programme has been suggested to relieve pain and depression and to improve quality of life.[16,17] In cancer patients, a systematic review judged the evidence for pain control as promising.[18] A systematic review included two RCTs on labour pain;[19] both trials found that massage provided pain relief and psychological support during labour. A number of RCTs have been conducted in perioperative pain.[20-24] Most of them suggest that massage is more effective for pain relief than no such treatment. For complex regional pain syndrome, a small RCT ($n = 35$) suggested better pain control with lymph drainage plus exercise compared with exercise alone.[25] Two RCTs for shoulder pain suggest that massage is more effective than no such treatment.[26,27] The safety of massage was systematically reviewed and it was found that the serious adverse events on record were associated mostly with massage techniques other than 'Swedish' massage.[28] The study concluded that, although massage is not entirely risk-free, serious adverse events are probably true rarities.

RISKS

CONTRAINDICATIONS

Phlebitis, deep vein thrombosis, burns, skin infections, eczema, open wounds, bone fractures and advanced osteoporosis.

PRECAUTIONS/WARNINGS

Cancer, myocardial infarction, osteoporosis and pregnancy. Massage should generally be considered as an adjunctive treatment, not as an alternative to conventional care.

ADVERSE EFFECTS

Adverse effects are extremely rare. Serious adverse events such as bone fractures and liver rupture have been reported.

INTERACTIONS

Interactions and adverse effects attributable to the oils that may be used are not considered in the assessment of risks involved in massage. The medical history should, however, include questions relating to any allergic predisposition.

RISK–BENEFIT ASSESSMENT

Massage appears to have beneficial effects in low back pain, musculoskeletal pain and peri-operative pain. Given the few risks involved when performed by a responsible, well-trained practitioner, it may be worth considering. Its comparative effectiveness against other complementary therapies or against conventional treatment approaches is unclear. Given its relaxing effects, massage may have some beneficial influence on the well-being of most pain patients.

REFERENCES

1. Furlan AD, Brosseau L, Imamura M, Irvin E. Massage for low-back pain: a systematic review within the framework of the Cochrane Collaboration Back Review Group. Spine 2002;27: 1896–1910
2. Ernst E. Massage therapy for low back pain: a systematic review. J Pain Symptom Manage 1999;17:65–69
3. Wang B, Wu JX, Wang J. Active exercise and massage for nonspecific low back pain: a clinical randomized controlled trial. Chin J Clin Rehab 2005;9:1–3
4. Chatchawan U, Thinkhamrop B, Kharmwan S, Knowles J, Eungpinichpong W. Effectiveness of traditional Thai massage versus Swedish massage among patients with back pain associated with myofascial trigger points. J Bodywork Mov Ther 2005;9: 298–309
5. Plews-Ogan M, Owens JE, Goodman M, Wolfe P, Schorling J. A pilot study evaluating mindfulness-based stress reduction and massage for the management of chronic pain. J Gen Intern Med 2005;20:1136–1138
6. Fernandez de Las Penas C, Alonso Blanco C, Fernandez Carnero J, Carlos Miangolarra Page J. The immediate effect of ischemic compression technique and transverse friction massage on tenderness of active and latent myofascial trigger points: a pilot study. J Bodywork Mov Ther 2006;10:3–9
7. Verhagen AP, Bierma-Zeinstra SMA, Feleus A, Karels C, Dahaghin S, Burdorf L, de Vet HCW, Koes BW. Ergonomic and physiotherapeutic interventions for treating upper extremity work related disorders in adults. The Cochrane Database of Systematic Reviews 2003, Issue 3. Art. No.: CD003471
8. Brosseau L, Casimiro L, Milne S, Robinson V, Shea B, Tugwell P, Wells G. Deep transverse friction massage for treating tendinitis. The Cochrane Database of Systematic Reviews 2002, Issue 4. Art. No.: CD003528
9. Bronfort G, Assendelft WJ, Evans R, Haas M, Bouter L. Efficacy of spinal manipulation for chronic headache: a systematic review. J Manipulative Physiol Ther 2001;24: 457–466
10. Biondi DM. Physical treatments for headache: a structured review. Headache 2005;45:738–746
11. Fernandez de Las Penas C, Alonso Blanco C, Cuadrado ML, Miangolarra JC, Barriga FJ, Pareja JA. Are manual therapies effective in reducing pain from tension-type headache?: a systematic review. Clin J Pain 2006;22:278–285
12. Mok E, Woo CP. The effects of slow-stroke back massage on anxiety and shoulder pain in elderly stroke patients. Complement Ther Nurs Midwifery 2004;10:209–216
13. Gottschild S, Kröling P. Vibrationsmassage. Eine Literaturübersicht zu physiologischen Wirkungen und therapeutischer Wirksamkeit. Phys Med Rehab Kuror 2003;13:85–95
14. Jonhagen S, Ackermann P, Eriksson T, Saartok T, Renstrom PA. Sports massage after eccentric exercise. Am J Sports Med 2004;32:1499–1503
15. Mancinelli CA, Davis DS, Aboulhosn L, Brady M, Eisenhofer J, Foutty S. The effects of massage on delayed onset muscle soreness and physical performance in female athletes. Phys Ther Sport 2006;7:5–13
16. Brattberg G. Connective tissue massage in the treatment of fibromyalgia. Eur J Pain 1999;3: 235–245

17. Lemstra M, Olszynski WP. The effectiveness of multidisciplinary rehabilitation in the treatment of fibromyalgia: a randomized controlled trial. Clin J Pain 2005;21:166–174
18. Corbin L. Safety and efficacy of massage therapy for patients with cancer. Cancer Control 2005;12:158–164
19. Huntley AL, Coon JT, Ernst E. Complementary and alternative medicine for labor pain: a systematic review. Am J Obstet Gynecol 2004;191:36–44
20. Hulme J, Waterman H, Hillier VF. The effect of foot massage on patients' perception of care following laparoscopic sterilisation as day case patients. J Adv Nurs 1999;30: 460–468
21. Le Blanc-Louvry I, Costaglioli B, Boulon C, Leroi AM, Ducrotte P. Does mechanical massage of the abdominal wall after colectomy reduce postoperative pain and shorten the duration of ileus? Results of a randomized study. J Gastrointest Surg 2002;6:43–49
22. Taylor AG, Galper DI, Taylor P, Rice LW, Andersen W, Irvin W, Wang XQ, Harrell FE Jr. Effects of adjunctive Swedish massage and vibration therapy on short-term postoperative outcomes: a randomized, controlled trial. J Altern Complement Med 2003;9:77–89
23. Piotrowski MM, Paterson C, Mitchinson A, Kim HM, Kirsh M, Hinshaw DB. Massage as adjuvant therapy in the management of acute postoperative pain: a preliminary study in men. J Am Coll Surg 2003;197:1037–1046
24. Forchuk C, Baruth P, Prendergast M, Holliday R, Bareham R, Brimner S, Schulz V, Chan YC, Yammine N. Postoperative arm massage: a support for women with lymph node dissection. Cancer Nurs 2004;27:25–33
25. Uher EM, Vacariu G, Schneider B, Fialka V. Comparison of manual lymph drainage with physical therapy in complex regional pain syndrome, type I. A comparative randomized controlled therapy study. [In German.] Wien Klin Wochenschr 2000;112:133–137
26. Mok E, Woo CP. The effects of slow-stroke back massage on anxiety and shoulder pain in elderly stroke patients. Complement Ther Nurs Midwifery 2004;10:209–216
27. van den Dolder PA, Roberts DL. A trial into the effectiveness of soft tissue massage in the treatment of shoulder pain. Aust J Physiother 2003;49:183–188
28. Ernst E. The safety of massage therapy. Rheumatology (Oxford) 2003;42:1101–1106

MEDITATION

Peter H Canter

SYNONYMS

Transcendental meditation (TM), Sahaja yoga/meditation, mindfulness meditation (MM).

DEFINITION

Meditation is a very diverse range of techniques based on listening to the breath, repeating a mantra and detaching from the thought process or other self-directed mental practices; this focuses attention and brings about a state of self-awareness and inner calm.

RELATED TECHNIQUES

Bensons' relaxation response, qigong.

BACKGROUND

Most forms of meditation originated within the major religions, particularly those of the East where the aim is to bring about altered consciousness or 'enlightenment'. Meditation became popular in the West during the 1960s and 1970s when it became associated with the hippie and pop culture of the time. In addition to its spiritual goals, meditation has been increasingly promoted as a means to achieve relaxation, deal with stress and promote general health and well-being. Meditation continues to be taught in religious, cultic and non-cultic contexts. The last includes forms developed for research or therapeutic purposes.

SCIENTIFIC RATIONALE

Numerous studies appear to demonstrate changes in physiological parameters such as oxygen consumption, respiration rate, heart rate and brain activity[1] during meditation, which could be considered characteristic of a state of deep relaxation. This is not the same thing as proving that regular practice of meditation has prophylactic or therapeutic effects. It is feasible that physiological changes that occur during the state of relaxation could have positive health effects, but specific mechanisms remain unknown.

PRACTITIONERS

Meditation is taught mainly by religious or quasi-religious groups. TM, one of the more popular forms, is promoted by a worldwide organisation and instruction is paid for. In contrast, MM was developed within a health-care context and has been researched and used with a variety of patient groups.

CONDITIONS FREQUENTLY TREATED

Anxiety, asthma, stress, drug and alcohol addiction, epilepsy, heart disease and hypertension.

TYPICAL SESSION

After initial instruction carried out over several sessions either in a group or individually with a teacher, the meditator is expected to practise regularly on a daily basis. In the case of TM, new meditators attend an introductory lecture, several group training sessions, an individual initiation ceremony with a teacher and then periodic follow-up sessions to check for correct practice. Expected daily practice is two 15- to 20-minute sessions.

COURSE OF TREATMENT

The prophylactic and therapeutic effects of meditation are expected to accrue from continuing daily practice.

CLINICAL EVIDENCE

Research on meditation has been beset by methodological problems, including highly selected study populations, uncontrolled or inappropriately controlled designs, high drop-out rates and designs using mixed interventions, which prevent the isolation of specific effects. Additionally, many studies have been carried out by researchers affiliated to the organisations promoting the particular technique in question. This is particularly so in the case of TM, the subject of over 800 research papers and reviews, many of which have not been peer-reviewed.[2,3] A recent review of the therapeutic effects of meditation techniques in general concluded that there is, at present, only weak evidence for the therapeutic effectiveness of any type of meditation and even less evidence for any specific effect above that of credible control interventions.[4]

There are two clinical trials of meditation specifically for pain and both of these relate to chronic low back pain. The first, a pilot trial, reports improvements in pain and psychological distress in the meditation group but not in a standard care control group.[5] However, a formal intergroup statistical comparison is not reported. The second compared a mixed modality intervention incorporating breath therapy, meditation, body awareness and movement with physical therapy.[6] There were no significant differences in pain or quality of life immediately after 6–8 weeks of treatment or at a 6-month follow-up.

RISKS

CONTRAINDICATIONS

There is a theoretical risk that meditation could create conditions in the brain conducive to epilepsy.[7]

PRECAUTIONS/WARNINGS

People with pre-existing mental health problems should only take up meditation under the supervision of a qualified psychiatrist or psychotherapist experienced in the use of such techniques in a therapeutic context. People diagnosed with epilepsy or at risk of developing epilepsy should consider the theoretical risk of precipitating attacks before proceeding.

ADVERSE EFFECTS

The safety of meditation has not been studied systematically. There are a few isolated reports of adverse events including exacerbation of pre-existing depression and anxiety, depersonalisation, an attempted suicide and precipitation of schizophrenic episodes.[8,9]

INTERACTIONS

None known.

RISK–BENEFIT ASSESSMENT

Meditation appears to be safe for most people and those with sufficient motivation to practise regularly will probably find it a pleasant and relaxing experience. Evidence for effectiveness in any indication is weak.

REFERENCES

1. Wallace R, Benson H. The physiology of meditation. Sci Am 1972;226:84–90
2. Canter PH, Ernst E. The cumulative effects of Transcendental Meditation on cognitive function – a systematic review of randomised controlled trials. Wien Klin Wochenschr 2003;115:758–766
3. Canter PH, Ernst E. Insufficient evidence to conclude whether or not Transcendental Meditation lowers blood pressure: results of a systematic review of randomised clinical trials. J Hypertension 2004;22:2049–2054
4. Canter PH. The therapeutic effects of meditation. BMJ 2003;326:1049–1050
5. Carson JW, Keefe FJ, Lynch TR, Carson KM, Goli V, Fras AM, Thorp SR. Loving-kindness meditation for chronic low back pain: results from a pilot trial. Holistic Nurs 2005;23:287–304
6. Mehling WE, Hamel KA, Acree M, Byl N, Hecht FM. Randomized controlled trial of breath therapy for patients with chronic low back pain. Altern Ther Health Med 2005;11:44–52
7. Jaseja H. Meditation may predispose to epilepsy: an insight into the alteration in brain environment induced by meditation. Med Hypotheses 2005;64:464–467
8. Lazarus AA. Psychiatric problems precipitated by transcendental meditation. Psychol Rep 1976;39:601–602
9. Sethi S, Bhargava SC. Relationship of meditation and psychosis: case studies. Aust NZ J Psychiatry 2003;37:382

MUSIC THERAPY

SYNONYMS

Acoustic or auditory stimulation.

DEFINITION

Music therapy is generally defined as the use of music by an accredited professional to achieve individualised therapeutic goals.

BACKGROUND

The 20th century discipline of music therapy began after World War I and World War II when community musicians of all types went to hospitals around the country to play for the thousands of veterans suffering physical and emotional trauma from the wars. Music therapy as a clinical profession started to be recognised in North and South America in the 1940s, with Austria and England following in 1958, and soon after that many other countries in Europe and elsewhere. Music therapy models practised today are most commonly based on psychoanalytical, humanistic, cognitive–behavioural or developmental theory.

TRADITIONAL CONCEPTS

There are many forms of music therapy depending on the patient's needs and aims. The most basic distinction is between receptive and active music therapy. Receptive music therapy includes listening to music played by the therapist for the patient or listening to recorded music selected by either therapist or patient. In active music therapy, which is most commonly used in mental health, patients are actively involved in the music making by playing of instruments of their choice, song writing, discussion of lyrics, and other activities related to music. A common misconception about music therapy is that patients need some level of musical ability; however, no musical talent or previous expertise are required for patients to benefit from this type of therapy.

SCIENTIFIC RATIONALE

There are wide variations in individual music preferences, which have a strong impact on the physiological effects of music. Sensations that accompany music therapy (e.g. the acoustic stimulation) may activate limbic or other areas of the brain related to the reward and motivation circuitry (limbic-cortical circuits). Secondary physiological changes and bodily reactions may follow, i.e. autoregulatory mind–body reactions such as an influence on hemispheric dominance, changes in autonomic nervous system activity, relaxation effects on vital functions such as breath, respiratory rate, blood pressure and cardiac output. Analgesic and anxiolytic properties of music are mainly the result of the lowering of stress levels and stress hormone production in a similar way to the relaxation response.

PRACTITIONERS

Music therapists will typically practise in a manner that incorporates music therapy techniques with broader clinical practices such as assessment, diagnosis, psychotherapy, rehabilitation and other practices. They work in a wide range of settings and must be trained to select and apply musical parameters adequately, tailored to a patient's needs and goals. Music therapists need the skills of both musicians and therapists. In the UK, music therapy is a state-registered profession and practitioners are required to hold a postgraduate qualification such as a Master's degree or postgraduate diploma in music therapy in addition to a music qualification. In the US, candidates who complete one of the approved college or university music therapy curricula are eligible to sit for the national examination to obtain the credential MT-BC (Music Therapy-Board Certified) necessary for professional practice.

CONDITIONS FREQUENTLY TREATED

Acute and chronic pain including mothers in labour, Alzheimer's disease, brain injuries, developmental and learning disabilities, mental-health needs, palliative care, physical disabilities and substance abuse problems.

TYPICAL SESSION

Since music therapists serve a wide variety of patients with many different types of needs there is no such thing as an overall typical session. In pain management, mainly receptive music therapy is used and patients listen to either self-selected music or music selected by the therapist. Sometimes it is combined with other relaxation therapies. For procedural pain, music is played either during or immediately after the intervention.

COURSE OF TREATMENT

The duration of receptive music therapy for pain can range from a single session, for example before, during or after surgery, to a series of sessions over several weeks for chronic pain patients. Patients might be instructed to listen to music in their own home.

CLINICAL EVIDENCE

A systematic review of the effectiveness of music as an intervention for hospital patients concluded that there was no effect when patients were asked to think about and rate the severity of their pain but it suggested that music may be an effective diversion.[1] Five RCTs found music therapy not to be superior to control interventions while only one RCT reported less narcotic analgesia administered during the procedure via a patient-controlled device in the music group.

Several RCTs assessed the effect of music on patients undergoing surgery. They found beneficial effects on pain parameters after gynaecological surgery,[2,3] intestinal surgery,[4] abdominal surgery,[5,6] heart surgery,[7] varicose vein or open inguinal hernia repair,[8,9] open hernia repair,[10] laceration repair,[11] hysterectomy,[12] open-heart surgery,[13] thyroid, parathyroid or breast surgery[14] and renal lithotripsy.[15] Similarly, music reduced pain during colposcopy,[16] colonoscopy,[17,18] tissue biopsy, or port placement or removal[19] and reduced intravenous insertion pain.[20] An RCT of 64 women receiving routine care plus music therapy versus routine care alone during Caesarean delivery found no differences between physiological measures in the women.[21]

Positive effects and verbal responses were noted in stroke patients while performing upper extremity exercises with both music and karaoke accompaniment music in a small RCT.[22] One RCT reported a reduction of chronic osteoarthritis pain in community-dwelling elderly.[23] Conflicting results exist for low back pain in hospitalised patients; one RCT reported improvement in pain in the music and relaxation group compared with relaxation only[24] while in another RCT the improvement observed in the group listening to music in addition to undergoing standard physical therapy was not significant when compared with physical therapy alone.[25] A systematic review including one RCT of music for pain management in labour found music not to be beneficial[26] while one RCT found that soft music provided greater pain relief during the active labour phase.[27] The effects of music-based imagery and musical alternate engagement in the management of pain and anxiety during debridement were tested in an RCT ($n = 25$) using a repeated measure design with patients serving as their own controls.[28] It found a reduction of self-reported pain in patients receiving music therapy. A small RCT found no difference between the music and no music groups for pain during the rehabilitation of patients with burns.[29]

RISKS

CONTRAINDICATIONS

None known.

PRECAUTIONS/WARNINGS

None known.

ADVERSE EFFECTS

None known.

INTERACTIONS

None known.

RISK–BENEFIT ASSESSMENT

Music seems to be a beneficial adjunct in the management of pain related to surgery or diagnostic procedures. It is associated with virtually no risks and little cost, therefore its use in addition to medication in these patients can be encouraged. It still needs to be established whether intra-operative versus post-operative or patient-selected versus therapist-selected music has additional beneficial effects. There is no compelling evidence for music therapy in any other pain condition.

REFERENCES

1. Evans D. The effectiveness of music as an intervention for hospital patients: a systematic review. J Adv Nurs 2002;37:8–18
2. Good M, Anderson GC, Stanton-Hicks M, Grass JA, Makii M. Relaxation and music reduce pain after gynecologic surgery. Pain Manag Nurs 2002;3:61–70
3. Laurion S, Fetzer SJ. The effect of two nursing interventions on the postoperative outcomes of gynecologic laparoscopic patients. J Perianesth Nurs 2003;18:254–261
4. Good M, Anderson GC, Ahn S, Cong X, Stanton-Hicks M. Relaxation and music reduce pain following intestinal surgery. Res Nurs Health 2005;28:240–251
5. Good M, Stanton-Hicks M, Grass JA, Anderson GC, Lai HL, Roykulcharoen V, Adler PA. Relaxation and music to reduce postsurgical pain. J Adv Nurs 2001;33:208–215
6. Good M, Stanton-Hicks M, Grass JA, Cranston Anderson G, Choi C, Schoolmeesters LJ, Salman A. Relief of postoperative pain with jaw relaxation, music and their combination. Pain 1999; 81:163–172
7. Kshettry VR, Carole LF, Henly SJ, Sendelbach S, Kummer B. Complementary alternative medical therapies for heart surgery patients: feasibility, safety, and impact. Ann Thorac Surg 2006;81:201–205
8. Nilsson U, Rawal N, Unosson M. A comparison of intra-operative or postoperative exposure to music — a controlled trial of the effects on postoperative pain. Anaesthesia 2003;58: 699–703
9. Nilsson U, Rawal N, Enqvist B, Unosson M. Analgesia following music and therapeutic suggestions in the PACU in ambulatory surgery; a randomized controlled trial. Acta Anaesthesiol Scand 2003;47:278–283
10. Nilsson U, Unosson M, Rawal N. Stress reduction and analgesia in patients exposed to calming music postoperatively: a randomized controlled trial. Eur J Anaesthesiol 2005;22:96–102
11. Menegazzi JJ, Paris PM, Kersteen CH, Flynn B, Trautman DE. A randomized, controlled trial of the use of music during laceration repair. Ann Emerg Med 1991;20:348–350
12. Nilsson U, Rawal N, Unestahl LE, Zetterberg C, Unosson M. Improved recovery after music and therapeutic suggestions during general anaesthesia: a double-blind randomised controlled trial. Acta Anaesthesiol Scand 2001;45:812–817
13. Voss JA, Good M, Yates B, Baun MM, Thompson A, Hertzog M. Sedative music reduces anxiety and pain during chair rest after open-heart surgery. Pain 2004;112:197–203
14. Heitz L, Symreng T, Scamman FL. Effect of music therapy in the postanesthesia care unit: a nursing intervention. J Post Anesth Nurs 1992;7:22–31
15. Cepeda MS, Diaz JE, Hernandez V, Daza E, Carr DB. Music does not reduce alfentanil requirement during patient-controlled analgesia (PCA) use in extracorporeal shock wave lithotripsy for renal stones. J Pain Symptom Manage 1998;16:382–387
16. Chan YM, Lee PW, Ng TY, Ngan HY, Wong LC. The use of music to reduce anxiety for patients undergoing colposcopy: a randomized trial. Gynecol Oncol 2003;91:213–217
17. Lee DW, Chan KW, Poon CM, Ko CW, Chan KH, Sin KS, Sze TS, Chan AC. Relaxation music decreases the dose of patient-controlled sedation during colonoscopy: a prospective randomized controlled trial. Gastrointest Endosc 2002;55:33–36
18. Uedo N, Ishikawa H, Morimoto K, Ishihara R, Narahara H, Akedo I, Ioka T, Kaji I, Fukuda S. Reduction in salivary cortisol level by music therapy during colonoscopic examination. Hepatogastroenterology 2004;51:451–453
19. Kwekkeboom KL. Music versus distraction for procedural pain and anxiety in patients with cancer. Oncol Nurs Forum 2003;30:433–440
20. Jacobson AF. Intradermal normal saline solution, self-selected music, and insertion difficulty effects on intravenous insertion pain. Heart Lung 1999;28:114–122

SECTION THREE

21. Chang SC, Chen CH. Effects of music therapy on women's physiologic measures, anxiety, and satisfaction during cesarean delivery. Res Nurs Health 2005;28:453–461

22. Kim SJ, Koh I. The effects of music on pain perception of stroke patients during upper extremity joint exercises. J Music Ther 2005;42:81–92

23. McCaffrey RG, Good M. The lived experience of listening to music while recovering from surgery. J Holist Nurs 2000;18:378–390

24. Kullich W, Bernatzky G, Hesse HP, Wendtner F, Likar R, Klein G. Music therapy – effect on pain, sleep and quality of life in low back pain. [In German.] Wien Med Wochenschr 2003;153:217–221

25. Guetin S, Coudeyre E, Picot MC, Ginies P, Graber-Duvernay B, Ratsimba D, Vanbiervliet W, Blayac JP, Herisson C. Effect of music therapy among hospitalized patients with chronic low back pain: a controlled, randomized trial. [In French.] Ann Readapt Med Phys 2005; 48:217–224

26. Smith CA, Collins CT, Cyna AM, Crowther CA. Complementary and alternative therapies for pain management in labour. The Cochrane Database of Systematic Reviews 2003, Issue 2. Art. No.: CD003521

27. Phumdoung S, Good M. Music reduces sensation and distress of labor pain. Pain Manag Nurs 2003;4:54–61

28. Fratianne RB, Prensner JD, Huston MJ, Super DM, Yowler CJ, Standley JM. The effect of music-based imagery and musical alternate engagement on the burn debridement process. J Burn Care Rehabil 2001;22:47–53

29. Ferguson SL, Voll KV. Burn pain and anxiety: the use of music relaxation during rehabilitation. J Burn Care Rehabil 2004;25:8–14

NATUROPATHY

DEFINITION

An eclectic system of health care that uses elements of complementary and conventional medicine to support and enhance self-healing processes.

RELATED TECHNIQUES

Hydrotherapy, *Kneippkur* (German), physical medicine, physiotherapy, *Naturheilverfahren* (German).

BACKGROUND

The 'healing power of nature' gained interest during the 18th and 19th centuries when the Germans Vinzenz Prießnietz (1799–1851) and Sebastian Kneipp (1821–1897) established complex hydrotherapeutic interventions as a cure for many ailments. A disciple of Kneipp, Benedict Lust (1870–1945), introduced hydrotherapy to the US and later used the term naturopathy to describe the concept that he developed.

TRADITIONAL CONCEPTS

Naturopathy is based on the belief that health can be influenced by what is called 'nature's own healing power' (*vis medicatrix naturae*), which is understood as an inherent property of the living organism. Ill health is viewed as a direct result of ignoring or violating general principles of a healthy lifestyle. These principles are thought to be determined by an internal and external environment that optimises the health of an individual. Naturopathy aims to correct and stabilise the conditions of the internal and external environment.

SCIENTIFIC RATIONALE

The general principles of a healthy lifestyle, including a diet with plenty of fresh fruit and vegetables and regular physical exercise, are now well recognised in mainstream medicine. The different therapeutic interventions and techniques that are used in naturopathy include herbal medicine, hydrotherapy and iridology as well as physical treatments such as spinal manipulation and others. The scientific rationale varies according to each individual treatment. For some interventions a plausible scientific rationale is lacking, while for others the rationale is supported by data from scientific investigations.

PRACTITIONERS

In the US, licensed naturopaths will have completed training that includes basic medical sciences and conventional diagnostic techniques. In the US and Canada, accredited colleges of naturopathic medicine exist offering 4-year training programmes, which may lead to licensing. Naturopaths are currently licensed in 13 US states.[1] In the UK, the number of registered naturopaths, a profession not regulated by statute, is about 500.

CONDITIONS FREQUENTLY TREATED

Naturopaths treat any condition but are trained to refer patients with serious medical conditions for conventional treatment.

TYPICAL SESSION

During an initial consultation the naturopath will usually take a detailed medical history of the patient to assess the medical status and screen for any serious conditions. This will include questions relating to lifestyle and diet and may be followed by a more conventional diagnostic evaluation. According to the diagnosed condition, the treatment plan will vary but often includes changes in lifestyle. The treatment of a particular condition may vary between practitioners. Follow-up appointments are arranged as necessary and the medicines and regimen are reviewed and changed if appropriate.

COURSE OF TREATMENT

Depends largely on the nature and severity of the condition but generally one or two appointments weekly for a treatment period of one to several weeks.

CLINICAL EVIDENCE

The clinical evidence has to be evaluated according to each individual therapy used in naturopathy (see respective chapters). There is clinical evidence from RCTs and systematic reviews for some of its elements, such as certain herbal extracts,[2,3] balneotherapy[4] and speleotherapy.[5] For other elements there is little evidence of effectiveness.[6] The effectiveness of the totality of the naturopathic approach has not been evaluated in RCTs.

RISKS

CONTRAINDICATIONS

Contraindications and precautions vary for each individual therapy (see respective chapters) and often include pregnancy and lactation (see p. 4).

PRECAUTIONS/WARNINGS

Precautions may vary for each individual therapy (see respective chapters).

ADVERSE EFFECTS

The risk of adverse effects exists. The reader is referred to the respective chapters in this book and the conventional medical literature.

INTERACTIONS

Possible interactions, for instance between different herbal preparations or with conventional drugs or with other interventions, should be considered (see respective chapters) and patients at risk should be closely monitored. Patients should be asked about self-prescribed drug use.

RISK–BENEFIT ASSESSMENT

The possibility of adverse effects exists and the risk–benefit ratio has to be assessed for each treatment individually (see respective chapters). Given a beneficial safety profile, elements of naturopathy may be worth considering when performed by a responsible, well-trained and licensed therapist.

REFERENCES

1. Atwood KC 4th. Naturopathy: a critical appraisal. Med Gen Med 2003;5:39
2. Pittler MH, Ernst E. Horse chestnut seed extract for chronic venous insufficiency. The Cochrane Database of Systematic Reviews 2004, Issue 2. Art. No.: CD003230
3. Thompson Coon J, Pittler MH, Ernst E. *Trifolium pratense* isoflavones in the treatment of menopausal hot flushes. A systematic review and meta-analysis. Phytomedicine 2007;14:153–159
4. Verhagen AP, Bierma-Zeinstra SMA, Cardoso JR, de Bie RA, Boers M, de Vet HCW. Balneotherapy for rheumatoid arthritis. The Cochrane Database of Systematic Reviews 2004, Issue 1. Art. No.: CD000518
5. Beamon S, Falkenbach A, Fainburg G, Linde K. Speleotherapy for asthma. The Cochrane Database of Systematic Reviews 2001, Issue 2. Art. No.: CD001741
6. Ernst E. Iridology. Arch Ophthalmol 2000;118:120–121

NEURAL THERAPY

DEFINITION

Therapy using injection of local anaesthetics into 'irritation zones' (*Störfelder*) in the hope of unblocking reflex pathways leading to diseased organs.

RELATED TECHNIQUES

Trigger-point injection, acupuncture.

BACKGROUND

The method was developed by the German physician Ferdinand Huneke. He noted that injection of local anaesthetics into certain points was followed by symptom relief – sometimes instantly (*Sekundenphänomen* = phenomenon of seconds).

TRADITIONAL CONCEPTS

Neural therapy is a reflex therapy that aims to stimulate reflector segments. It is believed to act via the autonomic nervous system on autoregulatory mechanisms.[1] The three principles of neural therapy can be summarised as follows:

- every chronic disease can be caused by 'irritation zones'
- every disease or injury generates an 'irritation zone'
- every 'irritation zone' condition can be treated by eliminating it with neural therapy.

SCIENTIFIC RATIONALE

Some elements of neural therapy are based on neurophysiological principles.

PRACTITIONERS

Neural therapy is not well known outside continental Europe. In Germany, it is practised by many physicians.

CONDITIONS FREQUENTLY TREATED

Chronic benign conditions, particularly those associated with pain.

TYPICAL SESSION

The practitioner would take a medical history and, using conventional diagnostic techniques and criteria, would try to define the problem. This would usually be followed by injection of local anaesthetics into various parts of the body.

COURSE OF TREATMENT

One treatment is rarely regarded as sufficient. One course of treatment might comprise six to 12 sessions. Frequently, repeat courses are recommended.

CLINICAL EVIDENCE

Several retrospective uncontrolled studies suggest that neural therapy is effective for a range of conditions, particularly musculoskeletal pain,[2,3] but there are very few CCTs. One small RCT suggested that a variation of neural therapy improves the functional status of patients suffering from multiple sclerosis.[4] Another small RCT implied that neural therapy reduces the symptoms of chronic back pain patients just as well as standard orthopaedic care.[5] Both these studies require independent replication in more rigorous RCTs.

RISKS

CONTRAINDICATIONS

Intolerance to local anaesthetics.

PRECAUTIONS/WARNINGS

Patients with needle phobia might find this approach difficult to accept.

ADVERSE EFFECTS

Hypersensitivity to local anaesthetics, puncture of inner organs.

INTERACTIONS

Those of the specific local anaesthetics used, e.g. hypersensitivity or allergy to lidocaine.

RISK–BENEFIT ASSESSMENT

To date there is no convincing evidence that neural therapy is effective for any indication. The risks of this treatment are relatively small. A risk–benefit assessment fails to arrive at a positive conclusion.

REFERENCES

1. Fischer L. Pathophysiology of pain and neural therapy. [In German.] Schweiz Rundsch Med Prax 2003;92:2051–2059
2. Barbagli P, Bollettin R. Therapy of articular and periarticular pain with local anesthetics (neural therapy of Huneke). Long and short term results. [In Italian.] Minerva Anestesiol 1998;64:35–43
3. Barbagli P, Bollettin R, Ceccherelli F. Acupuncture (dry needle) versus neural therapy (local anesthesia) in the treatment of benign back pain. Immediate and long-term results. [In Italian.] Minerva Med 2003;94(Suppl. 1):17–25

SECTION THREE

4. Gibson RG, Gibson SL. Neural therapy in the treatment of multiple sclerosis. J Altern Complement Med 1999;5:543–552

5. Dinter W, Thakkar S, Ullrich H, Busch M. Clinical investigation of Huneke's Neural Therapy. [In German.] Z Allg Med 1999;75:19–20

OSTEOPATHY

DEFINITION

Form of manual therapy (and diagnosis) involving the manipulation of soft tissues and the mobilisation or manipulation of peripheral and spinal joints.

RELATED TECHNIQUES

Craniosacral therapy, chiropractic, manual therapy, spinal manipulation and mobilisation.

BACKGROUND

Osteopathy was founded in the US by Andrew Taylor Still in 1874 and, since then, it has had a turbulent history. It is now an accepted form of conventional health care in the US. In the UK and most other countries, osteopathy is a well-established form of CAM.

TRADITIONAL CONCEPTS

Osteopaths believe that the primary role of the therapist is to facilitate the body's inherent ability to heal itself, that the structure and function of the body are closely related and that problems of one organ affect other parts of the body.[1] For osteopaths, an adequate alignment of the musculoskeletal system eliminates obstructions in blood and lymph flow, which, in turn, maximises health and function. To ensure alignment, osteopaths have developed a range of techniques. These can be grouped into the following five major categories:

- direct techniques: high-velocity, low-amplitude thrusts, articulatory, general osteopathic techniques, muscle energy techniques
- indirect techniques: functional techniques, counterstrain, balanced ligamentous tension, ligamentous articulatory strain
- combined techniques: myofascial/fascial release, visceral techniques, osteopathy in the cranial field, involuntary mechanism
- reflex-based techniques: Chapman's reflexes, trigger points, neuromuscular techniques
- fluid-based techniques: lymphatic pump techniques.[1]

SCIENTIFIC RATIONALE

Some of the traditional osteopathic concepts ring intuitively true, yet their scientific rationale is not firmly established. In particular, the theory of the overriding importance of alignment lacks a scientific rationale.

PRACTITIONERS

In the US, osteopaths today constitute the smaller of the two major schools of medicine. US osteopaths (doctors of osteopathy or DOs) use most allopathic therapeutic options alongside osteopathic manipulative techniques and are now regarded as mainstream health-care professionals. Outside the US, osteopaths mainly use spinal manipulation and mobilisation and are usually thought of as CAM practitioners. In the UK, osteopaths are now regulated by statute. In continental Europe, the title 'DO' has a different meaning than in the US and stands for 'diploma of osteopathy'.

CONDITIONS FREQUENTLY TREATED

Osteopaths mostly treat patients who are suffering from musculoskeletal problems, particularly back and neck pain. US osteopaths would treat many other conditions as well, combining allopathic treatments with manual osteopathic techniques. The majority of US osteopaths, however, no longer use manipulative techniques routinely.

TYPICAL SESSION

A visit to a US osteopath is usually very similar to a consultation with a conventional physician. Outside the US, an osteopath would take a medical history and perform a careful physical examination, particularly of the musculoskeletal system. In most cases this would be followed by treatment consisting of spinal manipulation and mobilisation.

COURSE OF TREATMENT

Depending on the condition and on clinical progress, three to six treatments would constitute a full course for acute conditions. More sessions are usually advised for chronic conditions.

CLINICAL EVIDENCE

There is some evidence to suggest that osteopathy is helpful for low back pain, particularly the acute and subacute stages.[1-3] A systematic review of six RCTs of osteopathic manipulative treatment for low back pain found greater pain reductions with osteopathy compared to active control treatment, placebo or no treatment.[4] A UK cost–utility analysis generated encouraging results for osteopathic treatment of subacute spinal pain.[5] A small ($n = 76$) CCT suggested that osteopathic treatment after knee or hip arthroplasty was superior to conventional care in speeding up post-operative rehabilitation.[6] A small RCT suggested that post-operative osteopathic manipulation enhanced perioperative morphine analgesia in the 48 hours after total elective hysterectomy.[7] Another study suggested that osteopathic manipulative treatments are beneficial for acute ankle injuries.[8]

These positive data require independent replication. Two small RCTs failed to generate convincing evidence that osteopathic approaches to treating shoulder pain[9] or tennis elbow[10] are superior to standard care. A Cochrane review found no reliable evidence that osteopathy is effective in the treatment of primary or secondary dysmenorrhea.[11] For other indications the clinical trial evidence is also sparse and not compelling.[1,2]

RISKS

CONTRAINDICATIONS

Osteoporosis, neoplasms, infections, bleeding disorders (depending on the approach used).

PRECAUTIONS/WARNINGS

None known.

ADVERSE EFFECTS

Spinal trauma after high-velocity thrusts, vertebral artery dissection, stroke.

INTERACTIONS

None known.

RISK–BENEFIT ASSESSMENT

Osteopathic spinal manipulation and mobilisation may be helpful in cases of low back pain. For all other pain syndromes the evidence is not convincing. Osteopathic techniques are typically gentler than those used by chiropractors; thus, the risk of spinal injury should be smaller. On balance, osteopathy may be worth trying for patients with low back pain. For all other conditions the evidence is insufficient for issuing definitive recommendations.

REFERENCES

1. Lesho EP. An overview of osteopathic medicine. Arch Fam Med 1999;8:477–483
2. Schwerla F, Hass-Degg K, Schwerla B. Evaluierung und kritische Bewertung von in der europäischen Literatur veröffentlichten, osteopathischen Studien im klinischen Bereich und im Bereich der Grundlagenforschung. Forsch Komplementärmed 1999;6:302–310
3. Williams NH, Wilkinson C, Russell I, Edwards RT, Hibbs R, Linck P, Muntz R. Randomized osteopathic manipulation study (ROMANS): pragmatic trial for spinal pain in primary care. Fam Pract 2003;20:662–669
4. Licciardone JC, Brimhall AK, King LN. Osteopathic manipulative treatment for low back pain: a systematic review and meta-analysis of randomized controlled trials. BMC Musculoskelet Disord 2005;6:43.
5. Williams NH, Edwards RT, Linck P, Muntz R, Hibbs R, Wilkinson C, Russell I, Russell D, Hounsome B. Cost–utility analysis of osteopathy in primary care: results from a pragmatic randomized controlled trial. Fam Pract 2004;21:643–650
6. Jarski RW, Loniewski EG, Williams J, Bahu A, Shafinia S, Gibbs K, Muller M. The effectiveness of osteopathic manipulative treatment as complementary therapy following surgery: a prospective match-controlled outcome study. Altern Ther Health Med 2000;6:77–81
7. Goldstein FJ, Jeck S, Nicholas AS, Berman MJ, Lerario M. Preoperative intravenous morphine sulfate with postoperative osteopathic manipulative treatment reduces patient analgesic use after total abdominal hysterectomy. J Am Osteopath Assoc 2005;105:273–279
8. Eisenhart AW, Gaeta TJ, Yens DP. Osteopathic manipulative treatment in the emergency department for patients with acute ankle injuries. J Am Osteopath Assoc 2003;103:417–421
9. Knebl JA, Shores JH, Gamber RG, Gray WT, Herron KM. An RCT of osteopathy for shoulder problems. J Am Osteopath Assoc 2002;102:387–396
10. Geldschläger S. Osteopathic versus orthopaedic interventions for chronic epicondylopathia humeri radialis: randomized controlled trial. Forsch Komplementärmed Klass Naturheildkd 2004; 11:93–97
11. Proctor ML, Hing W, Johnson TC, Murphy PA. Spinal manipulation for primary and secondary dysmenorrhoea. The Cochrane Database of Systematic Reviews 2001, Issue 4. Art. No.: CD002119

QIGONG

SYNONYMS

Chi gung, qui gong, ki gong, qi training, qi therapy

DEFINITION

An Asian healing art that uses gentle, focused, exercises for mind and body to increase and restore the flow of qi (life energy) or to accumulate qi with the aim of encouraging and accelerating the healing process.

RELATED TECHNIQUES

Tai chi, Danjun (Tantien) breathing, Zen meditation, Reiki, therapeutic touch, Johrei, spiritual healing.

BACKGROUND

Qigong has been described as 'a way of working with life energy'. It consists of two main types of practice: internal and external. Internal qigong is self-directed and involves the use of movements and meditation and sometimes chanting. It can be performed with or without a teacher and actively engages people in their own health and well-being. It is best practised daily to promote health maintenance and disease prevention. External qigong is performed by a Master or highly trained practitioner using the hands and any part of the body to direct qi energy onto the patient for the purpose of healing.

TRADITIONAL CONCEPTS

Both internal and external techniques of qigong often include five steps: meditation, cleansing, recharging/strengthening, and circulating and dispersing qi. Each step comprises specific exercises, meditations and sounds. Qigong aims to restore health through removing blockages of qi. Qigong is intended to be harmonious with the natural rhythms of the environment.

SCIENTIFIC RATIONALE

Qigong consists of two main aspects: controlled breathing (or deep breathing) with slow body movements as an aerobic exercise and relaxation. The qigong exercises are physical stimuli with effects on the cardiovascular and muscular systems. In addition to adaptation processes at the nervous system level, these effects produce better cardiovascular function and may enhance balance and coordination. This stimulation and relaxation activates and modulates the neurohormonal system to improve the psychological state and enhance immune function.

PRACTITIONERS

Practitioners should have some knowledge of the philosophy of Asian medicine and the Asian world view. Practitioners should have an understanding of human anatomy and physiology.

CONDITIONS FREQUENTLY TREATED

Internal qigong: chronic pain, chronic fatigue syndrome, osteoporosis, high blood pressure, stomach ulcers, asthma.
External qigong: acute pain, headache, fatigue, anxiety, depression.

TYPICAL SESSION

Qigong is taught on an individual basis or in groups. The student should maintain a level of concentration and should not be distracted by external influences. Qigong is a lifelong endeavour and regular practice is essential in achieving beneficial effects.

COURSE OF TREATMENT

Treatment may differ in duration but usually takes 30 minutes. Daily practice is ideal and at least twice weekly sessions are recommended. The best time for practice is said to be early in the morning and late in the evening. Usually, external qigong is for the beginner who cannot yet perform internal qigong, which is thought to be superior.

CLINICAL EVIDENCE
INTERNAL QIGONG

A non-randomised pilot study of internal qigong found improvement on the fibromyalgia impact questionnaire and reductions in pain[1] whereas no improvement was found for fibromyalgia symptoms or physical function in a small ($n = 36$) RCT.[2] A large ($n = 128$) RCT tested a mind–body intervention that combined training in mindfulness meditation with qigong movement therapy against an education support group for individuals with fibromyalgia.[3] It reported improvements over time for the fibromyalgia impact questionnaire and pain scores in the treatment group. There were no differences in either the rate or magnitude of these changes between the qigong group and the education control group. Single

SECTION THREE

RCTs or non-randomised trials of qigong, which require independent replication in rigorous trials, report positive effects for shoulder-arm pain in women,[4] in late-stage complex regional pain syndrome,[5] pain in patients with mild essential hypertension,[6] migraine and tension-type headache.[7]

EXTERNAL QIGONG

For elderly patients (mean age 64 years) with chronic pain of different origin, reductions in pain are reported after a single 10-minute qigong session compared with baseline.[8] These findings are supported by another RCT which reported differences compared with a no-treatment control group.[9] For patients with pre-menstrual syndrome, two RCTs of qigong reported beneficial effects on measures of pain compared with baseline and compared with waiting list controls.[10,11] For breast cancer patients, a non-randomised controlled trial reported reductions in pain compared with baseline.[12]

RISKS
CONTRAINDICATIONS

Contraindications and precautions are largely based on common sense (e.g. severe osteoporosis, severe heart conditions, acute back pain, knee problems, sprains and fractures). Usually, it can be safely practised during pregnancy and lactation.

PRECAUTIONS/WARNINGS

Before starting qigong older individuals should be carefully examined for any of the above or other contraindications. For external qigong, it is of importance, as with many other therapies, to find an experienced practitioner.

ADVERSE EFFECTS

Adverse effects are rare, but may include delayed-onset muscle soreness. When practised inappropriately, it may induce abnormal psychosomatic responses and even mental disorders.[13]

INTERACTIONS

None known.

RISK–BENEFIT ASSESSMENT

There is some encouraging yet limited evidence for the effectiveness of external qigong in elderly patients with chronic pain and women with pain related to premenstrual syndrome. When practised judiciously it might be a useful adjunct in managing pain in these patient groups. There is no convincing evidence for any other pain conditions.

REFERENCES
1. Singh BB, Berman BM, Hadhazy VA, Creamer P. A pilot study of cognitive behavioral therapy in fibromyalgia. Altern Ther Health Med 1998;4:67–70
2. Mannerkorpi K, Arndorw M. Efficacy and feasibility of a combination of body awareness therapy and qigong in patients with fibromyalgia: a pilot study. J Rehabil Med 2004;36:279–281
3. Astin JA, Berman BM, Bausell B, Lee WL, Hochberg M, Forys KL. The efficacy of mindfulness meditation plus Qigong movement therapy in the treatment of fibromyalgia: a randomized controlled trial. J Rheumatol 2003;30:2257–2262
4. Youn HM, Kim MY, Kim YS, Lim JS. Effects of the doing qigong exercise on the shoulder-arm pain in women. J Korean Acu Moxibust Soc 2005;22:177–190
5. Wu WH, Bandilla E, Ciccone DS, Yang J, Cheng SC, Carner N, Wu Y, Shen R. Effects of qigong on late-stage complex regional pain syndrome. Altern Ther Health Med 1999; 5:45–54

6. Cheung BM, Lo JL, Fong DY, Chan MY, Wong SH, Wong VC, Lam KS, Lau CP, Karlberg JP. Randomised controlled trial of qigong in the treatment of mild essential hypertension. J Hum Hypertens 2005;19:697–704

7. Friedrichs E. Qigong-yangsheng-Übungen als Begleittherapie bei Migräne und Spannungskopfschmerz – Ergebnisse einer multizentrischen prospectiven Pilotstudie. Chinesische Medizin 2004;19:16–30

8. Lee MS, Jang JW, Jang HS, Moon SR. Effects of Qi-therapy on blood pressure, pain and psychological symptoms in the elderly: a randomized controlled pilot trial. Complement Ther Med 2003;11:159–164

9. Yang KH, Kim YH, Lee MS. Efficacy of Qi-therapy (external Qigong) for elderly people with chronic pain. Int J Neurosci 2005;115:949–963

10. Jang HS, Lee MS, Kim MJ, Chong ES. Effects of Qi-therapy on premenstrual syndrome. Int J Neurosci 2004;114:909–921

11. Jang HS, Lee MS. Effects of qi therapy (external qigong) on premenstrual syndrome: a randomized placebo-controlled study. J Altern Complement Med 2004;10:456–462

12. Lee TI, Chen HH, Yeh ML. Effects of chan-chuang qigong on improving symptom and psychological distress in chemotherapy patients. Am J Chin Med 2006;34:37–46

13. Ng BY. Qigong-induced mental disorders: a review. Aust NZ J Psychiatry 1999;33:197–206

REFLEXOLOGY

SYNONYMS

Zone therapy, reflex zone therapy. Note that the term 'reflexology' is sometimes used to describe treatment of segmental nerve reflexes with needles. 'Reflexotherapy' was used historically to describe acupuncture in the former USSR.

DEFINITION

A therapeutic method that uses manual pressure applied to specific areas, or zones, of the feet (and sometimes the hands or ears) that are believed to correspond to other areas or organs of the body.

RELATED TECHNIQUES

Reflexology may be used together with other techniques by manual therapists of various disciplines. Other therapies that use the concept of correspondence to parts of the body include acupuncture techniques such as auriculotherapy and Korean hand acupuncture.

BACKGROUND

Egyptian papyri from about 2500 BCE show manual treatment of the feet and there is evidence that similar treatment was part of Chinese culture. Zone therapy is recorded in various ancient European medical systems and those of the North American Indians. In the early 20th century William Fitzgerald investigated the effects of pressure in inducing analgesia elsewhere in the body and concluded that the body was divided into 10 vertical zones, each represented by a part of the foot including one toe. From this concept, the charts of bodily correspondences evolved, initially drawn up by Eunice Ingham and published from the 1930s onwards.

TRADITIONAL CONCEPTS

The organs, glands and other components of each half of the body are believed to be represented at the foot on that side, mainly on the sole. It is assumed that the health of the body can be assessed by examining the feet to detect imbalances or obstructions to the flow of energy,

SECTION THREE

which are expressed as tenderness or feelings of grittiness or crystal formation. Bodily functions are believed to be influenced by stimulating these areas with pressure or massage. Reflexology is claimed to reduce pain and stress, improve circulation, eliminate toxins and promote metabolic homeostasis.

SCIENTIFIC RATIONALE

There is no known neurophysiological basis for connections between organs or other body parts and specific areas of the feet. Reflexologists' diagnoses were no better than chance in identifying medical conditions in one blinded study,[1] whereas in another their diagnostic success was better than chance but not clinically relevant.[2] A further study suggested that reflexologists' diagnoses correlate with some organ systems and not with others.[3] Pressure on the specific areas produced changes in renal and intestinal blood flow.[4,5] Foot massage may have general benefits regardless of any reflex correspondences.

PRACTITIONERS

Practitioners range from those who teach themselves from books to those who follow training courses and join professional associations. In most countries, no regulatory systems exist, as there are currently no state licensing or training requirements. Reflexology is sometimes used by other health professionals including conventionally trained nurses.

CONDITIONS FREQUENTLY TREATED

Various pain syndromes such as arthritis, back and neck pain, migraine and headaches, chronic fatigue, asthma, digestive problems such as irritable bowel syndrome and constipation, insomnia, postmenopausal symptoms, sinusitis and stress-related disorders.

TYPICAL SESSION

The reflexologist usually takes a history before examining the bare feet systematically, with the patient lying on a couch or semi-reclining in a chair. Tender or gritty areas will be massaged as soon as they are found. The strength of pressure used varies. For lubrication, therapists may use talc or oil. Some practitioners will use sticks or other instruments to treat the feet. The whole session usually lasts 45–60 minutes.

COURSE OF TREATMENT

This varies considerably between practitioners and the condition treated. Often, treatment is offered weekly for a course of six to eight sessions. For chronic conditions, follow-up treatments may be offered.

CLINICAL EVIDENCE

A large observational study of reflexology found that 81% of patients with headache reported themselves helped or cured at a 3-month follow-up[6] and an RCT found a positive trend in the same condition.[7] One RCT found reflexology to be superior to placebo reflexology for the treatment of premenstrual symptoms, but the protocol included foot, hand and ear treatment so no conclusions can be drawn about any one independently.[8] Other RCTs found no advantage of reflexology over non-specific foot massage in the treatment of irritable bowel syndrome.[9] For cancer pain control the evidence from two studies was contradictory.[10,11] It should be noted that the results of the above studies tended to be negative when placebo effects were adequately controlled for and positive when this was not the case.

RISKS

CONTRAINDICATIONS

Relevant conditions of the feet such as gout, ulceration or vascular disease.

PRECAUTIONS/WARNINGS

Individuals with bone or joint conditions of the feet or lower legs should be treated cautiously. Although professional reflexology associations insist that reflexologists should not make diagnostic claims, there have been incidents where reflexologists have made false-positive or false-negative diagnoses and thus interfered with medical management to the patient's detriment.

ADVERSE EFFECTS

Fatigue, changes in micturition or bowel function. Allergy to lubricants.

INTERACTIONS

Possible interference with the effects of some drugs, e.g. insulin.

RISK–BENEFIT ASSESSMENT

There is no convincing evidence that reflexology is an effective technique for pain control. However, in the hands of responsible practitioners, reflexology seems to do little harm and possibly some good in the management of many functional disorders. Reflexology should never be used to make, or suggest, a medical diagnosis.

REFERENCES

1. White AR, Williamson J, Hart A, Ernst E. A blinded investigation into the accuracy of reflexology charts. Complement Ther Med 2000;8:166–172
2. Baerheim A, Algroy R, Skogedal KR, Stephansen R, Sandvik H. Fottene – et diagnostisk hjelpemiddel? Tidsskr Nor Laegeforen 1998;5:753–755
3. Raz I, Rosengarten Y, Carasso R. Correlation study between conventional medical diagnosis and the diagnosis by reflexology (non-conventional). [In Hebrew.] Harefuah 2003;142:600–605
4. Sudmeier I, Bodner G, Egger I, Mur E, Ulmer H, Herold M. Änderung der Nierendurchblutung durch organassoziierte Reflexzonentherapie am Fuß gemessen mit farbkodierter Doppler-Sonographie. Forsch Komplementärmed 1999;6:129–134
5. Mur E, Schmidseder J, Egger I, Bodner G, Eibl G, Hartig F, Pfeiffer KP, Herold M. Influence of reflex zone therapy of the feet on intestinal blood flow measured by color Doppler sonography. Forsch Komplementärmed Klass Naturheilkd 2001;8:86–89
6. Launso L, Brendstrup E, Arnberg S. An exploratory study of reflexological treatment for headache. Alt Ther Health Med 1999;5:57–65
7. Lafuente A, Noguera M, Puy C, Molins A, Titus F, Sanz F. Effekt der Reflexzonenbehandlung am Fuss bezüglich der prophylaktischen Behandlung mit Funarizin bei an Cephalea-Kopfschmerzen leidenden Patienten. Erfahrungsheilkunde 1990;39:713–715
8. Oleson T, Flocco W. Randomised controlled study of premenstrual symptoms treated with ear, hand and foot reflexology. Obstet Gynaecol 1993;82:906–911
9. Tovey PA. A single-blind trial of reflexology for irritable bowel syndrome. Br J Gen Pract 2002;52:19–23
10. Hodgson H. Does reflexology impact on cancer patients' quality of life? Nurs Stand 2000; 14:33–38
11. Stephenson NL, Weinrich SP, Tavakoli AS. The effects of foot reflexology on anxiety and pain in patients with breast and lung cancer. Oncol Nurs Forum 2000;27:67–72

SECTION THREE

RELAXATION THERAPY

DEFINITION
Techniques for eliciting the 'relaxation response' of the autonomic nervous system.

RELATED TECHNIQUES
Autogenic training, biofeedback, hypnotherapy, meditation. Many CAM interventions include an element of relaxation.

BACKGROUND
Progressive muscle relaxation is one of the most common relaxation techniques, pioneered by the American physician Edmund Jacobson in 1930. Modified over time by others, it is still based on the original principles. Other relaxation techniques involve passive muscle relaxation, refocusing, breathing control or imagery.

TRADITIONAL CONCEPTS
Progressive muscle relaxation is based on the notion that it is impossible to be tense in any part of the body where the muscles are completely relaxed. In addition, tension in involuntary muscles can be reduced if the associated skeletal muscles are relaxed. The technique is taught by first tensing a muscle before relaxing it, to recognise the difference between tension and relaxation. Subsequently, it is possible to relax a limb without tensing it first. Passive muscle relaxation involves release of tension while focusing on muscle groups. Benson's relaxation response contains an attention control element where the focus is on slow rhythmical breathing combined with repetition of a single word or phrase. With imagery-based relaxation, the idea is to imagine oneself in a place or situation associated with relaxation and comfort using visualisation and involving all the other senses in creating a vivid image.

SCIENTIFIC RATIONALE
Progressive muscle relaxation appears to be effective in eliciting the relaxation response, resulting in the normalising of blood supply to the muscles, decreases in oxygen consumption, heart rate, respiration and skeletal muscle activity and increases in skin resistance and alpha brain waves. Other relaxation techniques have also been shown to be effective in diffusing muscle tension.

PRACTITIONERS
Relaxation techniques are taught by various complementary practitioners, physicians, psychotherapists, hypnotherapists, nurses, clinical psychologists and sports therapists. There is no formal credentialing for relaxation therapies.

CONDITIONS FREQUENTLY TREATED
Musculoskeletal pain, headaches, anxiety and stress disorders.

TYPICAL SESSION
During a session of progressive muscle relaxation, subjects usually lie on their back with arms by their sides in a quiet environment. Occasionally a sitting posture is adopted instead. Muscle groups are systematically contracted then relaxed in a predetermined order. In the early stages, an entire session will be devoted to a single muscle group. With practice it becomes possible to combine muscle groups and then eventually relax the entire body all at once.

COURSE OF TREATMENT

To evoke the relaxation response within seconds using progressive muscle relaxation, several months of daily practice is generally needed.

CLINICAL EVIDENCE

A Cochrane review assessed the effects of behavioural treatments for chronic low back pain.[1] Comparing behavioural treatment with waiting list control ($n = 134$) revealed evidence of a positive effect on pain in favour of a combined respondent–cognitive therapy; progressive relaxation also compared favourably with waiting list control ($n = 39$). It concluded that combined respondent–cognitive therapy and progressive relaxation therapy are more effective than waiting list control for short-term pain relief. This is supported by another systematic review, which reported that for chronic low back pain progressive relaxation is effective for short-term pain relief and improvement of function.[2]

A systematic review and additional trials suggested overall that relaxation therapy is beneficial for patients with headache.[3–6] Another systematic review included 27 CCTs of various relaxation techniques used as an adjunctive treatment in ischaemic heart disease.[7] Overall, the results suggest that relaxation improves exercise tolerance, anxiety and depression and reduces the frequency of ischaemic pain. A meta-analysis and additional RCTs suggest that relaxation is effective for migraine[8–11] although it might be inferior to biofeedback.[12] For patients with chronic cancer pain, an RCT reported positive effects of relaxation therapy using music on falling asleep.[13] An RCT testing imagery and progressive muscle relaxation for patients undergoing resections of colorectal cancer did not report differences for analgesic consumption and pain intensity compared with a no-treatment control group.[14] In patients after intestinal surgery, another RCT reported some beneficial effects for relaxation and music therapy.[15] No difference was reported when relaxation therapy was compared with an occlusal appliance in temporomandibular disorder pain.[16] For menopausal symptoms there is some encouraging evidence for the effectiveness of relaxation therapy,[17] whereas for irritable bowel syndrome relaxation therapy as an addition to routine clinical care was no different to clinical care alone.[18] For patients with rheumatoid arthritis, beneficial effects have been reported.[19,20]

RISKS

CONTRAINDICATIONS

Schizophrenic or actively psychotic patients.

PRECAUTIONS/WARNINGS

Techniques requiring inward focusing may intensify depressed mood.

ADVERSE EFFECTS

None known.

INTERACTIONS

Adjunctive relaxation therapy may reduce the required dosage of certain medications, i.e. antihypertensive or anxiolytic drugs.

RISK–BENEFIT ASSESSMENT

Relaxation techniques seem to be effective for short-term pain relief and cause improvement of function in patients with chronic low back pain. For conditions with a strong psychosomatic element, relaxation appears to have some potential benefits although these may not be long term. Since relaxation therapies are almost risk free, they can be recommended as an adjunctive therapy.

REFERENCES

1. Ostelo RW, van Tulder MW, Vlaeyen JW, Linton SJ, Morley SJ, Assendelft WJ. Behavioural treatment for chronic low-back pain. The Cochrane Database of Systematic Reviews 2005, Issue 1. Art. No.: CD002014

2. van Tulder MW, Koes B, Malmivaara A. Outcome of non-invasive treatment modalities on back pain: an evidence-based review. Eur Spine J 2006;15(Suppl. 1):S64–81

3. Bogaards MC, ter Kuile MM. Treatment of recurrent tension headache: a meta-analytic review. Clin J Pain 1994;10:174–190

4. Larsson B, Melin L. Chronic headaches in adolescents: treatment in a school setting with relaxation training as compared with information-contact and self-registration. Pain 1986;25:325–336

5. Engel JM, Rapoff MA, Pressman AR. Long-term follow-up of relaxation training for pediatric headache disorders. Headache 1992;32:152–156

6. Passchier J, Van Den Bree MB, Emmen HH, Osterhaus SO, Orlebeke JF, Verhage F. Relaxation training in school classes does not reduce headache complaints. Headache 1990;30:660–664

7. van Dixhoorn J, White A. Relaxation therapy for rehabilitation and prevention in ischaemic heart disease: a systematic review and meta-analysis. Eur J Cardiovasc Prev Rehabil 2005;12:193–202

8. Holroyd KA, Penzien DB. Pharmacological versus non-pharmacological prophylaxis of recurrent migraine headache: a meta-analytic review of clinical trials. Pain 1990;42:1–13

9. Fichtel A, Larsson B. Relaxation treatment administered by school nurses to adolescents with recurrent headaches. Headache 2004;44:545–554

10. Larsson B, Carlsson J, Fichtel A, Melin L. Relaxation treatment of adolescent headache sufferers: results from a school-based replication series. Headache 2005;45:692–704

11. Hermann C, Kim M, Blanchard EB. Behavioral and prophylactic pharmacological intervention studies of pediatric migraine: an exploratory meta-analysis. Pain 1995;60:239–256

12. NIH Technology Assessment Statement. Integration of behavioral and relaxation approaches into the treatment of chronic pain and insomnia. NIH Technol Assess Statement 1995;16–18:1–34

13. Reinhardt U. Investigations into synchronisation of heart rate and musical rhythm in a relaxation therapy in patients with cancer pain. [In German.] Forsch Komplementärmed 1999;6:135–141

14. Haase O, Schwenk W, Hermann C, Muller JM. Guided imagery and relaxation in conventional colorectal resections: a randomized, controlled, partially blinded trial. Dis Colon Rectum 2005;48:1955–1963

15. Good M, Anderson GC, Ahn S, Cong X, Stanton-Hicks M. Relaxation and music reduce pain following intestinal surgery. Res Nurs Health 2005;28:240–251

16. Wahlund K, List T, Larsson B. Treatment of temporomandibular disorders among adolescents: a comparison between occlusal appliance, relaxation training, and brief information. Acta Odontol Scand 2003;61:203–211

17. Irvin JH, Domar AD, Clark C, Zuttermeister PC, Friedman R. The effects of relaxation response training on menopausal symptoms. J Psychosom Obstet Gynecol 1996;17: 202–207

18. Boyce PM, Talley NJ, Balaam B, Koloski NA, Truman G. A randomized controlled trial of cognitive behavior therapy, relaxation training, and routine clinical care for the irritable bowel syndrome. Am J Gastroenterol 2003;98:2209–2218

19. Lundgren S, Stenstrom CH. Muscle relaxation training and quality of life in rheumatoid arthritis. A randomized controlled clinical trial. Scand J Rheumatol 1999;28:47–53

20. Carroll D, Seers K. Relaxation for the relief of chronic pain: a systematic review. J Adv Nurs 1998;27:476–487

SHIATSU

SYNONYMS

Acupressure.

DEFINITION

Therapy of Japanese origin in which pressure is applied with mainly the fingers or hands to certain points of the body.

RELATED TECHNIQUES

Bodywork therapy, massage.

BACKGROUND

Applying finger pressure to specific acupuncture points throughout the body has long been used in Japan and other Asian countries. In Japanese the term shiatsu literally means finger (*shi*) pressure (*atsu*). It can, however, also involve palm or elbow pressure, stretching, massaging and other manual techniques.

TRADITIONAL CONCEPTS

Health is viewed to be a state of balance, which is maintained by the flow of life energy along specific meridians. A disease state is believed to occur when the energy flow is blocked, deficient or in excess. A goal of shiatsu is to restore the normal flow of life energy using finger and palm pressure, stretching, massaging and other bodywork techniques.

SCIENTIFIC RATIONALE

The soft-tissue manipulation of cutaneous and subcutaneous structures may improve blood circulation and may reduce muscle pain and tension. The acupuncture points to which pressure is applied are sites at which nerves can be stimulated. Shiatsu could thus be a method of affecting the nervous and muscular systems, similar to massage and acupuncture.

PRACTITIONERS

Shiatsu is practised by a number of different health-care professionals. There are training courses but most practitioners are not medically qualified.

CONDITIONS FREQUENTLY TREATED

Musculoskeletal and psychological conditions, including neck pain, shoulder pain and lower back pain, arthritis, depression and anxiety.[1]

TYPICAL SESSION

Normally patients remain fully clothed during a treatment session. It typically lasts about an hour. A practitioner will generally take details of a client's health before giving a treatment.

COURSE OF TREATMENT

Depending on the condition being treated, one treatment or a series of treatments may be recommended.

CLINICAL EVIDENCE

Uncontrolled studies report pain relief in patients treated with shiatsu.[2,3] Very few CCTs exist. In patients with fibromyalgia, water shiatsu was reported to reduce pain whereas massage did not.[4]

RISKS

CONTRAINDICATIONS

Phlebitis, deep vein thrombosis, burns, skin infections, eczema, open wounds, bone fractures and advanced osteoporosis.

PRECAUTIONS/WARNINGS

Cancer, myocardial infarction, osteoporosis and pregnancy. Shiatsu should generally be considered as an adjunctive treatment, not as an alternative to conventional care.

SECTION THREE

ADVERSE EFFECTS

Adverse effects are extremely rare. Serious adverse events such as jugular vein thrombosis[5] and stroke[6] have been reported. Mild to moderate pain during application of pressure is reported by most patients.

INTERACTIONS

None known.

RISK–BENEFIT ASSESSMENT

There are not sufficient data available from rigorous trials to suggest that shiatsu is effective for reducing pain of any origin. Adverse events have been reported and therefore the risk–benefit ratio has to be negative.

REFERENCES

1. Harris PE, Pooley N. What do shiatsu practitioners treat? A nationwide survey. Complement Ther Med 1998;6:30–35
2. Inagaki J, Yoneda J, Ito M, Nogaki H. Psychophysiological effect of massage and shiatsu while in the prone position with face down. Nurs Health Sci 2002;4(3 Suppl.):A5–6
3. Brady LH, Henry K, Luth JF 2nd, Casper-Bruett KK. The effects of shiatsu on lower back pain. J Holist Nurs 2001;19:57–70
4. Faull K. A pilot study of the comparative effectiveness of two water-based treatments for fibromyalgia syndrome: Watsu and Aix massage. J Bodywork Mov Ther 2005;9: 202–210
5. Wada Y, Yanagihara C, Nishimura Y. Internal jugular vein thrombosis associated with shiatsu massage of the neck. J Neurol Neurosurg Psychiatry 2005;76:142–143
6. Elliott MA, Taylor LP. 'Shiatsu sympathectomy': ICA dissection associated with a shiatsu massage. Neurology 2002;58:1302–1304

SPIRITUAL HEALING

SYNONYMS/SUBCATEGORIES

Distant healing, faith healing, intercessory prayer, paranormal healing, psychic healing, Reiki, therapeutic touch.

DEFINITION

The direct interaction between one individual (the healer) and a second (sick) individual with the intention of bringing about an improvement or cure of the illness.[1]

RELATED TECHNIQUES

All types of energy healing systems.

TRADITIONAL CONCEPTS

Spiritual healing can be traced as far back as the Bible (New Testament, *1 Corinthians* 12:9) where it was listed among the gifts bestowed on the faithful. It has always had its adherents and, in recent years, has gained widespread popularity in the US, the UK and other countries. Spiritual healers believe that the therapeutic effect results from the channelling of healing 'energy' from an assumed source via the healer to the patient. The central claim of healers is that they promote or facilitate self-healing in the patient.

SCIENTIFIC RATIONALE

There is no scientific evidence to support the existence of this 'energy', nor is there a scientific rationale for any other concept underlying spiritual healing.

PRACTITIONERS

In the UK around 14,000 members are today registered in nine separate healing organisations. In the US its related therapies, therapeutic touch and Reiki, boast many thousands of healers. Therapeutic touch was developed in the early 1970s by Dora Kunz and Dolores Krieger and the technique is taught at numerous US institutions and universities. Krieger claims she has personally taught therapeutic touch to more than 48,000 health-care professionals in 75 countries. Most healers are not medically qualified and there is no mandatory training. Members of the UK Confederation of Healing Organisations have, however, a minimum of 2 years training. Most US practitioners of therapeutic touch are trained nurses.

CONDITIONS FREQUENTLY TREATED

Healers do not usually relate to the disease entities of conventional medicine. Their aim is to help the patient in more general terms, for instance by increasing well-being. Many healers treat patients with chronic pain or emotional problems. Patients suffering from chronic pain are more likely to engage in religious practices than healthy individuals.[2]

TYPICAL SESSION

The healer discusses the problem with the patient to gain some understanding of it. Subsequently, the patient may be asked to lie or sit down and the therapist may scan the patient's body with his or her hands at a distance and channel healing 'energy' through his or her body towards the patient.

COURSE OF TREATMENT

A typical course may consist of eight or more single sessions. Often, several courses of treatment are given within a year.

CLINICAL EVIDENCE

A systematic review[3] of all types of healing included 23 placebo-controlled RCTs involving almost 3000 patients, many of them suffering from chronic pain. About half of these studies yielded a positive result, suggesting that spiritual healing is effective. However, these trials had numerous methodological limitations so no firm conclusions could be drawn. An update of this review included eight further non-randomised and nine randomised clinical trials.[4] These additional data collectively shifted the weight of the evidence against the notion that healing is more than a placebo. Cochrane reviews found no convincing evidence that intercessory prayer alleviates ill health of any type.[5] The largest RCT of intercessory prayer failed to show that healing is associated with specific therapeutic effects.[6] A recent RCT with 20 chronic pain patients showed that spiritual healing has no effects on pain over and above placebo.[7]

RISKS

CONTRAINDICATIONS

Psychiatric illness.

PRECAUTIONS/WARNINGS

None known.

ADVERSE EFFECTS

Sensations like heat or tingling are often reported in areas under the hands of the healer. If patients are led to believe in 'supernatural' powers or 'energies', which, in fact, do not exist, healing might undermine rational thinking in general with detrimental effects far beyond health care.

INTERACTIONS

None known.

RISK–BENEFIT ASSESSMENT

The best evidence available to date fails to demonstrate that spiritual healing is associated with specific therapeutic effects. Healing is not entirely free of risks. Thus, the risk–benefit balance is not positive. Healing cannot be recommended as a reliable method for pain control, particularly not as a substitute for conventional therapies.

REFERENCES

1. Hodges RD, Scofield AM. Is spiritual healing a valid and effective therapy? J R Soc Med 1995;88:203–207
2. Rippentrop EA, Altmaier EM, Chen JJ, Found EM, Keffala VJ. The relationship between religion/spirituality and physical health, mental health, and pain in a chronic pain population. Pain 2005;116:311–321
3. Astin J, Harkness E, Ernst E. The efficacy of spiritual healing: a systematic review of randomised trials. Ann Intern Med 2000;132:903–910
4. Ernst E. Distant healing – an 'update' of a systematic review. Wien Klin Wochenschr 2003; 115:241–245
5. Roberts L, Ahmed I, Hall S. Intercessory prayer for the alleviation of ill health. The Cochrane Database of Systematic Reviews 2000, Issue 2. Art. No.: CD000368
6. Krucoff MW, Crater SW, Gallup D, Blankenship JC, Cuffe M, Guarneri M, Krieger RA, Kshettry VR, Morris K, Oz M, Pichard A, Sketch MH Jr, Koenig HG, Mark D, Lee KL. Music, imagery, touch, and prayer as adjuncts to interventional cardiac care: the Monitoring and Actualisation of Noetic Trainings (MANTRA) II randomised study. Lancet 2005;366:211–217
7. Lyvers M, Barling N, Harding-Clark J. Effect of belief in 'psychic healing' on self-reported pain in chronic pain sufferers. J Psychosom Res 2006;60:59–61

STATIC MAGNETS

DEFINITION

Magnets produce energy in the form of magnetic fields. Two main types of magnets exist:

- static or permanent magnets where the magnetic field is unchanging and is generated by the spin of the electrons of the material itself
- electromagnets where a magnetic field is generated only when an electric current runs through them.[1]

The magnetic field generated by the latter can be oscillating while the former is constant.

RELATED TECHNIQUES

Electromagnetic field therapy.

BACKGROUND

The majority of magnets marketed to consumers for health purposes are static magnets with varying strengths, typically between 30 and 500 mTesla. Magnets have been incorporated into arm and leg wraps, belts, mattress pads, necklaces, shoe inserts and bracelets. They are usually made from iron, steel or alloys. Today, the market for magnets for pain relief amounts to an estimated US$5 billion worldwide.[1]

TRADITIONAL CONCEPTS

Magnets have long been used in attempts to treat pain. Their use probably began when the presence of naturally magnetised stones, also called lodestones, was first noticed. Later, healers claimed that magnetic fields existed in the blood, organs and other parts of the body and that people became ill when their magnetic fields were depleted. Thus, healers marketed magnets as a means of restoring a person's magnetic fields. More recently, magnets have been marketed for a wide range of diseases and conditions, including pain.

SCIENTIFIC RATIONALE

None of the theories or claims put forward for static magnets have been conclusively proven. It is conceivable that magnets might increase the temperature of the area of the body being exposed to them and some experiments suggest that magnets might have effects on cell function.

PRACTITIONERS

The vast majority of static magnets are marketed to consumers directly via health-product outlets or the internet. CAM practitioners might recommend magnets for a large number of different conditions.

CONDITIONS FREQUENTLY TREATED

Pain of any type, arthritis, respiratory problems, high blood pressure, circulatory problems and stress.

TYPICAL SESSION

Static magnets are usually bought and used by patients directly, often without consulting a health-care professional. Typically, the magnets are placed directly on the skin or placed inside clothing with close contact to the body.

COURSE OF TREATMENT

Depending on the condition, treatment with static magnets may vary; it may comprise days or weeks of continuous or interrupted use.

CLINICAL EVIDENCE

A Cochrane review of non-surgical treatment for carpal tunnel syndrome reported that magnet therapy did not demonstrate symptom benefit when compared to placebo.[2] For plantar heel pain, a Cochrane review reported that there is no evidence of effectiveness for insoles with magnetic foil,[3] which is supported by the results of a further double-blind RCT[4] ($n = 101$) and another double-blind RCT ($n = 83$) of non-specific foot pain.[5] For chronic knee pain, a double-blind RCT ($n = 43$) reported that wearing pads containing magnets appears to reduce pain and enhance physical function.[6] In patients with osteoarthritis of the knee, a small ($n = 29$) double-blind RCT showed a decrease of visual analogue scale pain scores compared with placebo at 4 hours of treatment. There were no differences in any measures of effectiveness after 6 weeks of self-treatment.[7] Pain from osteoarthritis of the knee and hip ($n = 194$) was found to decrease when wearing magnetic bracelets for 12 weeks, but whether this response was the result of specific or non-specific effects remained uncertain.[8] For patients with rheumatoid arthritis of the knee, a magnetic device demonstrated pain reduction in comparison to baseline, but no difference compared to a weak magnetic control device.[9] Sleeping on magnetic mattresses resulted in a decrease in pain and fatigue compared with baseline in fibromyalgia patients,[10] which is supported by the results of another RCT.[11] Two pilot studies assessing patients with chronic low back pain found no differences when magnet therapy was compared with placebo and a weak magnetic device.[12,13] For delayed-onset muscle soreness the evidence from RCTs shows no effect of magnet therapy compared with placebo.[14,15] Other single RCTs, which require independent replication, reported positive results for chronic pelvic pain,[16] diabetic neuropathy,[17] shoulder pain[18] and dysmenorrhoea,[19] whereas negative reports exist for wrist pain.[20]

RISKS

CONTRAINDICATIONS

Pregnancy and lactation (see p. 4). Pacemakers, insulin pumps.

PRECAUTIONS/WARNINGS

Wounds, acute sprains, inflammation.

ADVERSE EFFECTS

Static magnets are generally considered to be safe. Adverse effects are rare but a reddening of the skin on the area of application has been observed.

INTERACTIONS

None known.

INDIRECT RISKS

The possibility of indirect harm exists if treatment with magnets delays access to effective health care.

RISK–BENEFIT ASSESSMENT

The evidence is not compelling for the effectiveness of static magnets for reducing any type of pain above non-specific effects. However, given that adverse events are rare, magnets may be worth trying.

REFERENCES

1. http://nccam.nih.gov/health/magnet/magnet.htm 6 Dec 2005
2. O'Connor D, Marshall S, Massy-Westropp N. Non-surgical treatment (other than steroid injection) for carpal tunnel syndrome. The Cochrane Database of Systematic Reviews 2003, Issue 1. Art. No.: CD003219
3. Crawford F, Thomson C. Interventions for treating plantar heel pain. The Cochrane Database of Systematic Reviews 2003, Issue 3. Art. No.: CD000416
4. Winemiller MH, Billow RG, Laskowski ER, Harmsen WS. Effect of magnetic vs sham-magnetic insoles on plantar heel pain: a randomized controlled trial. JAMA 2003;290: 1474–1478
5. Winemiller MH, Billow RG, Laskowski ER, Harmsen WS. Effect of magnetic vs sham-magnetic insoles on nonspecific foot pain in the workplace: a randomized, double-blind, placebo-controlled trial. Mayo Clin Proc 2005;80:1138–1145

6. Hinman MR, Ford J, Heyl H. Effects of static magnets on chronic knee pain and physical function: a double-blind study. Altern Ther Health Med 2002;8:50–55

7. Wolsko PM, Eisenberg DM, Simon LS, Davis RB, Walleczek J, Mayo-Smith M, Kaptchuk TJ, Phillips RS. Double-blind placebo-controlled trial of static magnets for the treatment of osteoarthritis of the knee: results of a pilot study. Altern Ther Health Med 2004;10:36–43

8. Harlow T, Greaves C, White A, Brown L, Hart A, Ernst E. Randomised controlled trial of magnetic bracelets for relieving pain in osteoarthritis of the hip and knee. BMJ 2004;329:1450–1454

9. Segal NA, Toda Y, Huston J, Saeki Y, Shimizu M, Fuchs H, Shimaoka Y, Holcomb R, McLean MJ. Two configurations of static magnetic fields for treating rheumatoid arthritis of the knee: a double-blind clinical trial. Arch Phys Med Rehabil 2001;82:1453–1460

10. Colbert AP, Markov MS, Banerji M, Pilla AA. Magnetic mattress pad use in patients with fibromyalgia: a randomized double-blind pilot study. J Back Muskuloskelet Rehabil 1999;13:19–31

11. Alfano AP, Taylor AG, Foresman PA, Dunkl PR, McConnell GG, Conaway MR, Gillies GT. Static magnetic fields for treatment of fibromyalgia: a randomized controlled trial. J Altern Complement Med 2001;7:53–64

12. Collacott EA, Zimmerman JT, White DW, Rindone JP. Bipolar permanent magnets for the treatment of chronic low back pain: a pilot study. JAMA 2000;283:1322–1325

13. Langford J, McCarthy PW. Randomised controlled clinical trial of magnet use in chronic low back pain; a pilot study. Clin Chiropractic 2005;8:13–19

14. Reeser JC, Smith DT, Fischer V, Berg R, Liu K, Untiedt C, Kubista M. Static magnetic fields neither prevent nor diminish symptoms and signs of delayed onset muscle soreness. Arch Phys Med Rehabil 2005;86:565–570

15. Mikesky AE, Hayden MW. Effect of static magnetic therapy on recovery from delayed onset muscle soreness. Phys Ther Sport 2005;6:188–194

16. Brown CS, Ling FW, Wan JY, Pilla AA. Efficacy of static magnetic field therapy in chronic pelvic pain: a double-blind pilot study. Am J Obstet Gynecol 2002;187:1581–1587

17. Weintraub MI, Wolfe GI, Barohn RA, Cole SP, Parry GJ, Hayat G, Cohen JA, Page JC, Bromberg MB, Schwartz SL; Magnetic Research Group. Static magnetic field therapy for symptomatic diabetic neuropathy: a randomized, double-blind, placebo-controlled trial. Arch Phys Med Rehabil 2003;84:736–746

18. Kanai S, Taniguchi N, Kawamoto M, Endo H, Higashino H. Effect of static magnetic field on pain associated with frozen shoulder. Pain Clinic 2004;16:173–179

19. Eccles NK. A randomized, double-blinded, placebo-controlled pilot study to investigate the effectiveness of a static magnet to relieve dysmenorrhea. J Altern Complement Med 2005;11:681–687

20. Carter R, Aspy CB, Mold J. The effectiveness of magnet therapy for treatment of wrist pain attributed to carpal tunnel syndrome. J Fam Pract 2002;51:38–40

TAI CHI

DEFINITION

A system of movements and postures rooted in ancient Chinese philosophy and martial arts used to enhance mental and physical health.

RELATED TECHNIQUES

Qigong.

BACKGROUND

Tai chi has a long history in China and is widely practised there. It has also become increasingly popular in many Western countries. A number of different styles and forms were developed from the original 13 postures, believed to have been created in the early 12th century. The various forms of tai chi comprise a series of postures linked by gentle and graceful movements.

TRADITIONAL CONCEPTS

Influenced by Confucian and Buddhist philosophy, tai chi is based on the principles of the two opposing life forces, yin and yang. Ill health is viewed as an imbalance between yin, the female, receptive principle, and yang, the male, creative principle. The alternating movements and postures are thought to stabilise these flowing energies, creating inner and outer harmony and emotional balance.

SCIENTIFIC RATIONALE

The slow movements between different postures that are normally held for a short period of time are physical stimuli with effects on the cardiovascular and muscular systems. These stimuli, much like other physical exercise, result in muscular adaptation, which ultimately leads to increased muscle strength if performed regularly and with adequate intensity. In addition to adaptation processes, these effects produce better cardiovascular function,[1] and may enhance strength, balance and coordination.[2]

PRACTITIONERS

Teachers should have a basic understanding of human anatomy and physiology and should have some knowledge of the philosophy and historical background of tai chi. Ideally, teachers have had at least 5 years of experience and have studied with a master before undertaking independent teaching. There are, however, no generally acknowledged minimum requirements.

CONDITIONS FREQUENTLY TREATED

Osteoporosis, depression, stress-related conditions and high or low blood pressure.

TYPICAL SESSION

Tai chi is usually taught in classes of five people to 10 or more. The atmosphere during practice is quiet and relaxed but intense. The student should maintain a level of concentration and should not be distracted by external influences. The movements are performed simultaneously by the group, responding to advice and corrections by the teacher. Tai chi is a lifelong endeavour and regular practice is essential in achieving beneficial effects.

COURSE OF TREATMENT

The various forms take between 5 and 30 minutes to complete. Daily practice is ideal but at least twice-weekly exercises are recommended. The best time for practice is said to be early in the morning.

CLINICAL EVIDENCE

A systematic review of health outcomes in patients with chronic conditions identified nine RCTs.[3] It concluded that, although tai chi appears to have physiological and psychosocial benefits and also appears to be safe and effective in promoting balance control, flexibility and cardiovascular fitness in older patients with chronic conditions, limitations or biases exist in most studies, and it is difficult to draw firm conclusions about the benefits reported. As an option for treating rheumatoid arthritis, a Cochrane review suggested that tai chi is beneficial for lower extremity range of motion, particularly ankle range of motion, and does not exacerbate the symptoms of rheumatoid arthritis.[4] Two RCTs also report beneficial effects in patients with osteoarthritis.[5,6]

RISKS

CONTRAINDICATIONS

Contraindications and precautions are largely based on common sense (e.g. severe osteoporosis, severe heart conditions, acute back pain, knee problems, sprains and fractures). Usually it can be safely practised during pregnancy and lactation.

PRECAUTIONS/WARNINGS

Before starting tai chi, older individuals should be carefully examined for any of the above or other contraindications.

ADVERSE EFFECTS

Adverse effects are rare, but may include delayed-onset muscle soreness, pulled ligaments or ankle sprains.

INTERACTIONS

None known.

INDIRECT RISK

Tai chi should be viewed as an adjunctive treatment, not as an alternative to conventional medical care.

RISK–BENEFIT ASSESSMENT

There is only limited evidence from rigorous clinical trials to suggest that tai chi is effective for reducing pain. However, it appears that it has a range of psychological effects similar to those established for other physical exercise, which may be beneficial for patients with pain. Given the mild nature and the rare occurrence of adverse events when instructed by a responsible teacher, it is also worth considering as a general measure for promoting a healthy lifestyle.

REFERENCES

1. Taylor-Piliae RE, Froelicher ES. Effectiveness of Tai Chi exercise in improving aerobic capacity: a meta-analysis. J Cardiovasc Nurs 2004;19:48–57
2. Wolfson L, Whipple R, Derby C, Judge J, King M, Amerman P, Schmidt J, Smyers D. Balance and strength in older adults: intervention gains and tai chi maintenance. J Am Geriatr Soc 1996;44:498–506
3. Wang C, Collet JP, Lau J. The effect of Tai Chi on health outcomes in patients with chronic conditions: a systematic review. Arch Intern Med 2004;164:493–501
4. Han A, Robinson V, Judd M, Taixiang W, Wells G, Tugwell P. Tai chi for treating rheumatoid arthritis. The Cochrane Database of Systematic Reviews 2004, Issue 3. Art. No.: CD004849
5. Song R, Lee EO, Lam P, Bae SC. Effects of tai chi exercise on pain, balance, muscle strength, and perceived difficulties in physical functioning in older women with osteoarthritis: a randomized clinical trial. J Rheumatol 2003;30:2039–2044
6. Hartman CA, Manos TM, Winter C, Hartman DM, Li B, Smith JC. Effects of T'ai Chi training on function and quality of life indicators in older adults with osteoarthritis. J Am Geriatr Soc 2000;48:1553–1559

YOGA

DEFINITION

A mind–body intervention including gentle stretching, exercises for breath control and meditation.

RELATED TECHNIQUES

Meditation, breathing, exercise.

BACKGROUND

The word yoga is derived from the Sanskrit word *yuj*, which means 'to yoke', reflecting its purpose in joining mind and body in harmonious relaxation. Indian symbols dating from 3000

BCE suggest that yoga was in existence at that time. Records of the Yoga Sutras, the eight aspects of spiritual enlightenment, date from about 2300 years ago and include principles of ethical behaviour. Most widely used in the West is hatha yoga, which includes the poses (*asanas*), breath control (*pranayama*) and meditation that are aimed at bringing the body to a state of perfect health and stillness, thus achieving heightened awareness. Yoga devotees practice regularly and increase their skills and techniques throughout their lifetime. Today yoga is widely practised around the world; it does not require spiritual or religious beliefs.

TRADITIONAL CONCEPTS

Yoga is believed to increase the vital energy (*prana*) and to facilitate its flow. The body becomes a 'fit vehicle for the spirit'. Poor diet, stress and other factors are believed to block the natural flow of prana, leaving the body vulnerable.

SCIENTIFIC RATIONALE

The regular practice of yoga induces a deep sense of relaxation which may be beneficial. Physical benefits of regular practice include bodily suppleness and muscular strength. Mental benefits include feelings of well-being and, possibly, reduction of sympathetic drive. Yoga breathing exercises counter the rapid breathing that accompanies the stress response and may, in addition, reduce muscular spasm and expand the available lung capacity.

PRACTITIONERS

Although yoga can be self-taught, it is preferable to learn with supervision. Practitioners or teachers should have the knowledge and experience to ensure that benefit is obtained without harm, e.g. overstretching joints and muscles. No uniform credentialing exists and no licensing is currently required to teach yoga.

CONDITIONS FREQUENTLY TREATED

Pain syndromes such as arthritis, back pain and headaches as well as anxiety, cardiovascular problems, gastrointestinal complaints, insomnia, premenstrual syndrome, respiratory problems and stress. Also used in pregnancy as a preparation for childbirth. Yoga can also be used by healthy people to gain self-mastery.

TYPICAL SESSION

Classes last about 1 hour and involve some theoretical introduction, supervised postures and breathing exercises usually leading to a period of deep relaxation or sometimes meditation. Precise content and form vary considerably.

COURSE OF TREATMENT

Yoga is probably best practised daily for maximum benefit. It should be regarded as a long-term commitment.

CLINICAL EVIDENCE

According to a large UK consumer survey, yoga leads to more patient satisfaction than any other CAM modality.[1] RCTs suggested that yoga is an effective symptomatic therapy for back pain[2-4] and carpal tunnel syndrome.[5] Controlled trials suggest that yoga may reduce joint stiffness in osteoarthritis.[6] Unfortunately, the methodological quality of many yoga studies is poor.

RISKS

CONTRAINDICATIONS

No absolute contraindications exist but extreme postures are contraindicated in pregnancy. Meditation may precipitate feelings of unreality and depersonalisation and should therefore not be used by people with a history of psychotic or personality disorder.

PRECAUTIONS/WARNINGS

Physical damage can occur from overstretching either healthy or, more particularly, diseased joints and ligaments. Those learning yoga for treatment of medical conditions are advised to inform their doctors and to seek supervision by an experienced and knowledgeable teacher who will adapt the postures in appropriate ways.

ADVERSE EFFECTS

Drowsiness may occur and one case is documented where Kapalabhati pranayama has been associated with pneumothorax.[7]

INTERACTIONS

None known. Possible additive effects on antihypertensive medication.

RISK–BENEFIT ASSESSMENT

Regular practice of yoga is a largely safe method of improving general health and well-being. Its role as an adjunct to the management of some pain syndromes, e.g. back pain, is reasonably well established. Risks are not normally serious provided yoga is practised in accordance with accepted principles. Thus, for some conditions, the benefits of this approach can outweigh the risks.

REFERENCES

1. Anonymous. Healing power. Which 2001;Dec:35–37
2. Galantino ML, Bzdewka TM, Eissler-Russo JL, Holbrook ML, Mogck EP, Geigle P, Farrar JT. The impact of modified hatha yoga on chronic low back pain: a pilot study. Altern Ther Health Med 2004;10:56–59
3. Williams KA, Petronis J, Smith D, Goodrich D, Wu J, Ravi N, Doyle EJ Jr, Gregory Juckett R, Munoz Kolar M, Gross R, Steinberg L. Effect of Iyengar yoga therapy for chronic low back pain. Pain 2005;115:107–117
4. Sherman KJ, Cherkin DC, Erro J, Miglioretti DL, Deyo RA. Comparing yoga, exercise, and a self-care book for chronic low back pain: a randomized, controlled trial. Ann Intern Med 2005;143:849–856
5. Garfinkel MS, Singhal A, Katz WA, Allan DA, Reshetar R, Schumacher HR Jr. Yoga-based intervention for carpal tunnel syndrome: a randomized trial. JAMA 1998;280: 1601–1603
6. Garfinkel MS, Schumacher HR, Husain A, Levy M, Reshetar RA. Evaluation of a yoga based regimen for treatment of osteoarthritis of the hands. J Rheumatol 1994;21: 2341–2343
7. Johnson DB, Tierney MJ, Sadighi PJ. Kapallabhati pranayama: breath of fire or cause of pneumothorax? A case report. Chest 2004;125:1951–1952

SECTION THREE

SECTION THREE

Table 3.3 **Other complementary therapies which have been tested for effectiveness or are used frequently**

Therapy	Description	Conditions frequently treated	Safety concerns
Anthroposophical medicine	An approach that integrates conventional medicine with an exploration of inner feelings and the meaning of illness. Treatment may involve both conventional and CAM interventions	Any condition including cancer	None other than those of the individual therapies
Back school	A structured educational programme, usually in a group setting, designed to inform patients about low back problems	Back pain	None known
Breath therapy	A Western mind–body therapy integrating body awareness, breathing, meditation and movement	Proprioception and low back pain	None known
Chelation therapy	A method for removing toxins, minerals and metabolic wastes from the bloodstream and vessel walls using intravenous ethylene diamine tetraacetic acid (EDTA) infusions.	To induce regression of arteriosclerotic lesions, e.g. in ischaemic heart disease, and intermittent claudication or for stroke prevention or as an alternative to bypass surgery (in conventional medicine, it is an accepted intervention for heavy metal poisoning)	Faintness, gastrointestinal symptoms, proteinuria, renal failure, arrhythmias, tetany, hypocalcaemia, hypoglycaemia, hypotension, bone marrow depression, prolonged bleeding time, convulsions, respiratory arrest and autoimmune diseases, phlebitis and pain
CO_2 applications	Subcutaneous CO_2 insufflations or immersion in CO_2-containing water used as vasodilator	Intermittent claudication due to peripheral arterial occlusive disease	Infection, risk of cardiac decompensation
Cranial electrotherapy	The use of low-level electrical current applied to the head for therapeutic purposes	Pain, anxiety, depression, insomnia, substance abuse	None known
Distraction therapy	Various methods of distraction aimed at taking the patient's mind off a painful or difficult procedure by concentrating on something else	Painful and difficult procedures	None known

Enzyme therapy	Plant-derived and pancreatic enzymes given orally with the aim of improving the digestive and immune system	A wide variety of conditions including chronic digestive disorders, inflammatory and viral diseases, multiple sclerosis and cancer	Increased risk of bleeding
Exercise	Aerobic or anaerobic physical exercise sometimes with specific targets under physiotherapeutic supervision	Many conditions including cardiovascular problems, musculoskeletal conditions, depression	Injuries, ischaemia
Homotoxicology	A form of therapy that uses homeopathically diluted remedies with a view to eliminating toxins from the body, following concepts that differ from those of homeopathy	Any condition	None known
Low-level laser therapy	Applying wavelengths of light at certain intensities delivered by laser or other monochromatic sources	Soft-tissue injuries, chronic pain, wound healing, nerve regeneration	None known
Magnetic field therapy	Permanent or pulsed magnetic fields applied to head or other part of body; often used with acupuncture	Mainly pain control but also other purposes, e.g. healing of wounds, fractures and other injuries	Contraindicated in pregnancy, pacemakers, myasthenia gravis, bleeding disorders
Mind–body therapies	A range of therapies focusing on the interactions between the brain, mind, body and behaviour. See also Autogenic training (p. 106), Biofeedback (p. 110), Hypnosis (p. 130), Imagery (p. 132), Meditation (p. 140), Qigong (p. 152), Relaxation (p. 158), Tai chi (p. 167), Yoga (p. 169)	Any condition	See respective chapters
Mobilisation	Manual treatments aimed at freeing soft tissue around a joint; includes traction or stretching and rotation of a joint within its range of motion	Pain	Pulled muscles and ligaments, bruises
Ornish programme	Intensive lifestyle (e.g. smoking cessation) and dietary changes, exercise and stress management	Heart disease	Malnutrition

table continues

SECTION THREE

Therapy	Description	Conditions frequently treated	Safety concerns
Oxygen therapy	Use of oxygen injections; use of hyperbaric oxygen for unconventional indications (sometimes used for ozone therapy)	Stroke and other brain injury; many conditions, especially chronic; physical fitness enhancement	Excess free radicals, peroxidation; risk of embolism or infection with intravenous injection
Prolotherapy	Injections of dextrose solutions, which cause a localised inflammation, increase the blood supply and are thought to stimulate tissue repair and pain relief	Spinal pain	Exaggerated inflammatory response with pain increase
Reiki	A form of spiritual healing (see p. 162)	Chronic pain, emotional problems	None known
Stress management	An umbrella term for psychological interventions to reduce stress	Stress	None known
Tragerwork	Use of a therapist's hands and mind to communicate lightness and encourage 'playfulness'	Many chronic physical and psychological conditions	None known
Transcutaneous electrical nerve stimulation; percutaneous electrical nerve stimulation	Electrical stimulation of the skin to relieve pain by interfering with the neural transmission of signals from underlying pain receptors	Pain (mostly chronic)	None known
Vedic vibration technology	The use a refined impulse of Vedic sound or Vedic vibration to restore functioning	Any condition	None known
Vegetarian diet	Nutrition without meat or fish products	Rheumatic problems, cardiovascular disease, cancer	Malnutrition
Water immersion	Immersion in water during, for example, labour and/or delivery or used to treat musculoskeletal conditions	Labour pain, back pain	Infection, neonate inhaling water
Water injection	Subcutaneous injection of sterile water over trigger points	Painful conditions, particularly due to myofascial trigger points	Local pain, bruising, infection

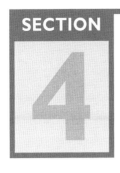

Medicines

ARNICA
(Arnica montana)

SOURCE
Flowers.

MAIN CONSTITUENTS
Sesquiterpene lactones (helenalin), volatile oil, flavonoids.

BACKGROUND
Arnica is a perennial herbaceous plant native to the mountainous regions of Europe. The plant is rare and protected in several countries. The arnica plant has a bright yellow, daisy-like flower that blooms around July. Preparations made from the flowering heads are commonly used in homeopathic medicine. The name *arnica* means 'lamb's skin', which refers to its soft, hairy leaves.

EXAMPLES OF TRADITIONAL USES
Symptomatic relief of bruised tissue, joints and muscles, reduction of pain and swelling, arthritis, burns, ulcers, eczema, acne, to stimulate blood circulation and raise blood pressure. Arnica is used medicinally in homeopathic dilutions (usually oral administration) and as a herbal treatment. Undiluted arnica is toxic so the herbal version is applied topically.

PHARMACOLOGICAL ACTION
Anti-inflammatory, antimicrobial.

CONDITIONS FREQUENTLY TREATED
Pain after trauma, bruising and sprains, muscle soreness caused by exercise, post-operative ileus.

CLINICAL EVIDENCE
A systematic review of 49 prospective controlled trials of homeopathic arnica found all trials highly heterogeneous and concluded that the hypothesis that homeopathic arnica is effective could neither be proved nor rejected.[1] An earlier systematic review of homeopathic arnica with stricter inclusion criteria including eight trials found that most of the studies were burdened with severe methodological flaws and do not suggest that it is more efficacious than placebo.[2] A subsequent double-blind randomised clinical trial (RCT) ($n = 64$) found no advantage of homeopathic arnica over placebo in reducing post-operative pain, bruising and swelling in patients undergoing elective hand surgery.[3] A double-blind RCT ($n = 37$) testing a combination of homeopathic arnica and (undiluted) herbal arnica ointment after carpal-tunnel release surgery reported pain reduction compared with placebo.[4] In a double-blind RCT of 60 patients undergoing varicose vain surgery, no reduction of haematoma and pain during the post-operative course were noted with homeopathic arnica compared to placebo.[5] In a non-randomised controlled trial of 40 patients undergoing surgery following hip fractures, homeopathic arnica reduced post-operative swelling but not bleeding or pain.[6] A double-blind RCT of 93 patients undergoing total abdominal hysterectomy found no beneficial effects of homeopathic arnica on post-operative recovery compared to placebo.[7] A double-blind crossover trial found a reduction of oedema with homeopathic arnica but no effect on trismus and pain compared to placebo in patients submitting to extraction of impacted third molars.[8] Pooled results from two double-blind studies suggest that homeopathic arnica has a positive effect on muscle soreness after marathon running, but not on cell damage as measured by enzymes.[9] Two double-blind RCTs, however, found no difference in muscle soreness

scales in 50 healthy volunteers[10] and 519 marathon runners[11] receiving homeopathic arnica or placebo. Topical arnica gel was not efficacious in the prevention or resolution of laser-induced bruises compared to vehicle-only gel.[12]

DOSAGE

Arnica is toxic when taken by mouth unless diluted in homeopathic preparations.

- *Tincture*: 1:5, 45% application of 2–4 ml.
- *Poultice*: 2–3 g arnica covered with 150 ml hot water and strained after 10 min.

RISKS

CONTRAINDICATIONS

Pregnancy and lactation (see p. 4).

PRECAUTIONS/WARNINGS

Arnica is toxic by mouth unless extremely diluted (homeopathic preparations). Safe use for more than 2 weeks has not been well studied. Avoid using topical arnica on open wounds or near the eyes and mouth. Theoretically, arnica may increase the risk of bleeding.

ADVERSE EFFECTS

Allergies, stomach discomfort, nausea and vomiting, liver and kidney damage, skin rashes, eczema or lesions in the mouth. Other side effects may include muscle weakness, organ damage, coma and death. Irregular heart rhythms, rapid heartbeat, high blood pressure or failure of the heart to beat may occur when arnica is taken by mouth, especially in large doses. These adverse reactions apply to non-homeopathic preparations or to low homeopathic potencies.

OVERDOSE

Organ failure may occur from high doses.

INTERACTIONS

Anticoagulants or antiplatelet drugs.

RISK–BENEFIT ASSESSMENT

There is no convincing evidence that homeopathic arnica is useful in relieving pain after trauma or for other indications. The evidence for its usefulness in delayed-onset muscle soreness is conflicting. Arnica is safe in highly diluted homeopathic doses but toxic if undiluted. Its use can, at present, not be recommended.

REFERENCES

1. Lüdtke R, Hacke D. On the effectiveness of the homeopathic remedy *Arnica montana*. Wien Med Wschr 2005;155:482–490
2. Ernst E, Pittler MH. Efficacy of homeopathic arnica: a systematic review of placebo-controlled clinical trials. Arch Surg 1998;133:1187–1190
3. Stevinson C, Devaraj VS, Fountain-Barber A, Hawkins S, Ernst E. Homeopathic arnica for prevention of pain and bruising: randomized placebo-controlled trial in hand surgery. J R Soc Med 2003;96:60–65
4. Jeffrey SL, Belcher HJ. Use of Arnica to relieve pain after carpal-tunnel release surgery. Altern Ther Health Med 2002;8:66–68
5. Wolf M, Tamaschke C, Mayer W, Heger M. Efficacy of Arnica in varicose vein surgery: results of a randomized, double-blind, placebo-controlled pilot study. [In German.] Forsch Komplementarmed Klass Naturheilkd 2003;10:242–247

6. Wolf M, Lüdtke R, Rose O. Adjuvante Arnica-Medikation zur schwellungs- und schmerzre-duzierenden Wirkung bei operativ versorgten hüftgelenksnahen Frakturen – Kontrollierte, nicht randomisierte Therapiestudie. Allgem Hom Ztg 2002;247:141–145

7. Hart O, Mullee MA, Lewith G, Miller J. Double-blind, placebo-controlled, randomized clinical trial of homoeopathic arnica C30 for pain and infection after total abdominal hysterectomy. J R Soc Med 1997;90:73–78

8. Macedo SB, Carvalho JCT, Ferreira LR, Santos-Pinto R. Effect of *Arnica montana* on edema, tris-mus and pain after impacted molars extraction. J Dent Res 2000;79:573–577

9. Tveiten D, Bruset S. Effect of Arnica D30 in marathon runners. Pooled results from two double-blind placebo controlled studies. Homeopathy 2003;92:187–189

10. Jawara N, Lewith GT, Vickers AJ, Mullee MA, Smith C. Homoeopathic *Arnica* and *Rhus toxico-dendron* for delayed onset muscle soreness. Br Homeopath J 1997;86:10–15

11. Vickers AJ, Fisher P, Smith C, Wyllie SE, Rees R. Homeopathic Arnica 30 × is ineffective for muscle soreness after long-distance running: a randomized, double-blind, placebo-controlled trial. Clin J Pain 1998;14:227–231

12. Alonso D, Lazarus MC, Baumann L. Effects of topical arnica gel on post-laser treatment bruises. Dermatol Surg 2002;28:686–688

AVOCADO/SOYBEAN UNSAPONIFIABLES

SOURCE
Oil from avocado fruit and soy.

MAIN CONSTITUENTS
Fraction of oils (soy:avocado oil = 3:1) which, after hydrolysis, do not produce soap (e.g. sterols, volatile acids).

BACKGROUND
Avocado/soybean unsaponifiables (ASU) are a mixture of oils left over after hydrolysis. They are not chemically characterised and their pharmacologically active principles are not clearly defined. ASUs are sold as a food supplement in most countries.

EXAMPLES OF TRADITIONAL USES
Avocado has traditionally been used for a range of medicinal purposes, e.g. aphrodisiac, emmenagogue, promotion of hair growth, wound healing. However, ASU have no traditional use.

PHARMACOLOGICAL ACTION
Inhibition of interleukin-1 synthesis, stimulation of collagen synthesis, protective effects on chondrocytes, anti-inflammatory effects and anabolic effects.

CONDITIONS FREQUENTLY TREATED
Osteoarthritis pain.

CLINICAL EVIDENCE
A systematic review included four high-quality RCTs.[1] Three of these studies showed effi-cacy of ASU in the symptomatic treatment of osteoarthritis pain. One RCT showed no dif-ference between ASU and placebo in terms of joint space in osteoarthritic hip joints. In a

subgroup analysis, however, such a structural change was apparent in patients with advanced disease.[2] The structure-modifying effect of ASU is also supported by *in vitro* studies on isolated chondrocytes.[3]

DOSAGE
300–600 mg/day.

RISKS
CONTRAINDICATIONS
Pregnancy and lactation (see p. 4).

PRECAUTIONS/WARNINGS
None known.

ADVERSE EFFECTS
None known; in the RCTs adverse effect rates were similar to those of placebo.

INTERACTIONS
None known.

QUALITY ISSUES
Quality could vary from product to product.

RISK–BENEFIT ASSESSMENT
The available evidence suggests efficacy of ASU for pain relief in osteoarthritis. Whether ASU have disease-modifying properties is presently not clear. As the risks seem to be minor, the risk–benefit balance is positive and ASU are a treatment worth considering for osteoarthritis.

REFERENCES
1. Ernst E. Avocado-soybean unsaponifiables (ASU) for osteoarthritis – a systematic review. Clin Rheumatol 2003;22:285–288
2. Lequesne M, Maheu E, Cadet C, Dreiser RL. Structural effect of avocado/soybean unsaponifiables on joint space loss in osteoarthritis of the hip. Arthritis Rheum 2002; 47:50–58
3. Henrotin YE, Sanchez C, Deberg MA, Piccardi N, Guillou GB, Msika P, Reginster JY. Avocado/soybean unsaponifiables increase aggrecan synthesis and reduce catabolic and proinflammatory production by human osteoarthritic chondrocytes. J Rheumatol 2003; 30:1825–1834

CANNABIS
(Cannabis sativa)

SOURCE
Flower, leaf.

MAIN CONSTITUENTS
Cannabinoids [δ-9-tetrahydrocannabinol (δ-9-THC) and cannabidiol], flavonoids.

BACKGROUND

Cannabis or marijuana is believed to have originated in central Asia. It has a long history of both therapeutic and recreational use. It was employed as the primary pain reliever until aspirin was developed. In the past 10 years, cannabinoids and the endocannaboinoid system have come under intense scrutiny following the discovery of CB1 and CB2 receptors and the development of specific cannabinoid receptor agonist and antagonist ligands.[1] There is currently much debate about wider access to cannabis-based medicines as analgesics in chronic painful conditions or for treating spasticity in multiple sclerosis. The widespread illegal use of cannabis as a recreational drug makes its legal or licensed use in medicine a controversial issue in most countries.

EXAMPLES OF TRADITIONAL USES

Headache, migraine, childbirth and other pain syndromes, insomnia, gastrointestinal disorders, melancholia, appetite loss, and recreationally as a euphoriant.

PHARMACOLOGICAL ACTION

Analgesic, muscle relaxant, anti-emetic, appetite stimulant, reduces intra-ocular pressure.

CONDITIONS FREQUENTLY TREATED

Various forms of pain, tremor and spasticity associated with multiple sclerosis, chemotherapy-induced nausea and vomiting, glaucoma.

CLINICAL EVIDENCE

A systematic review including nine RCTs ($n = 222$) tested cannabinoids in cancer pain, chronic non-malignant pain and acute post-operative pain.[2] It concluded that cannabinoids are no more effective than codeine in controlling pain and have depressant effects on the central nervous system that limit their use. A double-blind RCT of 66 patients with multiple sclerosis found a whole-plant cannabis-based medicine containing δ-9-THC delivered via an oromucosal spray to be superior to placebo in reducing the intensity of central pain.[3] A further RCT of 630 multiple sclerosis patients suggested improved patient-reported pain in the group receiving δ-9-THC compared with a cannabis extract and placebo, although the authors noted that there was a degree of unmasking among patients in the active treatment groups.[4] The follow-up study found pain reduction with both the synthetic δ-9-THC extract and the cannabis extract at 12 months.[5] A series of double-blind single-patient crossover trials investigating whether sublingually administered whole-plant cannabis extracts can improve intractable neurogenic symptoms in patients with multiple sclerosis, spinal cord injury, brachial plexus damage and limb amputation as a result of neurofibromatosis concluded that pain relief with δ-9-THC and cannabidiol was superior to placebo.[6] Forty-eight patients receiving oromucosal spray preparations of a δ-9-THC and cannabidiol combination or a mainly δ-9-THC-containing preparation reported improvement in the severity of pain associated with central neuropathic pain from brachial plexus avulsion compared to placebo.[7] For chronic pain, three extracts (δ-9-THC, cannabidiol and their combination) for sublingual use were tested in 34 double-blind 'n of 1' studies.[8] THC was found to be most effective for pain symptom control. A cannabis-based medicine was assessed in a double-blind RCT of 58 patients with rheumatoid arthritis and improvements in pain on movement and pain at rest were noted compared with placebo.[9] A double-blind RCT of 40 women undergoing abdominal hysterectomy demonstrated no evidence of an analgesic effect of orally administered δ-9-THC on post-operative pain.[10] Similarly, no synergistic or even additive anti-nociceptive interaction between 9-THC and the μ-opioid agonist piritramide was found in patients undergoing radical retropubic prostatectomy with regional lymphadenectomy.[11] No reduction of experimentally induced pain with δ-9-THC was reported in a double-blind, placebo-controlled RCT of 12 healthy volunteers receiving δ-9-THC, morphine or a combination of both.[12]

DOSAGE

- *Oral*: five to 15 drops of tincture or one to three drops of fluid extract. Dronabinol, the prescription product for cancer chemotherapy-induced nausea and vomiting, is used in doses of 5–15 mg/m^2 body surface area every 2–4 hours.
- *Inhalation*: 65–195 mg for smoking.

RISKS

CONTRAINDICATIONS

Pregnancy and lactation (see p. 4), cardiovascular disease, respiratory disease (long-term use), seizure disorders.

PRECAUTIONS/WARNINGS

Has addictive potential.

ADVERSE EFFECTS

Xerostomia, nausea, vomiting, reddening of the conjunctiva, tachycardia, hypotension or hypertension, syncope, palpitations and vasodilatation. Intoxicating doses impair reaction time, motor coordination and visual perception; they can produce panic reactions, hallucinations, flashbacks, depression and other emotional disturbances. Long-term use is associated with mental problems, e.g. schizophrenia. Chronic use can cause laryngitis, bronchitis, apathy, psychic decline, sexual dysfunction, abnormal menstruation and bullous emphysema.

OVERDOSE

Nausea, vomiting, lacrimation, hacking cough, disturbed cardiac function, limb numbness.

INTERACTIONS

Barbiturates, fluoxetine or disulfiram, theophylline. Additive or synergistc effects with amphetamines, anticholinergics, antihistamines, cocaine, hypnotics, psychomimetics, sedatives and sympathomimetics.

QUALITY ISSUES

Not to be confused with hemp, a distinct variety of *C. sativa*, which contains less than 1% THC. A synthetic version of THC, dronabinol, is readily available as a prescription drug.

RISK–BENEFIT ASSESSMENT

There is encouraging evidence for the use of cannabinoid δ-9-THC for the relief of pain associated with multiple sclerosis and neuropathic pain when compared to placebo. However, there is no evidence of its analgesic effects being more powerful than conventional options. In view of the considerable risks associated with cannabis, its use remains controversial and it should only be considered in carefully selected cases where conventional treatment is not an option. There is no evidence for its usefulness in pain associated with any other conditions.

REFERENCES

1. Pertwee RG. Cannabinoid receptors and pain. Prog Neurobiol 2001;63:569–611
2. Campbell FA, Tramer MR, Carroll D, Reynolds DJ, Moore RA, McQuay HJ. Are cannabinoids an effective and safe treatment option in the management of pain? A qualitative systematic review. BMJ 2001;323:13–16
3. Rog DJ, Nurmikko TJ, Friede T, Young CA. Randomized, controlled trial of cannabis-based medicine in central pain in multiple sclerosis. Neurology 2005;65:812–819
4. Zajicek J, Fox P, Sanders H, Wright D, Vickery J, Nunn A, Thompson A; UK MS Research Group. Cannabinoids for treatment of spasticity and other symptoms related to multiple sclerosis (CAMS study): multicentre randomised placebo-controlled trial. Lancet 2003; 362:1517–1526
5. Zajicek JP, Sanders HP, Wright DE, Vickery PJ, Ingram WM, Reilly SM, Nunn AJ, Teare LJ, Fox PJ, Thompson AJ. Cannabinoids in multiple sclerosis (CAMS) study: safety and efficacy data for 12 months follow up. J Neurol Neurosurg Psychiatry 2005;76:1664–1669
6. Wade DT, Robson P, House H, Makela P, Aram J. A preliminary controlled study to determine whether whole-plant cannabis extracts can improve intractable neurogenic symptoms. Clin Rehabil 2003;17:21–29
7. Berman JS, Symonds C, Birch R. Efficacy of two cannabis based medicinal extracts for relief of central neuropathic pain from brachial plexus avulsion: results of a randomized controlled trial. Pain 2004;112:299–306
8. Notcutt W, Price M, Miller R, Newport S, Phillips C, Simmons S, Sansom C. Initial experiences with medicinal extracts of cannabis for chronic pain: results from 34 'N of 1' studies. Anaesthesia 2004;59:440–452
9. Blake DR, Robson P, Ho M, Jubb RW, McCabe CS. Preliminary assessment of the efficacy, tolerability and safety of a cannabis-based medicine (Sativex) in the treatment of pain caused by rheumatoid arthritis. Rheumatology (Oxford) 2006;45:50–52
10. Buggy DJ, Toogood L, Maric S, Sharpe P, Lambert DG, Rowbotham DJ. Lack of analgesic efficacy of oral delta-9-tetrahydrocannabinol in postoperative pain. Pain 2003;106: 169–172
11. Seeling W, Kneer L, Buchele B, Gschwend JE, Maier L, Nett C, Simmet T, Steffen P, Schneider M, Rockemann M. (9)-tetrahydrocannabinol and the opioid receptor agonist piritramide do not act synergistically in postoperative pain. [In German.] Anaesthesist 2006;55:391–400
12. Naef M, Curatolo M, Petersen-Felix S, Arendt-Nielsen L, Zbinden A, Brenneisen R. The analgesic effect of oral delta-9-tetrahydrocannabinol (THC), morphine, and a THC-morphine combination in healthy subjects under experimental pain conditions. Pain 2003;105:79–88

CAT'S CLAW
(Uncaria tomentosa, Uncaria guianensis)

SOURCE
Root and bark.

MAIN CONSTITUENTS
Alkaloids, glycosides, organic acids, procyanidins, triterpenes. The active constituents found in cat's claw may be dependent on climate and soil.

BACKGROUND
Cat's claw is a vine that grows wild in the Amazon rainforest and other areas in South and Central America. Its medicinal use allegedly dates back to the Inca civilisation: cat's claw was considered to possess great powers and life-giving properties by the Ashaninka priests of Peru.

Today it is widely used in the US and Europe. Several plant species other than *Uncaria tomentosa* or *U. guianensis* are marketed under the name cat's claw. In some countries, such as Germany and Austria, cat's claw is a registered pharmaceutical requiring a prescription.

EXAMPLES OF TRADITIONAL USES

Arthritis and other rheumatic complaints, asthma, birth control, cancer, 'cleansing' of kidneys, colitis, diverticulitis, gastritis, haemorrhoids, parasites, peptic ulcers, viral infections, wound healing.

PHARMACOLOGICAL ACTION

Antihypertensive, anti-inflammatory, antimutagenic, antioxidant, antiviral, contraceptive, immunostimulant, inhibition of platelet aggregation.

CONDITIONS FREQUENTLY TREATED

Inflammation, rheumatic diseases, arthritis.

CLINICAL EVIDENCE

An RCT of 45 patients with osteoarthritis of the knee found freeze-dried extracts of *U. guianensis* to be superior to placebo in reducing pain associated with activity but not in reducing knee pain at rest or knee circumference.[1] Sierrasil, a natural mineral supplement, administered alone or in combination with cat's claw improved joint health and function within 1–2 weeks of treatment but benefits over placebo were not sustained.[2] One double-blind RCT ($n = 40$) of an extract from the pentacyclic alkaloid-chemotype of *U. tomentosa* in the treatment of rheumatoid arthritis reported a modest reduction of the number of painful joints compared to placebo.[3]

DOSAGE

Products should be standardised to contain 3% alkaloids and 15% phenols per dose or 1.3% pentacyclic oxindole alkaloids.

- *Capsules*: 250–1000 mg daily.
- *Tincture*: 1–2 ml two or three times daily.
- *Tea*: 1–25 g of root bark added to 250 ml water three times daily.

RISKS

CONTRAINDICATIONS

Pregnancy and lactation (see p. 4); cat's claw has historically been used to prevent pregnancy and to induce abortion.

PRECAUTIONS/WARNINGS

May theoretically increase the risk of bleeding and decrease estrogen or progesterone levels. Many tinctures contain a high level of alcohol.

ADVERSE EFFECTS

Allergies to plants in the Rubiaceae family. Possibly stomach discomfort, nausea, diarrhoea, bradycardia, arrhythmia and kidney failure.

INTERACTIONS

Anticoagulants; caution with anti-arrhythmic drugs, blood pressure drugs and immunosuppressants.

QUALITY ISSUES

Products may be contaminated with other *Uncaria* species. Reports exist of a potentially toxic plant, *Acacia gregii*, being substituted for cat's claw in commercial preparations.

RISK–BENEFIT ASSESSMENT

There is encouraging yet very limited evidence for its efficacy in the treatment of rheumatoid arthritis and osteoarthritis. Few adverse effects have been reported from using cat's claw at recommended doses. Further trials are required before any recommendations can be made.

REFERENCES

1. Piscoya J, Rodriguez Z, Bustamante SA, Okuhama NN, Miller MJ, Sandoval M. Efficacy and safety of freeze-dried cat's claw in osteoarthritis of the knee: mechanisms of action of the species *Uncaria guianensis*. Inflamm Res 2001;50:442–448
2. Miller MJ, Mehta K, Kunte S, Raut V, Gala J, Dhumale R, Shukla A, Tupalli H, Parikh H, Bobrowski P, Chaudhary J. Early relief of osteoarthritis symptoms with a natural mineral supplement and a herbomineral combination: a randomized controlled trial. J Inflamm (Lond) 2005;2:11
3. Mur E, Hartig F, Eibl G, Schirmer M. Randomized double blind trial of an extract from the pentacyclic alkaloid-chemotype of *Uncaria tomentosa* for the treatment of rheumatoid arthritis. J Rheumatol 2002;29:678–681

CHILLI

(Capsicum spp.)

SOURCE

The fruits from *Capsicum* species are used.

MAIN CONSTITUENTS

Capsaicin.

BACKGROUND

The powerful irritant action of chilli fruits has been traditionally used for culinary and medicinal purposes.

EXAMPLES OF TRADITIONAL USES

Topical use for local pain syndromes. Stimulation of digestion, antiflatulent, for colic, diarrhoea, toothache, peripheral vascular disease, seasickness (internal use).

PHARMACOLOGICAL ACTION

Release of substance P after topical application, stimulation of unmyelinated C-fibres, antibacterial.

CONDITIONS FREQUENTLY TREATED

Used in pain management.

CLINICAL EVIDENCE

Systematic reviews of RCTs have found topical application of capsaicin, the main constituent of chilli, to be effective for chronic neuropathic and musculoskeletal pain,[1] post-herpetic neuralgia,[2] post-mastectomy syndrome, cluster headache and pruritus of psoriasis,[3] as well as complex regional pain syndromes.[4] It was, however, shown to be ineffective in relieving pain associated with human immunodeficiency virus (HIV)-related peripheral neuropathy.[5] Recent RCTs indicate that topical capsaicin may be effective for osteoarthritis pain,[6,7] back pain[8,9] and neuropathic cancer pain.[10] It was not effective for localised temporomandibular pain.[11] Another systematic review demonstrated intravesical application of capsaicin to be effective for neurogenic hyperreflexic bladder.[12]

DOSAGE

Three or four times/day topically. Cream or plaster containing 0.025–0.075% capsaicin is applied in the area of pain.

RISKS

CONTRAINDICATIONS

Pregnancy and lactation (see p. 4).

PRECAUTIONS/WARNINGS

Inflammatory skin conditions and wounds, do not use near the eyes or on sensitive skin.

ADVERSE EFFECTS

About one-third of all patients receiving topical capsaicin experience local adverse events, e.g. a burning sensation.[1] Systematic use of capsaicin frequently causes major gastrointestinal adverse effects.[13]

OVERDOSE

First-degree or second-degree burns.

INTERACTIONS

None.

QUALITY ISSUES

Creams and plasters containing less than 0.025–0.075% capsaicin are less effective. Higher concentrations should be used with caution only.

RISK–BENEFIT ASSESSMENT

Topical capsaicin preparations are effective in treating a range of pain syndromes. There are only a few risks. The risk–benefit profile of topically applied capsaicin can therefore be positive.

REFERENCES

1. Mason L, Moore RA, Derry S, Edwards JE, McQuay HJ. Systematic review of topical capsaicin for the treatment of chronic pain. BMJ 2004;328:991
2. Hempenstall K, Nurmikko TJ, Johnson RW, A'Hern RP, Rice AS. Analgesic therapy in postherpetic neuralgia: a quantitative systematic review. PLoS Med 2005;2:e164
3. Hautkappe M, Roizen MF, Toledano A, Roth S, Jeffries JA, Ostermeier AM. Review of the effectiveness of capsaicin for painful cutaneous disorders and neural dysfunction. Clin J Pain 1998;14:97–106
4. Kingery WS. A critical review of controlled clinical trials for peripheral neuropathic pain and complex regional pain syndromes. Pain 1997;73:123–139
5. Liu JP, Manheimer E, Yang M. Herbal medicines for treating HIV infection and AIDS. The Cochrane Database of Systematic Reviews 2005, Issue 3. Art. No.: CD003937

6. McKay-L, Gemmell-H, Jacobson-B, Hayes-B. Effect of a topical herbal cream on the pain and stiffness of osteoarthritis: a randomized double-blind, placebo-controlled clinical trial. J Clin Rheumatol 2003;9:164–169

7. McCleane G. The analgesic efficacy of topical capsaicin is enhanced by glyceryl trinitrate in painful osteoarthritis: a randomized, double blind, placebo controlled study. Eur J Pain 2000;4: 355–360

8. Frerick H, Keitel W, Kuhn U, Schmidt S, Bredehorst A, Kuhlmann M. Topical treatment of chronic low back pain with a capsicum plaster. Pain 2003;106:59–64

9. Keitel W, Frerick H, Kuhn U, Schmidt U, Kuhlmann M, Bredehorst A. Capsicum pain plaster in chronic non-specific low back pain. Arzneimittelforschung 2001;51:896–903

10. Ellison N, Loprinzi CL, Kugler J, Hatfield AK, Miser A, Sloan JA, Wender DB, Rowland KM, Molina R, Cascino TL, Vukov AM, Dhaliwal HS, Ghosh C. Phase III placebo-controlled trial of capsaicin cream in the management of surgical neuropathic pain in cancer patients. J Clin Oncol 1997;15:2974–2980

11. Winocur E, Gavish A, Halachmi M, Eli I, Gazit E. Topical application of capsaicin for the treatment of localized pain in the temporomandibular joint area. J Orofac Pain 2000;14:31–36

12. De Seze M, Wiart L, Ferriere JM, De Seze MP, Joseph PA, Barat M. Intravesical instillation of capsaicin in urology: a review of the literature. Eur Urol 1999;36:267–277

13. Petruzzi M, Lauritano D, De Benedittis M, Baldoni M, Serpico R. Systemic capsaicin for burning mouth syndrome: short-term results of a pilot study. J Oral Pathol Med 2004;33:111–114

CHONDROITIN

SOURCE

Bovine tracheal cartilage.

MAIN CONSTITUENTS

Glycosaminoglycans, principally chondroitin-4-sulphate and chondroitin-6-sulphate, and disaccharide polymers composed of equimolar amounts of D-glucuronic acid, N-acetylgalactosamine and sulphates in 30–100 disaccharide units.

BACKGROUND

Chondroitin is thought to rebuild cartilage and is promoted as a treatment for conditions associated with cartilage degeneration.

EXAMPLES OF TRADITIONAL USES

Joint pain, osteoarthritis.

PHARMACOLOGICAL ACTION

Chondroitin has anti-inflammatory activity, controls the formation of new cartilage matrix, and inhibits leukocyte elastase and hyaluronidase. It also stimulates the production of highly polymerised hyaluronic acid in synovial cells, thus increasing synovial viscosity and possibly contributing to a 'lubrication effect' in the joint. Furthermore, it reduces inflammatory activity by inhibiting the recognition process of complement. These actions are believed to work in concert and constitute chondroitin's complex mechanisms of action.

CONDITIONS FREQUENTLY TREATED

Osteoarthritis pain.

CLINICAL EVIDENCE

Several good-quality trials of chondroitin suggest symptomatic improvement in patients suffering from osteoarthritis pain.[1] A meta-analysis of seven RCTs, including 372 patients in total, came to a cautiously positive conclusion.[2] Yet it also pointed to the lack of long-term data. Three further meta-analyses of chondroitin and glucosamine for treatment of osteoarthritis all arrived at positive conclusions.[3–5] Further trials suggest positive long-term effects on osteoarthritis pain[6,7] and confirm that chondroitin has structure-modulating properties in osteoarthritic joints.[8] This notion was also confirmed in two RCTs ($n = 100$ and $n = 300$) showing that long-term medication with chondroitin and glucosamine sulphate prevents joint space narrowing in patients with knee osteoarthritis.[9,10] One RCT also suggested that a preparation of topical chondroitin and glucosamine is effective in relieving pain of knee osteoarthritis.[11] However, a further large ($n = 1229$), high-quality RCT failed to confirm that chondroitin is better than placebo in reducing the pain of knee osteoarthritis.[12] Other indications for chondroitin might be erosive osteoarthritis of the hands,[13] low back pain[14] and temperomandibular joint disorder.[15]

DOSAGE

800–1200 mg of chondroitin sulphate daily in divided doses.

RISKS

CONTRAINDICATIONS

Pregnancy and lactation (see p. 4).

PRECAUTIONS/WARNINGS

Bleeding disorders, asthma can be exacerbated.

ADVERSE EFFECTS

Dyspepsia, headache, euphoria, nausea.

INTERACTIONS

Potentiation of anticoagulants is theoretically possible.

QUALITY ISSUES

Many commercially available products do not contain the stated dosage.

RISK–BENEFIT ASSESSMENT

The efficacy of chondroitin is well documented and risks seem to be minor. The risk–benefit balance is therefore positive. Chondroitin can hence be recommended as an adjuvant to other interventions for osteoarthritis.

REFERENCES

1. Morreale P, Manopulo R, Galati M, Boccanera L, Saponati G, Bocchi L. Comparison of the anti-inflammatory efficacy of chondroitin sulfate and diclofenac sodium in patients with knee osteoarthritis. J Rheumatol 1996;23:1385–1391
2. Leeb BF, Scweitzer H, Montag K, Smolen JS. A metaanalysis of chondroitin sulfate in the treatment of osteoarthritis. J Rheumatol 2000;27:205–211
3. McAlindon TE, LaValley MP, Gulin JP, Felson DT. Glucosamine and chondroitin for treatment of osteoarthritis. A systematic quality assessment and meta-analysis. JAMA 2000;283:1469–1475
4. Häuselmann HJ. Nutripharmaceuticals for osteoarthritis. Best Pract Res Clin Rheumatol 2001; 15:595–607

5. Richy F, Bruyere O, Ethgen O, Cucherat M, Henrotin Y, Reginster JY. Structural and symptomatic efficacy of glucosamine and chondroitin in knee osteoarthritis: a comprehensive meta-analysis. Arch Intern Med 2003;163:1514–1522

6. Uebelhart D, Malaise M, Marcolongo R, DeVathaire F, Piperno M, Mailleux E, Fioravanti A, Matoso L, Vignon E. Intermittent treatment of knee osteoarthritis with oral chondroitin sulfate: a one-year, randomized, double-blind, multicenter study versus placebo. Osteoarthritis Cartilage 2004;12:269–276

7. Alekseeva LI, Chichasova NV, Benevolenskaia LI, Nasonov EL, Mendel' OI. Combined medication ARTRA in the treatment of osteoarthrosis. [In Russian.] Ter Arkh 2005;77:69–75.

8. Mathieu P. Radiological progression of internal femoro-tibial osteoarthritis in gonarthrosis. Chondro-protective effect of chondroitin sulfates ACS4-ACS6. Presse Med 2002;31: 1386–1390

9. Rai J, Pal SK, Gul A, Senthil R, Singh H. Efficacy of chondroitin sulfate and glucosamine sulfate in the progression of symptomatic knee osteoarthritis: a randomized, placebo-controlled, double blind study. Bull Postgrad Inst Med Educ Res Chandigarh 2004; 38:18–22

10. Michel BA, Stucki G, Frey D, De Vathaire F, Vignon E, Bruehlmann P, Uebelhart D. Chondroitins 4 and 6 sulfate in osteoarthritis of the knee: a randomized, controlled trial. Arthritis Rheum 2005;52:779–786

11. Cohen M, Wolfe R, Mai T, Lewis D. A randomized, double blind, placebo controlled trial of a top-ical cream containing glucosamine sulfate, chondroitin sulfate, and camphor for osteoarthritis of the knee. J Rheumatol 2003;30:2512

12. Clegg DO, Reda DJ, Harris CL, Klein MA, O'Dell JR, Hooper MM, Bradley JD, Bingham CO 3rd, Weisman MH, Jackson CG, Lane NE, Cush JJ, Moreland LW, Schumacher HR Jr, Oddis CV, Wolfe F, Molitor JA, Yocum DE, Schnitzer TJ, Furst DE, Sawitzke AD, Shi H, Brandt KD, Moskowitz RW, Williams HJ. Glucosamine, chondroitin sulfate, and the two in combination for painful knee osteoarthritis. N Engl J Med 2006;354:795–808

13. Rovetta G, Monteforte P, Molfetta G, Balestra V. Chondroitin sulfate in erosive osteoarthritis of the hands. Int J Tissue React 2002;24:29–32

14. Leffler CT, Philippi AF, Leffler SG, Mosure JC, Kim PD. Glucosamine, chondroitin, and man-ganese ascorbate for degenerative joint disease for the knee or low back: a randomized, double-blind, placebo-controlled pilot study. Mil Med 1999;164:85–91

15. Nguyen P, Mohamed SE, Gardiner D, Salinas T. A randomized double-blind clinical trial of the effect of chondroitin sulfate and glucosamine hydrochloride on temporomandibular joint disor-ders: a pilot study. Cranio 2001;19:130–139

COMFREY
(Symphytum officinale)

SOURCE
Leaf, rhizome, root.

MAIN CONSTITUENTS
Allantoin, derivatives of rosmarinic acids, saponins, tannins.

BACKGROUND
Comfrey is a perennial herb of the Boraginaceae family and is native to Europe and Asia. Its name is derived from the Latin word for 'grow together'. Comfrey has been cultivated since about 400 BCE as a medicinal herb for wound healing and broken bones and to stop bleeding. There are concerns about its toxicity, caused by pyrrolizidine alkaloids, so it is recom-mended for external use only.

EXAMPLES OF TRADITIONAL USES
Angina, bloody urine, bronchitis, cancer, diarrhoea, excessive menstrual flow, gum disease, persistent cough, pharyngitis, pleuritis, rheumatism and ulcers.

PHARMACOLOGICAL ACTION

Analgesic, anti-inflammatory, anti-oedematous, wound healing.

CONDITIONS FREQUENTLY TREATED

Bruises and sprains, fractures, ulcers and wounds.

CLINICAL EVIDENCE

Topically applied comfrey in the treatment of ankle distortions was tested in several RCTs. One single-blind RCT ($n = 164$) found comfrey ointment to be non-inferior to diclofenac with regards the pain reaction to pressure on the injured area, swelling and pain at rest and at movement.[1] The same comfrey ointment was found to be superior to placebo in a double-blind RCT ($n = 142$) in reducing pain, ankle oedema and in increasing ankle mobility.[2] Two different concentrations of comfrey were compared in a double-blind RCT ($n = 104$), which found the higher concentration to be far more effective than the lower one at decreasing pain and improving functional impairment.[3] One double-blind RCT compared two concentrations of a topical comfrey product with placebo in the treatment of myalgia patients and found better overall efficacy and faster onset of effects with the high-concentration product on pain in the lower and upper back.[4]

DOSAGE

Ointments and other external preparations are commonly made with 5–20% of comfrey.

RISKS

CONTRAINDICATIONS

Broken skin, pregnancy and lactation (see p. 4).

PRECAUTIONS/WARNINGS

Products, particularly those prepared from the roots, may contain liver-toxic pyrrolizidine alkaloids and are not recommended for internal use. Should not be used for more than 6 weeks a year.

ADVERSE EFFECTS

Veno-occlusive disease, liver damage (oral usage).

OVERDOSE

Daily use should not exceed 100 µg of the pyrrolizidine alkaloids.

INTERACTIONS

Risk of additive toxicity with concomitant use of other pyrrolizidine alkaloid-containing herbs.

QUALITY ISSUES

Only products with reduced toxicity levels should be used. Some products labelled comfrey or *Symphytum officinale* instead contain the more toxic prickly comfrey.

RISK–BENEFIT ASSESSMENT

There is encouraging yet limited evidence for the effectiveness of comfrey ointment in the treatment of ankle distortions. Cautiously used on unbroken skin only, it might be a useful adjunct in this indication but further evidence is required to make any firm recommendations.

REFERENCES

1. Predel HG, Giannetti B, Koll R, Bulitta M, Staiger C. Efficacy of a comfrey root extract ointment in comparison to a diclofenac gel in the treatment of ankle distortions: results of an observer-blind, randomized, multicenter study. Phytomedicine 2005;12:707–714

2. Koll R, Buhr M, Dieter R, Pabst H, Predel HG, Petrowicz O, Giannetti B, Klingenburg S, Staiger C. Efficacy and tolerance of a comfrey root extract (Extr. Rad. Symphyti) in the treatment of ankle distorsions: results of a multicenter, randomized, placebo-controlled, double-blind study. Phytomedicine 2004;11:470–477

3. Kucera M, Barna M, Horacek O, Kovarikova J, Kucera A. Efficacy and safety of topically applied Symphytum herb extract cream in the treatment of ankle distortion: results of a randomized controlled clinical double blind study. Wien Med Wochenschr 2004;154: 498–507

4. Kucera M, Barna M, Horacek O, Kalal J, Kucera A, Hladikova M. Topical symphytum herb concentrate cream against myalgia: a randomized controlled double-blind clinical study. Adv Ther 2005;22:681–692

DEVIL'S CLAW   (*Harpagophytum procumbens*)

SOURCE

Tuberous roots.

MAIN CONSTITUENTS

The major active ingredient is harpagoside. Other compounds are β-sitosterol, flavonoids, procumbides, stigmasterol, triterpenes.

BACKGROUND

The name devil's claw is derived from the plant's unique fruits, which are covered with claw-like hooks. It grows wild in southern Africa and the recent popularity of devil's claw has resulted in it nearly becoming an endangered species.

EXAMPLES OF TRADITIONAL USES

Dysmenorrhoea, headaches, rheumatic conditions, digestive problems, gastrointestinal complaints, liver and kidney diseases, malaria, menopausal symptoms, nicotine poisoning and skin cancer.

PHARMACOLOGICAL ACTION

Anti-inflammatory, analgesic, negative chronotropic, positive inotropic, anti-arrhythmic.

CONDITIONS FREQUENTLY TREATED

Arthritic and musculoskeletal pain.

CLINICAL EVIDENCE

A systematic review of RCTs, quasi-randomised clinical trials and controlled clinical trials assessed devil's claw in the treatment of various forms of musculoskeletal pain. It included five placebo- or reference-controlled RCTs of 385 patients with osteoarthritis of the hip or the knee, four placebo- or reference-controlled RCTs of 505 patients with acute exacerbations of chronic non-specific low back pain, and three placebo-controlled trials including 215 patients with various forms of musculoskeletal pain.[1] The review reported positive evidence from placebo-controlled or conventional treatment-controlled trials for an aqueous extract of devil's claw in the treatment of acute exacerbations of chronic non-specific low back pain; the best results were obtained with a daily dose equivalent to 50 mg harpagosides.

It also showed encouraging evidence for devil's claw powder at a dose of 60 mg harpago-sides in the treatment of osteoarthritis of the spine, hip and knee.

DOSAGE
400–500 mg of dried extract three times daily.

RISKS

CONTRAINDICATIONS
Pregnancy, because of the uterus-stimulating effects of devil's claw, lactation (see p. 4), gastric or duodenal ulcer, gallstones.

PRECAUTIONS/WARNINGS
There is insufficient reliable information available about the safety of topical or long-term oral use. Might lower blood sugar levels.

ADVERSE EFFECTS
Gastrointestinal symptoms, allergic skin reactions.

OVERDOSE
Cardiac effects.

INTERACTIONS
May increase the anticoagulation effects of warfarin; theoretically, it could interact with cardiac drugs.

QUALITY ISSUES
The harpagoside content and pharmacokinetic profile have been shown to vary considerably between commercial preparations.

RISK–BENEFIT ASSESSMENT
The effectiveness of devil's claw in the management of musculoskeletal pain related to osteoarthritis and non-specific low back pain is reasonably well documented and only mild adverse effects are on record. It has been compared to conventional treatment options (e.g. non-steroidal anti-inflammatory drugs) in four of the trials, suggesting that it is better than or equal to conventional medications. Thus, devil's claw can be tried in selected cases but the risks of herb–drug interactions should be considered.

REFERENCES
1. Gagnier JJ, Chrubasik S, Manheimer E. *Harpagophytum procumbens* for osteoarthritis and low back pain: a systematic review. BMC Complement Altern Med 2004;4:13

EVENING PRIMROSE   (*Oenothera biennis*)

SOURCE
Oil from seeds.

MAIN CONSTITUENTS
The seeds contain 14% fixed oil comprising approximately 70% *cis*-linoleic acid (LA), 9% *cis*-γ-linolenic acid (GLA), 2–16% oleic acid, 7% palmitic acid, 3% stearic acid.

SECTION FOUR

BACKGROUND

Evening primrose is not actually a primrose but belongs to the fuchsia (Onagraceae) family. It is native to North America and has become naturalised in western Europe and parts of Asia. The plant blooms in early summer, producing large yellow flowers that open in the evenings – hence its name. Originally the root was used as a vegetable and the whole plant was used for its medicinal properties to treat a wide range of conditions. Today it is mainly the oil that is employed for therapeutic purposes. It is popular, particularly with menopausal women.[1]

EXAMPLES OF TRADITIONAL USES

Neuralgia, asthma, gastrointestinal disorders, whooping cough.

PHARMACOLOGICAL ACTION

Through its effects on the prostaglandin system, evening primrose oil is thought to have anti-inflammatory effects that, in turn, have the potential to reduce pain. For individuals in whom the conversion of LA to GLA by the enzyme δ-6-desaturase is impaired, the rich GLA content of evening primrose oil allows this conversion to be bypassed.

CONDITIONS FREQUENTLY TREATED

Rheumatoid arthritis, mastalgia, cardiovascular conditions, atopic eczema, psoriasis, pre-menstrual syndrome, menopausal complaints, multiple sclerosis, schizophrenia, hyperactivity, dementia.

CLINICAL EVIDENCE

A large range of conditions has been investigated, including psoriatic or rheumatoid arthritis[2–4] and mastalgia.[5–8] Results have not been convincingly positive. In particular, there were no prominent effects on pain. In an RCT ($n = 90$) with patients suffering from Sjögren's syndrome, no pain reduction was noted compared to placebo.[9] For diabetic neuropathy, however, the results indicated that pain can effectively be reduced with evening primrose oil.[10,11] An RCT ($n = 120$) suggested that, for breast pain, evening primrose oil is not more effective than placebo;[12] a further review agrees with this conclusion.[13]

DOSAGE

3–8 g daily in divided doses.

RISKS

CONTRAINDICATIONS

Pregnancy and lactation (see p. 4), mania, epilepsy.

PRECAUTIONS/WARNINGS

There is a risk of undiagnosed temporal lope epilepsy being manifested in schizophrenics or other patients taking epileptogenic agents.

ADVERSE EFFECTS

Gastrointestinal symptoms, headache.

OVERDOSE

Gastrointestinal symptoms have been observed with large doses.

INTERACTIONS

Theoretically, interactions with anti-inflammatory drugs, corticosteroids, β-blockers, antipsychotics and anticoagulants are possible. Concomitant use with epileptogenic agents such as phenothiazines may increase the risk of seizures.

QUALITY ISSUES

Standardised preparations usually contain 8% GLA. Some products contain a combination of evening primrose oil and fish oil (omega-3 fatty acids).

RISK–BENEFIT ASSESSMENT

Despite having been subjected to a relatively large number of clinical trials, evening primrose oil has not been established as an efficacious treatment for any condition. It appears to be generally safe. Some encouraging data exist to suggest that it may be helpful for reducing pain in diabetic neuropathy. For this condition it may therefore merit consideration.

REFERENCES

1. Mahady GB, Parrot J, Lee C, Yun GS, Dan A. Botanical dietary supplement use in peri- and post-menopausal women. Menopause 2003;10:65–72
2. Veale DJ, Torley HI, Richards IM, O'Dowd A, Fitzsimons C, Belch JJ, Sturrock RD. A double-blind placebo-controlled trial of Efamol Marine on skin and joint symptoms of psoriatic arthritis. Br J Rheumatol 1994;33:954–958
3. Brzeski M, Madhok R, Capell HA. Evening primrose oil in patients with rheumatoid arthritis and side effects of non-steroidal anti-inflammatory drugs. Br J Rheumatol 1991;30:370–372
4. Belch JJ, Ansell D, Madhok R, O'Dowd A, Sturrock RD. Effects of altering dietary essential fatty acids on requirements for non-steroidal anti-inflammatory drugs in patients with rheumatoid arthritis: a double-blind placebo-controlled study. Ann Rheum Dis 1988;47:96–104
5. Gateley CA, Miers M, Mansel RE, Hughes LE. Drug treatments for mastalgia: 17 years experience in the Cardiff mastalgia clinic. J R Soc Med 1992;85:12–15
6. Gateley CA, Maddox PR, Pritchard GA, Sheridan W, Harrison BJ, Pye JK, Webster DJ, Hughes LE, Mansel RE. Plasma fatty acid profiles in benign breast disorders. Br J Surg 1992; 79:407–409
7. Mansel RE, Harrison BJ, Melhuish J, Sheridan W, Pye JK, Pritchard G, Maddox PR, Webster DJ, Hughes LE. A randomized trial of dietary intervention with essential fatty acids in patients with categorised cysts. Ann NY Acad Sci 1990;586:288–294
8. Blommers J, de Lange-De Klerk E, Kuik DJ, Bezemer PD, Meijer S. Evening primrose oil and fish oil for severe chronic mastalgia: a randomized, double-blind, controlled trial. Am J Obstet Gynecol 2002;187:1389–1394
9. Theander E, Horrobin DF, Jacobsson LTH, Manthorpe R. Gammalinolenic acid treatment of fatigue associated with primary Sjögren's syndrome. Scand J Rheumatol 2002;31: 72–79
10. Jamal GA, Carmichael H, Weir AI. Gamma-linolenic acid in diabetic neuropathy. Lancet 1986;1:1098
11. Keen H, Payan J, Allawi J, Walker J, Jamal GA, Weir AI, Henderson LM, Bissessar EA, Watkins PJ, Sampson M. Treatment of diabetic neuropathy with gamma-linolenic acid. Diabetes Care 1993;16:8–15
12. Blommers J, De Lange de Klerk ESM, Kuik DJ, Bezemer PD, Meijer S. Evening primrose oil and fish oil for severe chronic mastalgia: a randomized, double-blind, controlled trial. Am J Obstet Gynecol, 2002;187:1389–1394
13. Rosolowich V, Saettler E, Szuck B, Lea RH, Levesque P, Weisberg F, Graham J, McLeod L, Rosolowich V. Use of hormonal replacement therapy after treatment of breast cancer. J Obstet Gynaecol Can 2006;28:49–57

FEVERFEW *(Tanacetum parthenium)*

SOURCE
Leaves.

MAIN CONSTITUENTS
Camphor, chrysanthenyl acetate and flavonoids. Parthenolide is thought to be the active principle.

BACKGROUND
Feverfew is a perennial plant, native to Asia Minor. It is widely naturalised throughout much of Europe, North America and Canada. Its use as a herbal remedy goes back to ancient times when it was employed for many aches and pains, in particular for conditions associated with fevers and women's ailments. Today, extract of feverfew is predominantly used for the prevention of migraine attacks and to alleviate the accompanying symptoms.

EXAMPLES OF TRADITIONAL USES
General aches, headaches, colds, fevers, rheumatism and women's ailments.

PHARMACOLOGICAL ACTION
Analgetic, anti-inflammatory, antithrombotic, cytotoxic, spasmolytic. It has been suggested that parthenolide exerts inhibiting effects on serotonin release by human platelets *in vitro*. Other evidence suggests that chrysanthenyl acetate, which has been shown to inhibit prostaglandin synthesis *in vitro* and which seems to possess analgesic properties, may be important.

CONDITIONS FREQUENTLY TREATED
Migraine and rheumatoid arthritis.

CLINICAL EVIDENCE
A Cochrane review included five double-blind RCTs ($n = 343$) of feverfew for preventing migraine.[1] While the two studies with high methodological quality showed no beneficial effects, three others were in favour of feverfew. Of the four trials with a sample size of 50 or above, two studies reported feverfew to be superior to placebo, while two did not. An additional double-blind RCT ($n = 170$) showed a reduction of migraine frequency which was of borderline significance compared with placebo after a 4-month treatment period.[2] Overall, the data do not convincingly establish that feverfew is efficacious for preventing migraine. A combination preparation of 400 mg riboflavin, 300 mg magnesium and 100 mg feverfew daily generated no difference compared with placebo for the reduction in migraine attacks.[3] One double-blind RCT of feverfew as a treatment for rheumatoid arthritis found no relevant differences for clinical variables including pain compared with placebo.[4]

DOSAGE
50–140 mg of powdered or granulated dried leaf preparation daily in divided doses.

RISKS
CONTRAINDICATIONS
Pregnancy and lactation (see p. 4), hypersensitivity to members of the Asteraceae family.

PRECAUTIONS/WARNINGS

Should not be used for longer than 4 months because there is a lack of long-term toxicity data.

ADVERSE EFFECTS

Allergic reactions, contact dermatitis, mouth ulceration and soreness, gastrointestinal complaints, 'post-feverfew syndrome' including rebound of migraine symptoms, anxiety, dizziness, insomnia, muscle and joint stiffness.

INTERACTIONS

May potentiate the effects of anticoagulants.

QUALITY ISSUES

The amount of active constituents may vary according to the origin of the plant and the plant parts used.

RISK–BENEFIT ASSESSMENT

The evidence from rigorous clinical trials is encouraging but not convincing enough to suggest an effect of feverfew over and above placebo for preventing migraine attacks. However, given that feverfew presents no major safety problems, the limited number of available options for preventing migraine and the severity of the condition, this option may be worth considering in some cases. There are too few studies for any firm judgement on the effectiveness of feverfew in rheumatoid arthritis.

REFERENCES

1. Pittler MH, Ernst E. Feverfew for preventing migraine. The Cochrane Database of Systematic Reviews 2004, Issue 1. Art. No.: CD002286
2. Diener HC, Pfaffenrath V, Schnitker J, Friede M, Henneicke-von Zepelin HH. Efficacy and safety of 6.25 mg t.i.d. feverfew CO_2-extract (MIG-99) in migraine prevention – a randomized, double-blind, multicentre, placebo-controlled study. Cephalalgia 2005;25: 1031–1041
3. Maizels M, Blumenfeld A, Burchette R. A combination of riboflavin, magnesium, and feverfew for migraine prophylaxis: a randomized trial. Headache 2004;44:885–890
4. Pattrick M, Heptinstall S, Doherty M. Feverfew in rheumatoid arthritis: a double-blind, placebo-controlled study. Ann Rheum Dis 1989;48:547–549

GINGER

(Zingiber officinale)

SOURCE

Rhizome.

MAIN CONSTITUENTS

Niacin, non-pungent substances, non-volatile pungent principles, starch, triglycerides, vitamins and volatile oil.

BACKGROUND

Ginger is a perennial plant native to southern Asia. It has a long history of use as a food and for medicinal purposes, particularly to treat ailments such as stomach ache, diarrhoea and nausea.

In the 16th century, ginger was introduced to the Caribbean and Central America by the Spanish and was later cultivated for export. German and European monographs are available and, in 1997, the US Pharmacopoeia approved ginger and powdered ginger monographs for inclusion in the National Formulary.

EXAMPLES OF TRADITIONAL USES

Osteoarthritis, gastrointestinal complaints, diarrhoea, dyspepsia, nausea, vomiting and respiratory disorders.

PHARMACOLOGICAL ACTION

Anti-emetic, anti-inflammatory, positive inotropic, carminative, promotes secretion of saliva and gastric juices, cholagogue, inhibition of platelet aggregation.

CONDITIONS FREQUENTLY TREATED

Dyspepsia, loss of appetite, prevention of motion sickness.

CLINICAL EVIDENCE

Three double-blind RCTs tested whether ginger was effective for reducing pain associated with osteoarthritis of the knee.[1-3] Different preparations of ginger were administered for treatment periods from 3 to 12 weeks. All trials assessed pain on visual analogue scales and reported beneficial effects compared with placebo. The largest RCT[2] ($n = 261$) concluded that '… ginger extract had a statistically significant effect on reducing symptoms of osteoarthritis of the knee. This effect was moderate'. The three extracts used were from different plant genera.[4] Another double-blind RCT included 120 outpatients with osteoarthritis of moderate to severe pain and compared ginger with ibuprofen and placebo.[5] Overall symptom improvement was superior in the ginger and ibuprofen groups compared with the placebo group. Pain visual analogue scale scores and gelling or regressive pain after rising were higher in the placebo group than in the ginger and ibuprofen groups 1 month after the treatment, while there were no differences in visual analogue scores and gelling pain scores between the ginger and the ibuprofen groups.

DOSAGE

1–4 g of powdered extract daily.

RISKS

CONTRAINDICATIONS

Pregnancy and lactation (see p. 4). A clinical review found no scientific or medical evidence for the contraindication of ginger during pregnancy.[6] Preclinical safety data, however, do not rule out potential toxicity[7] and there is a theoretical risk of congenital deformity in neonates. Allergy to members of the Zingiberaceae family.

PRECAUTIONS/WARNINGS

Children under 6 years of age; gallstones. Patients using anticoagulants, patients before surgery.

ADVERSE EFFECTS

Heartburn, belching, bloating, flatulence, nausea; its mutagenic potential shown in *in vitro* studies requires further systematic research.

INTERACTIONS

Increased effects of anticoagulants; may interfere with cardiac and antidiabetic therapies; may enhance the effects of central nervous system depressants.

QUALITY ISSUES

The term ginger used in the studies might relate to different plant genera.[4] The principal components of ginger may vary greatly depending on the country of origin.

RISK–BENEFIT ASSESSMENT

For pain associated with osteoarthritis of the knee, the evidence is encouraging but not convincing because of the heterogeneity of the plant extracts used. However, given the reported low frequency of risks involved, ginger may be worth trying for this condition.

REFERENCES

1. Bliddal H, Rosetzky A, Schlichting P, Weidner MS, Andersen LA, Ibfelt HH, Christensen K, Jensen ON, Barslev J. A randomized, placebo-controlled, cross-over study of ginger extract and Ibuprofen in osteoarthritis. Osteoarthritis Cartilage 2000;8:9–12
2. Altman RD, Marcussen KC. Effects of a ginger extract on knee pain in patients with osteoarthritis. Arthritis Rheum 2001;44:2531–2538
3. Wigler I, Grotto I, Caspi D, Yaron M. The effects of Zintona EC (a ginger extract) on symptomatic gonarthritis. Osteoarthritis Cartilage 2003;11:783–789
4. Canter P. Ginger – do we know what we are talking about? Focus Altern Complement Ther 2004;9:184–185
5. Haghighi M, Khalvat A, Toliat T, Jallaei S. Comparing the effects of ginger (*Zingiber officinale*) extract and ibuprofen on patients with osteoarthritis. Arch Iran Med 2005;8:267–271
6. Fulder S, Tenne M. Ginger as an anti-nausea remedy in pregnancy: the issue of safety. Herbalgram 1996;38:47–50
7. Chrubasik S, Pittler MH, Roufogalis BD. *Zingiberis rhizoma*: a comprehensive review on the ginger effect and efficacy profiles. Phytomedicine 2005;12:684–701

SECTION FOUR

GLUCOSAMINE

SOURCE

Glucosamine is an amino-monosaccharide that occurs naturally in cartilage. It is produced synthetically for the food supplements market.

BACKGROUND

Glucosamine sulphate is the sulphate salt of 2-amino-2-deoxy-D-chitin glucopyranose, which is a constituent of joint cartilage. It was therefore hypothesised that its oral supplementation might stimulate cartilage formation and enhance cartilage repair. Glucosamine has since become a popular 'natural' treatment for arthritis.

EXAMPLES OF TRADITIONAL USES

Joint pain, osteoarthritis.

PHARMACOLOGICAL ACTION

Increased mucopolysaccharide and collagen production in fibroblasts *in vitro*, inhibition of enzymes which break down cartilage (e.g. elastase), similar actions to chondroitin (see p. 186).

CONDITIONS FREQUENTLY TREATED

Osteoarthritis.

CLINICAL EVIDENCE

Numerous trials have investigated the effect of glucosamine in the treatment of osteoarthritis in general and osteoarthritis of the knee in particular. Earlier systematic reviews concluded that glucosamine is superior to placebo[1,2] but results from more recent studies are no longer uniformly positive.[3–5] A Cochrane review[3] assessed 20 studies including 2570 patients. Collectively, the 20 analysed RCTs found glucosamine to be superior to placebo with a 28% improvement in pain and a 21% improvement in function from baseline using the Lequesne index. Meta-analysis of Western Ontario and McMaster Universities osteoarthritis index (WOMAC™) pain, function and stiffness outcomes did not reach statistical significance. When only the studies with adequate allocation concealment ($n = 8$) or those not using preparations of the Rotta brand were analysed, the results failed to show any benefit of glucosamine for pain and WOMAC function. Those studies evaluating a Rotta preparation showed glucosamine to be superior to placebo ($n = 10$) and superior ($n = 2$) or equivalent ($n = 2$) to non-steroidal anti-inflammatory drugs in the treatment of pain and functional impairment resulting from symptomatic osteoarthritis. WOMAC outcomes of pain, stiffness and function did not show a superiority of glucosamine over placebo. Glucosamine was as safe as placebo. One systematic review of long-term glucosamine treatment of knee osteoarthritis ($n = 2$) found glucosamine sulphate to be effective and safe in delaying progression and improving symptoms.[5] Subsequent RCTs have yielded contradictory results for knee osteoarthritis. One ($n = 90$) found glucosamine hydrochloride and glucosamine sulphate administered in addition to diclofenac more effective in decreasing pain and improving joint function than diclofenac alone[6] and a further RCT ($n = 142$) found glucosamine hydrochloride and glucosamine sulphate to be equally effective in reducing pain.[7] A high-quality RCT ($n = 1229$), however, failed to confirm that glucosamine and chondroitin sulphate alone or in combination are better than placebo in reducing pain; yet it suggested that the combination of both may be effective in a subgroup of patients with moderate-to-severe knee pain.[8]

Two RCTs investigated the effect of glucosamine in the treatment of temporomandibular joint disorders; one found glucosamine to be at least as effective as analgesic doses of ibuprofen for function and pain,[9] the other trial using a glucosamine/chondroitin combination was inconclusive.[10]

DOSAGE

500 mg of oral glucosamine sulphate three times daily.

RISKS

CONTRAINDICATIONS

Pregnancy and lactation (see p. 4).

PRECAUTIONS/WARNINGS

Avoid use in children under the age of 2 years, in patients with asthma or with shell-fish allergies (products derived from marine exoskeletons). Although initial concerns about use in diabetic patients based on *in vitro* and rat studies were not confirmed in human studies it is advisable to monitor these patients closely.

ADVERSE EFFECTS

Mild gastrointestinal complaints including nausea, heartburn, diarrhoea and constipation; drowsiness, dyspepsia, headache and rash.

INTERACTIONS

None known.

QUALITY ISSUES

Both glucosamine sulphate and glucosamine hydrochloride are used; it is unclear which is superior. Glucosamine is not required to be tested for quality in the US; in parts of Europe it is available as a prescription drug of defined chemical nature.

RISK–BENEFIT ASSESSMENT

There is some evidence from RCTs that glucosamine (sulphate) is superior to placebo in the treatment of osteoarthritis although more recent results are no longer unanimously positive. A number of studies also suggest that glucosamine and ibuprofen are similarly effective but longer treatment periods are needed (e.g. 4 weeks and more) for a clinical benefit to become manifest. The size of the clinical effect is usually moderate. Glucosamine seems to be well tolerated for up to 3 years and no major safety problems are on record. Thus, glucosamine can be recommended as an adjuvant therapy for osteoarthritis.

REFERENCES

1. Richy F, Bruyere O, Ethgen O, Cucherat M, Henrotin Y, Reginster JY. Structural and symptomatic efficacy of glucosamine and chondroitin in knee osteoarthritis: a comprehensive meta-analysis. Arch Intern Med 2003;163:1514–1522
2. McAlindon TE, LaValley MP, Gulin JP, Felson DT. Glucosamine and chondroitin for treatment of osteoarthritis: a systematic quality assessment and meta-analysis. JAMA 2000;283:1469–1475
3. Towheed TE, Maxwell L, Anastassiades TP, Shea B, Houpt J, Robinson V, Hochberg MC, Wells G. Glucosamine therapy for treating osteoarthritis. The Cochrane Database of Systematic Reviews 2005, Issue 2. Art. No.: CD002946
4. Bazian Ltd. Glucosamine for osteoarthritis: systematic review. Evid Based Health Care Public Health 2005;9:322–331
5. Poolsup N, Suthisisang C, Channark P, Kittikulsuth W. Glucosamine long-term treatment and the progression of knee osteoarthritis: systematic review of randomized controlled trials. Ann Pharmacother 2005;39:1080–1087
6. Alekseeva LI, Chichasova NV, Benevolenskaia LI, Nasonov EL, Mendel' OI. Combined medication ARTRA in the treatment of osteoarthrosis. [In Russian.] Ter Arkh 2005;77:69–75.
7. Qiu GX, Weng XS, Zhang K, Zhou YX, Lou SQ, Wang YP, Li W, Zhang H, Liu Y. A multi-central, randomized, controlled clinical trial of glucosamine hydrochloride/sulfate in the treatment of knee osteoarthritis. [In Chinese.] Zhonghua Yi Xue Za Zhi 2005;85: 3067–3070
8. Clegg DO, Reda DJ, Harris CL, Klein MA, O'Dell JR, Hooper MM, Bradley JD, Bingham CO 3rd, Weisman MH, Jackson CG, Lane NE, Cush JJ, Moreland LW, Schumacher HR Jr, Oddis CV, Wolfe F, Molitor JA, Yocum DE, Schnitzer TJ, Furst DE, Sawitzke AD, Shi H, Brandt KD, Moskowitz RW, Williams HJ. Glucosamine, chondroitin sulfate, and the two in combination for painful knee osteoarthritis. N Engl J Med 2006;354:795–808
9. Thie NM, Prasad NG, Major PW. Evaluation of glucosamine sulfate compared to ibuprofen for the treatment of temporomandibular joint osteoarthritis: a randomized double blind controlled 3 month clinical trial. J Rheumatol 2001;28:1347–1355
10. Nguyen P, Mohamed SE, Gardiner D, Salinas T. A randomized double-blind clinical trial of the effect of chondroitin sulfate and glucosamine hydrochloride on temporomandibular joint disorders: a pilot study. Cranio 2001;19:130–139

GREEN-LIPPED MUSSEL   (*Perna canaliculus*)

SOURCE

Tissue from the New Zealand green-lipped mussel (*Perna canaliculus*).

SECTION FOUR

MAIN CONSTITUENTS

Omega-3 fatty acids.

BACKGROUND

The coastal Maori population of New Zealand traditionally enjoyed green-lipped mussels as food. It was believed to promote good health and keep arthritic problems at bay.

EXAMPLES OF TRADITIONAL USES

Arthritis.

PHARMACOLOGICAL ACTION

Anti-inflammatory properties of omega-3 fatty acids, e.g. inhibition of pro-inflammatory prostaglandins.

CONDITIONS FREQUENTLY TREATED

Arthritis.

CLINICAL EVIDENCE

A systematic review included five RCTs of a freeze-dried preparation of green-lipped mussel as a treatment of rheumatoid arthritis or osteoarthritis.[1] Two of them suggested efficacy but the totality of this evidence was judged inconclusive.

DOSAGE

1 mg per day.

RISKS

CONTRAINDICATIONS

Pregnancy and lactation (see p. 4), coagulation abnormalities.

PRECAUTIONS/WARNINGS

As per omega-3 fatty acids; green-lipped mussel preparations may be cyclooxygenase 2 inhibitors.

ADVERSE EFFECTS

None known.

OVERDOSE

Bleeding tendency.

INTERACTIONS

Might enhance the effects of anticoagulants.

QUALITY ISSUES

Use only high-quality preparations.

RISK–BENEFIT ASSESSMENT

The benefits of green-lipped mussel preparations are not well documented. There are few risks associated with them but the risk–benefit balance is not demonstrably positive.

REFERENCES
1. Cobb CS, Ernst E. Systematic review of a marine nutriceutical supplement in clinical trials for arthritis: the effectiveness of the New Zealand green-lipped mussel *Perna canaliculus*. Clin Rheumatol 2006;25:275–284

HORSE CHESTNUT   (*Aesculus hippocastanum*)

SOURCE
Seeds.

MAIN CONSTITUENTS
Fatty acids, flavonoids, quinones, saponins, sterols, tannins and triterpenes.

BACKGROUND
The horse chestnut tree is native to south-east Europe and was allegedly first introduced to northern Europe in the mid-16th century by the botanist Charles de l'Écluse, from seeds brought from Constantinople. Today the tree is widely distributed all over the world. The genus name *Aesculus* derives from the Latin *esca* meaning 'food' and the Latin *hippocastanum* is reported to derive from the practice of feeding the seeds to horses to treat respiratory ailments.

EXAMPLES OF TRADITIONAL USES
Varicose veins, diarrhoea, haemorrhoids, malaria and respiratory diseases.

PHARMACOLOGICAL ACTION
Anti-exudative, anti-inflammatory and immunomodulatory activity. Escin, the principal active component of horse chestnut seed extract (HCSE), constricts veins and reduces the permeability of venous capillaries *in vitro*. It has been suggested to inhibit the activity of elastase and hyaluronidase, both involved in enzymatic proteoglycan degradation. Studies have shown increased levels of leukocytes in affected limbs and suggested a possible subsequent activation with release of such enzymes. Other studies reported an increased serum activity of proteoglycan hydrolases in patients with chronic venous insufficiency, which were reduced with HCSE use.

CONDITIONS FREQUENTLY TREATED
Symptoms (e.g. pain) or trophic changes linked to chronic venous insufficiency, haematoma.

CLINICAL EVIDENCE
A systematic review and meta-analysis[1] assessed the efficacy and safety of oral HCSE mono-preparations and concluded that, overall, there appeared to be an improvement in chronic venous insufficiency-related signs and symptoms with HCSE compared with placebo. Leg pain was assessed in seven placebo-controlled trials. Six reported a reduction of leg pain in the HCSE groups compared with the placebo groups, while another reported an improvement compared with baseline. Leg volume was assessed in seven placebo-controlled trials. Meta-analysis of six trials ($n = 502$) showed results that were in favour of HCSE compared with placebo. One trial ($n = 240$) indicated that HCSE may be as effective as compression stockings at reducing leg volume.[2] These results are corroborated by an earlier, independent meta-analysis.[3] For its topical use and for other indications there seems to be no evidence from rigorous clinical trials.

SECTION FOUR

DOSAGE

- *Internal use*: extract standardised to 100–150 mg escin daily in divided doses.
- *External use*: apply several times daily.

RISKS

CONTRAINDICATIONS

Pregnancy and lactation (see p. 4), bleeding disorders, allergy to any of its constituents.

PRECAUTIONS/WARNINGS

Open wounds, weeping eczema (external use), intravenous administration.

ADVERSE EFFECTS

Pruritus, nausea, gastrointestinal complaints, bleeding, dizziness, headache, nephropathy and allergic reactions.

INTERACTIONS

Increased effects of aspirin and other anticoagulants, antihyperglycaemics.

QUALITY ISSUES

Preparations are generally standardised to 50–75 mg escin per capsule. Quality of the extracts may vary between preparations.

RISK–BENEFIT ASSESSMENT

The available evidence suggests that HCSE is effective for treating patients with leg pain that is linked to chronic venous insufficiency. Given the nature and frequency of the reported adverse events and the relatively poor compliance with conventional treatments such as compression therapy, HCSE is worthy of consideration when treating patients with this condition.

REFERENCES

1. Pittler MH, Ernst E. Horse chestnut seed extract for chronic venous insufficiency. The Cochrane Database of Systematic Reviews 2006, Issue 1. Art. No.: CD003230
2. Diehm C, Trampisch HJ, Lange S, Schmidt C. Comparison of leg compression stocking and oral horse-chestnut seed extract therapy in patients with chronic venous insufficiency. Lancet 1996;347:292–294
3. Siebert U, Brach M, Sroczynski G, Berla K. Efficacy, routine effectiveness, and safety of horsechestnut seed extract in the treatment of chronic venous insufficiency. A meta-analysis of randomized controlled trials and large observational studies. Int Angiol 2002;21:305–315

INDIAN FRANKINCENSE   *(Boswellia serrata)*

SOURCE

Resin.

MAIN CONSTITUENTS

Boswellic acid, α-boswellic acid.

BACKGROUND

Indian frankincense is a branching tree found in India, northern Africa and the Middle East. When incisions are made in the bark of the trunk a resinous gum is exuded. Up to 16% of the resin is essential oil. Its use dates to ancient Egypt, where it was employed as an ingredient in embalming liquids for mummies. Indian frankincense has also been used to improve emotional well-being and as part of religious rituals. Extracts of Indian frankincense resin gum have traditionally been used in the Ayurvedic system of medicine as an anti-arthritic.

EXAMPLES OF TRADITIONAL USES

Rheumatism, painful menstruation, abdominal pain, sores, tumours, cancers, asthma, sore throat, syphilis, pimples, stomach complaints, nervous problems, as a stimulant, respiratory antiseptic, diuretic, and for stimulating menstrual flow.

PHARMACOLOGICAL ACTION

Analgesic, anti-inflammatory, inhibits the enzyme 5-lipoxygenase and glucosaminoglycan synthesis.

CONDITIONS FREQUENTLY TREATED

Arthritis, asthma and inflammatory bowel disease.

CLINICAL EVIDENCE

A double-blind crossover RCT of Indian frankincense extract including 30 patients with osteoarthritis of the knee reported decreased knee pain, increased knee flexion and increased walking distance compared with placebo.[1] Two RCTs tested combination products. RA-11, a combination of Indian frankincense, *Withania somnifera*, ginger (*Zingiber officinale*) and turmeric (*Curcuma longa*), was shown to reduce pain and improve WOMAC scores in 385 patients with osteoarthritis of the knee.[2] Articulin-F, a herbomineral formulation containing Indian frankincense, *Withania somnifera*, turmeric and zinc, reduced the severity of pain and disability scores in an RCT of 42 patients with osteoarthritis.[3] The effects of Indian frankincense alone are, however, not clear. A double-blind RCT of 182 patients with rheumatoid arthritis using RA-1, a standardised plant extract formulation of Indian frankincense, *Withania somnifera*, ginger and turmeric, reported that results were not superior to the high placebo response.[4] The results of an RCT testing Indian frankincense extract H15 in 37 patients with chronic polyarthritis reported no improvement in pain.[5]

DOSAGE

600–1200 mg of oral gum resin preparation daily have been used in clinical trials; 1500–3000 mg according to Ayurvedic medicine.

RISKS

CONTRAINDICATIONS

Pregnancy and lactation (see p. 4); according to reports in the Indian literature, resin from Indian frankincense may be an emmenagogue and cause abortion.

PRECAUTIONS/WARNINGS

Use cautiously in patients taking lipid-soluble medication and patients with gastritis or gastro-oesophageal reflux disease.

ADVERSE EFFECTS

Nausea, acid reflux, mild gastrointestinal upset.

SECTION FOUR

INTERACTIONS

May potentiate the action of leukotriene inhibitors, lipid-lowering agents, anti-neoplastic agents.

RISK–BENEFIT ASSESSMENT

Although the reported risks of Indian frankincense are generally of a mild and rare nature there is insufficient evidence to recommend for or against its use in osteoarthritis or rheumatoid arthritis.

REFERENCES

1. Kimmatkar N, Thawani V, Hingorani L, Khiyani R. Efficacy and tolerability of *Boswellia serrata* extract in treatment of osteoarthritis of knee – a randomized double blind placebo controlled trial. Phytomedicine 2003;10:3–7
2. Chopra A, Lavin P, Patwardhan B, Chitre D. A 32-week randomized, placebo-controlled clinical evaluation of RA-11, an Ayurvedic drug, on osteoarthritis of the knee. J Clin Rheumatol 2004; 10:236–245
3. Kulkarni RR, Patki PS, Jog VP, Gandage SG, Patwardhan B. Treatment of osteoarthritis with a herbomineral formulation: a double-blind, placebo-controlled, cross-over study. J Ethnopharmacol 1991;33:91–95
4. Chopra A, Lavin P, Patwardhan B, Chitre D. Randomized double blind trial of an ayurvedic plant derived formulation for treatment of rheumatoid arthritis. J Rheumatol 2000;27: 1365–1372
5. Sander O, Herborn G, Rau R. Is H15 (resin extract of *Boswellia serrata*, "incense") a useful supplement to established drug therapy of chronic polyarthritis? Results of a double-blind pilot study. [In German.] Z Rheumatol 1998;57:11–16

LAVENDER   (*Lavandula angustifolia*)

SOURCE

Flowering heads.

MAIN CONSTITUENTS

Camphor, cineole, flavonoids, hydroxycoumarins, limonene, perillyl alcohol, tannins, triterpenes, volatile oil (linalyl acetate, linalool).

BACKGROUND

The name lavender is derived from the Latin *lavare* (to wash). Native to the Mediterranean and common in southern Europe, lavender is widely cultivated for culinary, cosmetic and medicinal use. It has been used for centuries to treat various ailments.

EXAMPLES OF TRADITIONAL USES

Migraines, neuralgia and other pain syndromes, bruises, burns, cuts, wound healing, appetite stimulant, functional abdominal complaints, insomnia.

PHARMACOLOGICAL ACTION

Anxiolytic, spasmolytic, astringent, sedative, anticonvulsant, antioxidant, lipid-lowering.

CONDITIONS FREQUENTLY TREATED

Headaches, anxiety, insomnia.

SECTION FOUR

CLINICAL EVIDENCE

An RCT of acupoint stimulation followed by acupressure with aromatic lavender oil suggested that this treatment is effective for short-term low back pain relief compared with placebo.[1] Similar results were reported in an RCT of acupressure with aromatic lavender essential oil for subacute, non-specific neck pain;[2] the role of lavender in both trials was, however, unclear. No direct analgesic effect was found by an RCT of lavender aromatherapy in experimentally induced pain[3] and one RCT found no long-term benefit of aromatherapy massage with lavender oil on pain, anxiety or quality of life in 42 cancer patients.[4] A large RCT ($n = 635$) of postnatal perineal discomfort found no difference between lavender essential oil, synthetic lavender oil and an inert substance added to a bath.[5] A small controlled trial of lavender and lemon aromatherapies and two forms of music therapy found lavender or preferred music reduced pain after but not during dressing change of vascular wounds.[6]

DOSAGE

- *Oral*: one or two teaspoons of dried flowers in 150 ml hot water (lavender tea).
- *Aromatherapy*: two to four drops in two or three cups of boiling water for aromatherapy inhalation.
- *Topical*: six drops or up to half a cup of dried flowers as a bath additive.

RISKS

CONTRAINDICATIONS

Pregnancy and lactation (see p. 4); because of its alleged emmenagogic properties, excessive internal use should be avoided.

PRECAUTIONS/WARNINGS

The essential oil should be regarded as potentially poisonous if taken internally.

ADVERSE EFFECTS

Nausea, vomiting, headache and chills have been reported following inhalation or absorption through the skin. Contact allergy and phototoxicity are also possible.

OVERDOSE

Nausea, vomiting and anorexia have been reported after large doses of lavender. Large doses are also reported to exert 'narcotic-like' effects.

INTERACTIONS

Could potentiate effects of central nervous system depressants.

QUALITY ISSUES

Standardised preparations of the herb are rare, but lavender oil is often an ingredient in external rubs and massage oils and the essential oil is widely available.

RISK–BENEFIT ASSESSMENT

In recommended doses, lavender is generally well-tolerated with minimal adverse events. No positive effects have been reported for the treatment of pain with lavender on its own. Its use for this purpose therefore cannot be recommended.

REFERENCES

1. Yip YB, Tse SH. The effectiveness of relaxation acupoint stimulation and acupressure with aromatic lavender essential oil for non-specific low back pain in Hong Kong: a randomised controlled trial. Complement Ther Med 2004;12:28–37
2. Yip YB, Tse SH. An experimental study on the effectiveness of acupressure with aromatic lavender essential oil for sub-acute, non-specific neck pain in Hong Kong. Complement Ther Clin Pract 2006;12:18–26
3. Gedney JJ, Glover TL, Fillingim RB. Sensory and affective pain discrimination after inhalation of essential oils. Psychosom Med 2004;66:599–606
4. Soden K, Vincent K, Craske S, Lucas C, Ashley S. A randomized controlled trial of aromatherapy massage in a hospice setting. Palliat Med 2004;18:87–92
5. Dale A, Cornwell S. The role of lavender oil in relieving perineal discomfort following childbirth: a blind randomised clinical trial. J Adv Nurs 1994;19:89–96
6. Kane FM, Brodie EE, Coull A, Coyne L, Howd A, Milne A, Niven CC, Robbins R. The analgesic effect of odour and music upon dressing change. Br J Nurs 2004;13:S4–12

LEECHES

(Hirudo medicinalis)

SOURCE

Not applicable.

MAIN CONSTITUENTS

Leech saliva contains several pharmacologically active constituents, most importantly hirudin.

BACKGROUND

Leeches have been used medicinally in several cultures. The animals are applied to the skin where they bite, suck blood and secret saliva. When they have drawn sufficient blood, they eventually drop off.

EXAMPLES OF TRADITIONAL USES

Phlebitis, thrombotic states.

PHARMACOLOGICAL ACTION

Hirudin is a potent inhibitor of coagulation.

CONDITIONS FREQUENTLY TREATED

Today leeches are used in conventional medicine to relieve post-operative local congestion. In CAM, leeches are sometimes employed to reduce local musculoskeletal pain.

CLINICAL EVIDENCE

A small RCT compared leech therapy with topical diclofenac in 51 patients suffering from knee osteoarthritis.[1] The results indicated superiority of leech therapy in terms of function and pain. These findings require independent replication.

DOSAGE

Four to six leeches are applied per session with one session per day for several days; one session lasts around half an hour.

SECTION FOUR

RISKS
CONTRAINDICATIONS
>Pregnancy and lactation (see p. 4), hypocoagulability.

PRECAUTIONS/WARNINGS
>Long-term effects are unknown.

ADVERSE EFFECTS
>Theoretically, leeches could cause infection.

OVERDOSE
>Bleeding.

INTERACTIONS
>Anticoagulants.

QUALITY ISSUES
>A reliable source should be used to minimise the chance of infection.

RISK–BENEFIT ASSESSMENT
One RCT suggests benefit in knee osteoarthritis and the risks associated with leeches are relatively small. More data are required for a risk–benefit assessment.

REFERENCE
>1. Michalsen A, Klotz S, Lüdtke R, Moebus S, Spahn G, Dobos GJ. Effectiveness of leech therapy in osteoarthritis of the knee: a randomized, controlled trial. Ann Intern Med 2003;139:724–730

NETTLE (Urtica dioica)

SECTION FOUR

SOURCE
Leaves and roots.

MAIN CONSTITUENTS
- *Leaf*: minerals, flavonoids, sterols, tannins, vitamins.
- *Root*: coumarin, fatty acids, lectins, lignans, polysaccharides, sterols, tannins, terpenes.

BACKGROUND
The stinging nettle is a perennial herb, which grows throughout much of the temperate zones of both hemispheres. The genus name *Urtica* derives from the Latin verb *urere* ('to burn'), while the species name *dioica* ('two houses') refers to the flowers bearing male and female parts on separate plants. Nettles cause a characteristic itching rash upon contact with the skin. It has enjoyed a long history of medicinal use for a number of conditions such as asthma and disorders of the spleen.

EXAMPLES OF TRADITIONAL USES
Rheumatism, muscle relaxant during childbirth, kidney disorders, asthma, bleeding conditions, infantile and psychogenic eczema. Young stinging nettle is also eaten as a cooked vegetable.

PHARMACOLOGICAL ACTION

Analgesic, diuretic, antihypertensive, immunostimulatory and anti-inflammatory.

CONDITIONS FREQUENTLY TREATED

- *Leaf*: musculoskeletal pain, kidney gravel, lower urinary tract infections.
- *Root*: micturition disorders in benign prostatic hyperplasia.

CLINICAL EVIDENCE

One RCT investigated the effects of stinging nettle leaves for osteoarthritic pain of the base of the thumb or index finger and reported beneficial effects for pain and disability scores compared with deadnettle (*Laminum album*).[1] Stinging nettle has also been the subject of RCTs reporting positive effects in patients with acute arth-ritis.[2] A number of RCTs have also investigated nettle root extract for the treatment of benign prostatic hyperplasia[3-6] and reported improvements in symptom scores.

DOSAGE

- *Leaf*: 0.6–2.1 g of dry extract daily in divided doses.
- *Root*: 0.7–1.3 g of dry extract daily in divided doses.

RISKS

CONTRAINDICATIONS

Pregnancy and lactation (see p. 4).

PRECAUTIONS/WARNINGS

Children under the age of 2 years.

ADVERSE EFFECTS

Gastrointestinal complaints, diarrhoea, allergic reactions, urticaria, pruritus, oedema, decreased urine volume.

INTERACTIONS

May potentiate the effects of diuretics, antihypertensives, antihyperglycaemics and central nervous system antidepressants. Might decrease the effects of anticoagulant drugs.

RISK–BENEFIT ASSESSMENT

Encouraging findings are emerging for the use of nettle in arthritis but the evidence is not sufficiently strong to allow any firm recommendations.

REFERENCES

1. Randall C, Randall H, Dobbs F, Hutton C, Sanders H. Randomised controlled trial of nettle sting for treatment of base-of-thumb pain. J Roy Soc Med 2000;93:305–309
2. Chrubasik S, Enderlein W, Bauer R, Grabner W. Evidence of antirheumatic effectiveness of Herba Urticae dioicae in acute arthritis. A pilot study. Phytomedicine 1997;4:105–108
3. Engelmann U, Boos G, Kres H. Therapie der benignen Prostatahyperplasie mit Bazoton Liquidum. Urologe B 1996;36:287–291
4. Fischer M, Wilbert D. Wirkprüfung eines Phytopharmakons zur Behandlung der benignen Prostatahyperplasie. In: Rutishauser G, ed. Benigne Prostatahyperplasie III. München: Zuckerschwerdt; 1992:79
5. Dathe G, Schmid H. Phytotherapie der benignen Prostatahyperplasie (BPH). Doppelblindstudie mit Extraktum Radicis Urticae (ERU). Urologe B 1987;27:223–226
6. Vontobel HP, Herzog R, Rutishauser G, Kres H. Ergebnisse einer Doppelblindstudie über die Wirksamkeit von ERU-Kapseln in der konservativen Behandlung der benignen Prostatahyperplasie. Urologe A 1985;24:49–51

PEPPERMINT   *(Mentha x piperita)*

SOURCE
Leaves and oil.

MAIN CONSTITUENTS
- *Leaf*: caffeic, chlorogenic and rosmarinic acids, hesperidin, luteolin, rutin, volatile oil.
- *Oil*: cineol, isomenthone, limonene, menthofuran, menthol, menthone, menthyl acetate.

BACKGROUND
Peppermint is a perennial herb and is characterised by its smell and square stem, which is typical for members of the mint family. It is a natural hybrid of water mint (*Mentha aquatica*) and spearmint (*Mentha spicata*). Its genus name, *Mentha*, is derived from the Greek mythical nymph *Mintha*, who metamorphosed into this plant. Peppermint is mainly cultivated for its fragrant oil, which is obtained through steam distillation of the fresh aerial parts of the plant.

EXAMPLES OF TRADITIONAL USES
- *Leaf*: complaints of the gall bladder and bile duct, flatulence, gastrointestinal disorders.
- *Oil*: headache, myalgia, neuralgia, irritable bowel syndrome, inflammation of the oral mucosa, common cold.

PHARMACOLOGICAL ACTION
Antispasmodic, antimicrobial, antiseptic, carminative, cholagogue, cooling. The principal active constituent of peppermint oil is thought to be menthol, a cyclic monoterpene with calcium channel-blocking activity.

CONDITIONS FREQUENTLY TREATED
- *Leaf*: complaints of the gastrointestinal tract.
- *Oil*: headache, myalgia, irritable bowel syndrome, common cold.

DOSAGE
- *Leaf*: 3–6 g as infusion daily; 0.8–1.8 g of dry extract daily in divided doses.
- *Essential oil*: 0.6–1.2 ml in enteric-coated capsules daily; or three or four drops of oil three times daily in hot water internally (as inhalant). Apply as needed externally.

CLINICAL EVIDENCE
For children with recurrent abdominal pain, a systematic review identified evidence of effectiveness.[1] Antispasmodic effects for intraluminally administered peppermint oil have been reported during upper endoscopy.[2] RCTs from the same research group suggested positive effects of externally applied peppermint oil for patients with tension-type headache.[3,4] For irritable bowel syndrome, an earlier systematic review and meta-analysis suggested that, although the majority of RCTs report beneficial effects, methodological limitations prevent firm conclusions.[5] This was corroborated by a further independent systematic review.[6] For treating non-ulcer dyspepsia, a systematic review identified nine RCTs of combination preparations containing peppermint and caraway and concluded that they seem to have

effects with at least a similar magnitude to conventional therapies and encouraging safety profiles.[7] One RCT suggested peppermint tea as a possible adjuvant treatment for urinary tract infection.[8]

RISKS

CONTRAINDICATIONS

Pregnancy and lactation (see p. 4), children under the age of 12 years, obstruction of the bile duct, cholecystitis, allergy to any constituent of peppermint.

PRECAUTIONS/WARNINGS

Individuals with glucose-6-phosphate dehydrogenase deficiency; gallstones, hiatus hernia.

ADVERSE EFFECTS

Allergic reactions, skin irritation, contact dermatitis, laryngeal or bronchial spasm, mouth ulceration, eye irritation, heartburn, belching, perianal burning, gastrointestinal complaints, headache, dizziness, pruritus.

OVERDOSE

The fatal dose of menthol in humans is estimated to be 1 g per kg body weight.

INTERACTIONS

Might increase levels of drugs metabolised by CYP3A4, a member of the cytochrome p450 system

RISK–BENEFIT ASSESSMENT

The data for the external use of peppermint oil for treating headache are encouraging but require independent replication. For irritable bowel syndrome, some RCTs report positive effects, but the evidence is not convincing. For functional dyspepsia there seems to be good evidence of effectiveness for combination preparations of peppermint and caraway oil and their use can be recommended for this condition. Adverse effects exist but are usually transient and mild.

REFERENCES

1. Weydert JA, Ball TM, Davis MF. Systematic review of treatments for recurrent abdominal pain. Pediatrics 2003;111:e1–11
2. Hiki N, Kurosaka H, Tatsutomi Y, Shimoyama S, Tsuji E, Kojima J, Shimizu N, Ono H, Hirooka T, Noguchi C, Mafune KI, Kaminishi M. Peppermint oil reduces gastric spasm during upper endoscopy: a randomized, double-blind, double-dummy controlled trial. Gastrointest Endosc 2003;57:475–482
3. Göbel H, Fresenius J, Heinze A, Dworschak M, Soyka D. Effectiveness of peppermint oil and paracetamol in the treatment of tension type headache. Nervenarzt 1996;67:672–681
4. Göbel H, Heinze A, Dworschak M, Heinze-Kuhn K, Stolze H. Oleum menthae piperitae in the acute therapy of migraine and tension-type headache. Z Phytother 2004;25:129–139
5. Pittler MH, Ernst E. Peppermint oil for irritable bowel syndrome: a critical review and meta-analysis. Am J Gastroenterol 1998;93:1131–1135
6. Jailwala J, Imperiale TF, Kroenke K. Pharmacologic treatment of the irritable bowel syndrome: a systematic review of randomized, controlled trials. Ann Intern Med 2000;133:136–147
7. Thompson Coon J, Ernst E. Systematic review: herbal medicinal products for non-ulcer dyspepsia. Aliment Pharmacol Ther 2002:16:1689–1699
8. Ebbinghaus KD. A 'tea' containing various plant products as adjuvant to chemotherapy of urinary tract infections. Therapiewoche 1985;35:2041–2051

RED CLOVER
(Trifolium pratense)

SOURCE
Flower heads.

MAIN CONSTITUENTS
Carbohydrates, coumarins, flavonoids, isoflavonoids, saponins, volatile oil.

BACKGROUND
Red clover is a member of the Leguminosae family, native to most of Europe and naturalised in the US. It has a long history in agriculture and was considered a charm against witchcraft in the Middle Ages. It has also been used by traditional Chinese physicians and Russian folk healers for various medicinal purposes.

EXAMPLES OF TRADITIONAL USES
Mastalgia, cancer, chronic skin disease, tuberculosis, whooping cough.

PHARMACOLOGICAL ACTION
Estrogenic.

CONDITIONS FREQUENTLY TREATED
Mastalgia, cough, eczema, menopausal symptoms, psoriasis.

CLINICAL EVIDENCE
A systematic review included 11 RCTs.[1] Five studies tested the effects of red clover isoflavones on vasomotor symptoms in menopausal women and were suitable for inclusion in a meta-analysis. It indicated a small reduction in the frequency of hot flushes compared with placebo. Similar findings emerged from other systematic reviews.[2-4] The evidence that red clover reduces mastalgia pain is encouraging but not convincing.

DOSAGE
- *Dried extract*: 500 mg daily standardised to 40 mg isoflavones.
- *Liquid extract*: 1.5–3 ml (1:1 in 25% alcohol) three times daily.

RISKS
CONTRAINDICATIONS

Pregnancy and lactation (see p. 4), infants.

PRECAUTIONS/WARNINGS

Bleeding disorders, coagulation disorders. One long-term trial found no effect on mammographic breast density[5] but other authors are cautious regarding hormone-sensitive cancers.

ADVERSE EFFECTS

Breast tenderness, menstruation changes, weight gain, allergic reactions, myalgia, headache, nausea and vaginal spotting.[6]

INTERACTIONS

Theoretically, red clover may interfere with anticoagulants, hormonal therapies and tamoxifen. Red clover may inhibit the cytochrome P450 system and could thus increase blood levels of drugs metabolised by that system.[7]

QUALITY ISSUES

Red clover may appear in products combined with other herbs.

RISK–BENEFIT ASSESSMENT

There is reasonably strong evidence of a small effect of red clover in the short-term treatment of hot flushes in menopausal women. However, long-term effects are largely unknown. No serious adverse effects of short-term use are on record.

REFERENCES

1. Thompson Coon J, Pittler MH, Ernst E. *Trifolium pratense* isoflavones in the treatment of menopausal hot flushes. A systematic review and meta-analysis of randomized trials. Phytomedicine 2007;14:153–159
2. Hsu IP, Chia SL, Lin CT, Jou HJ. The effect of isoflavones from red clover on hot flushes in menopausal women – a systematic review of randomized, placebo-controlled trials. Nutr Sci J 2004;29:184–190
3. Krebs EE, Ensrud KE, MacDonald R, Wilt TJ. Phytoestrogens for treatment of menopausal symptoms: a systematic review. Obstet Gynecol 2004;104:824–836
4. Kashani L, Bathaei FS, Ojaghi M, Bathaei M, Akondzadeh S. A systematic review of herbal medical products for the treatment of menopausal symptoms. J Med Plants 2004;3:1–13
5. Atkinson C, Compston JE, Day NE, Dowsett M, Bingham SA. The effects of phytoestrogen isoflavones on bone density in women: a double-blind, randomized, placebo-controlled trial. Am J Clin Nutr 2004;79:326–333
6. Atkinson C, Oosthuizen W, Scollen S, Loktionov A, Day NE, Bingham SA. Modest protective effects of isoflavones from a red clover-derived dietary supplement on cardiovascular disease risk factors in perimenopausal women, and evidence of an interaction with ApoE genotype in 49–65-year-old women. J. Nutr 2004;6:170–179
7. Red clover monograph. Natural Medicines Comprehensive Database. Online. Available: http://www.natural database.com 5 Oct 2005

S-ADENOSYL-L-METHIONINE (SAM-E)

SOURCE

Naturally occurring molecule present in all parts of the human body. It is produced from methionine and adenosine triphosphate.

MAIN CONSTITUENTS

Not applicable.

BACKGROUND

Some people may have SAM-e levels that are too low, e.g. patients with vitamin B12 or folate deficiencies, HIV infections or liver disease. Supplementation with SAM-e is associated with low bioavailability because of its rapid hepatic metabolism. Its half-life is about 100 minutes. Excretion is via urine and faeces. SAM-e participates in complex ways with many biochemical reactions of the body. It is applied orally or by intravenous or intramuscular injections.

EXAMPLES OF TRADITIONAL USES
None.

PHARMACOLOGICAL ACTION
Contributes to the synthesis, activation or metabolism of hormones, neurotransmitters, nucleic acids, proteins, phospholipids and drugs. It has analgesic and anti-inflammatory effects, may stimulate articular cartilage growth, increases serotonin turnover and elevates dopamine and noradrenaline levels.

CONDITIONS FREQUENTLY TREATED
Osteoarthritis, fibromyalgia, other musculoskeletal pain syndromes, migraine, depression, heart disease, Alzheimer's disease, Parkinson's disease, multiple sclerosis and seizures.

CLINICAL EVIDENCE
Two meta-analyses agree that SAM-e is no better than placebo in reducing the pain of osteoarthritis.[1,2] One of these analyses[2] did, however, suggest that SAM-e is superior to placebo in improving function. Confusingly, both analyses implied that there is no significant difference between SAM-e and non-steroidal anti-inflammatory drugs in reducing pain but one points out that this cannot be seen as proof of equivalence.[1] More recent RCTs imply that SAM-e has a slower onset of action but is as effective as celecoxib in reducing the pain of osteoarthritis.[3] The trial data are contradictory as to the effects of SAM-e in fibromyalgia[4,5] and there is a suggestion that it might be helpful for migraine sufferers.[6]

DOSAGE
- *Oral*: 400–1600 mg/day
- *Intravenous or intramuscular injections*: 200–400 mg/day

RISKS
CONTRAINDICATIONS
Pregnancy and lactation (see p. 4).

PRECAUTIONS/WARNINGS
Anxiety, hypomania or mania have been reported in patients with depression or bipolar disorder.

ADVERSE EFFECTS
Flatulence, vomiting, diarrhoea, headache and nausea.

OVERDOSE
Not known.

INTERACTIONS
Serotonin syndrome in combination with selective serotonin reuptake inhibitor.

QUALITY ISSUES
SAM-e is administered orally as a salt, e.g. the sulphate or tosylate. The latter has only 1% bioavailability and low stability. Butanedisulphonate salt has 5% bioavailability and is stable for 2 years.

SECTION FOUR

RISK–BENEFIT ASSESSMENT

There is little compelling evidence that SAM-e is effective for any condition including pain control. There are only a few risks associated with it. On balance, a risk–benefit assessment fails to reach a positive balance.

REFERENCES

1. Witte S, Lasek R, Victor N. Meta-analysis of the efficacy of adenosylmethionine and oxaceprol in the treatment of osteoarthritis. [In German.] Orthopade 2002;31:1058–1065
2. Soeken KL, Lee WL, Bausell RB, Agelli M, Berman BM. Safety and efficacy of *S*-adenosylmethionine (SAMe) for osteoarthritis. J Fam Pract 2002;51:425–430
3. Najm WI, Reinsch S, Hoehler F, Tobis JS, Harvey PW. *S*-adenosyl methionine (SAMe) versus celecoxib for the treatment of osteoarthritis symptoms: a double-blind cross-over trial. BMC Musculoskelet Disord 2004;26:6
4. Volkmann H, Norregaard J, Jacobsen S, Danneskiold-Samsoe B, Knoke G, Nehrdich D. Double-blind, placebo-controlled cross-over study of intravenous *S*-adenosyl-L-methionine in patients with fibromyalgia. Scand J Rheumatol 1997;26:206–211
5. Jacobsen S, Danneskiold-Samsoe B, Andersen RB. Oral *S*-adenosylmethionine in primary fibromyalgia. Double-blind clinical evaluation. Scand J Rheumatol 1991;20:294–302
6. Gatto G, Caleri D, Michelacci S, Sicuteri F. Analgesizing effect of a methyl donor (*S*-adenosylmethionine) in migraine: an open clinical trial. Int J Clin Pharmacol Res 1986;6:15–17

SHARK CARTILAGE

SOURCE

Cartilage from the fin of the hammerhead shark (*Sphyrna lewini*) and the spiny dogfish shark (*Squalus acanthias*).

MAIN CONSTITUENTS

Sphyrastatin 1 and 2 (glycoproteins).

BACKGROUND

Based on the assumption that sharks never get cancer, it was hypothesised that shark cartilage might have anticancer properties in humans. As the result of much publicity and clever market-ing, shark cartilage became a popular food supplement in the 1990s. The debate over whether or not shark cartilage is associated with health benefits has developed into an ongoing and, at times, emotional controversy.[1–3]

EXAMPLES OF TRADITIONAL USES

None.

PHARMACOLOGICAL ACTION

Anti-angiogenic (starving tumours of essential nutrients) effects have been well documented in various test models and constitute the postulated mechanism of action. However, it seems debatable whether this is applicable to oral administration in humans because large macro-molecules like sphyrastatins are not usually absorbed in sufficiently large quantities by the intestinal tract.

CONDITIONS FREQUENTLY TREATED

Cancer, arthritis.

SECTION FOUR

CLINICAL EVIDENCE

There is no compelling evidence that shark cartilage alleviates arthritis pain. As most cancers are associated with pain, shark cartilage may have a role in the management of cancer pain. The best evidence available to date, however, fails to show that shark cartilage is helpful for cancer patients in any respect including pain.[4,5]

DOSAGE

Depending on the purity of the supplement, 500–4500 mg daily in divided doses.

RISK

CONTRAINDICATIONS

Pregnancy and lactation because of insufficient information (see p. 4).

PRECAUTIONS/WARNINGS

Liver diseases.

ADVERSE EFFECTS

Hepatitis, taste disturbances, nausea, vomiting, dyspepsia, constipation, hypotension, dizziness, hyperglycaemia, hypoglycaemia, hypocalcaemia, altered consciousness, decreased motor strength, decreased sensation, erythema, peripheral oedema, generalised weakness and fatigue.[6]

INTERACTIONS

None known.

QUALITY ISSUES

Large variations in the purity of commercially available preparations exist.

RISK–BENEFIT ASSESSMENT

According to the most reliable evidence to date, shark cartilage is not an effective treatment of any medical symptom or disease. In particular, it has no role in the management of pain. Serious safety concerns have been repeatedly voiced.[4,7] Its use should be discouraged.

REFERENCES

1. Lane IW, Comac L. Sharks don't get cancer. How shark cartilage can save your life. New York: Avery; 1992
2. Mathews J. Media feeds frenzy over shark cartilage as a cancer treatment. J Natl Cancer Inst 1993;85:1190–1191
3. Folkman J. What is the evidence that tumors are angiogenesis dependent? J Natl Cancer Inst 1990;82:2–4
4. Miller DR. Phase I/II trial of the safety and efficacy of shark cartilage in the treatment of advanced cancer. J Clin Oncol 1998;16:3649–3655
5. Loprinzi CL, Levitt R, Barton DL; North Central Cancer Treatment Group. Evaluation of shark cartilage in patients with advanced cancer: a North Central Cancer Treatment Group trial. Cancer 2005;104:176–182
6. Shark cartilage monograph. Natural Medicines Comprehensive Database. Online. Available: http://www.naturaldatabase.com 5 Oct 2005
7. Hunt TJ, Conelly JF. Shark cartilage for cancer treatment. Am J Health-Syst Pharm 1995;52:1756–1760

WILLOW   (*Salix* spp.)

SOURCE
Bark.

MAIN CONSTITUENTS
Derivatives of salicin, mainly salicortin, tannins, tremulacin.

BACKGROUND
Willow bark has been used as a remedy for inflammatory joint diseases and gout since 50 BCE. It was later rediscovered that willow bark extracts could be used as a remedy against pain and fever. Salicin was isolated as an active compound and eventually the compound was synthesised by Löwing, a German chemist working for Bayer. As he had used extracts from plants of the genus *Spirea*, he called the substance spiric acid, which appears in the brand name Aspirin (acetylsalicylic acid).

EXAMPLES OF TRADITIONAL USES
Pain, rheumatic complaints, fever.

PHARMACOLOGICAL ACTION
Salicin is metabolised to salicylic acid, which has analgesic and antipyretic effects.

CONDITIONS FREQUENTLY TREATED
Headache, rheumatic diseases, common cold.

CLINICAL EVIDENCE
A systematic review identified one RCT of willow bark extract for treating osteoarthritis.[1] This double-blind RCT ($n = 78$) reported the superiority of willow bark extract compared with placebo for the WOMAC pain dimension.[2] A double-blind RCT including 82 patients with chronic arthritic pain over a treatment period of 2 months confirmed these findings,[3] whereas another RCT including 127 patients with osteoarthritis did not.[4] An RCT in 210 patients with lower back pain using placebo and willow bark dry extracts equivalent to 120 mg salicin daily and 240 mg salicin daily, respectively, showed positive results.[5] When willow bark extract, equivalent to a daily dose of 240 mg salicin, was compared with 12.5 mg of the cyclo-oxygenase-2 inhibitor rofecoxib ($n = 228$) for low back pain, there was no difference as measured on a modified Arhus index, its pain component and the total pain index.[6]

DOSAGE
120–240 mg of total salicin daily in divided doses.

RISKS
CONTRAINDICATIONS

Pregnancy and lactation (see p. 4), patients with salicylate intolerance.

PRECAUTIONS/WARNINGS

Patients on anticoagulation treatment. Although there are data indicating that willow bark has no effect on coagulation time[7] and affects platelet aggregation to a lesser extent than acetylsalicylate,[8] patients on this kind of pharmacological therapy should use willow bark extracts only under careful supervision.

ADVERSE EFFECTS
Anaphylactic reactions, gastrointestinal complaints, skin rashes.

INTERACTIONS
Additive effects on anticoagulants and other salicylate-containing drugs.

QUALITY ISSUES
Preparations standardised to salicin should be used.

RISK–BENEFIT ASSESSMENT
The limited data suggest that willow bark extracts are efficacious for pain control. Whether they are superior to aspirin (or other non-steroidal anti-inflammatory drugs) is doubtful. However, the adverse effects profile appears to be more favourable. Therefore, willow bark extracts may be worthy of consideration for patients with mild pain who prefer a herbal remedy.

REFERENCES
1. Long L, Soeken K, Ernst E. Herbal medicines for the treatment of osteoarthritis: a systematic review. Rheumatology 2001;40:779–793
2. Schmid B, Lüdtke R, Selbmann HK, Kötter I, Tschirdewahn B, Schaffner W, Heide L. Efficacy and tolerability of a standardized willow bark extract in patients with osteoarthritis: randomized placebo-controlled, double blind clinical trial. Phytother Res 2001;15: 344–350
3. Mills SY, Jacoby RK, Chacksfield M, Willoughby M. Effect of a proprietary herbal medicine on the relief of chronic arthritic pain: a double-blind study. Br J Rheumatol 1996;35: 874–878
4. Biegert C, Wagner I, Ludtke R, Kotter I, Lohmuller C, Gunaydin I, Taxis K, Heide L. Efficacy and safety of willow bark extract in the treatment of osteoarthritis and rheumatoid arthritis: results of 2 randomized double-blind controlled trials. J Rheumatol 2004;31:2121–2130
5. Chrubasik S, Eisenberg E, Balan E, Weinberger T, Luzzati R, Conradt C. Treatment of low back pain exacerbations with willow bark extract: a randomised double-blind study. Am J Med 2000;109:9–14
6. Chrubasik S, Künzel O, Model A, Conradt C, Black A. Treatment of low back pain with a herbal or synthetic anti-rheumatic: a randomized controlled study. Willow bark extract for low back pain. Rheumatology 2001;40:1388–1393.
7. Krivoy N, Pavlotzky F, Eisenberg E, Chrubasik J, Chrubasik S, Brook G. *Salix cortex* (willow bark dry extract) effect on platelet aggregation. Drug Monit 1999;21:202
8. Krivoy N, Pavlotzky E, Chrubasik S, Eisenberg E, Brook G. Effect of salicis cortex extract on human platelet aggregation. Planta Med 2001;67:209–212

Table 4.1 **Other herbal and non-herbal medicines which have been tested for effectiveness or are used frequently**

Name	Description
Abana	Ayurvedic herbal preparation containing arjuna (*Terminalia arjuna*), billilotan (*Nepeta hindostana*), ashwagandha (*Withania somnifera*), guggul (*Commiphora mukul*), gotu Kola (*Centella asiatica*), amalaki (*Emblica officinalis*), haritaki (*Terminalia chebula*), liquorice (*Glycyrrhiza glabra*)
Aloe vera	Perennial succulent plant with antimicrobial, anti-inflammatory and antipruritic properties
Arginine; L-arginine	Essential amino acid, substrate for nitric oxide synthase
Arjuna (*Terminalia arjuna*)	A shade and ornamental tree, the bark is used and thought to have cardioprotective properties
Arthritis Relief Plus	Commercial product; see: http://www.arthritisreliefplus.com
Bitongxiao	A cream made from a number of traditional Chinese herbs for pain relief
Butterbur (*Petasites hybridus*)	A plant from the daisy family (Asteraceae) with antispasmodic and anti-inflammatory properties
Calendula (*Calendula officinalis*)	Perennial herbaceous plant with anti-inflammatory, immune stimulating and antimicrobial properties
Chamomile (*Matricaria recutita*)	Herbaceous plant with antibacterial, anti-inflammatory and antispasmodic properties
Chanlibao	Liquid made from a number of Chinese herbal medicines, including ginseng and dong quai (*Angelica sinensis*)
Chaste tree (*Vitex agnus-castus*)	A deciduous shrub with hypoprolactinaemic, dopaminergic, anti-inflammatory, anti-androgenic and antimicrobial properties
Co-enzyme Q10	Fat-soluble antioxidant produced in the body
Danggui-Shao-Yao-San	Classical traditional Chinese medicine combination that can be used as a decoction, granules or in tablet form, possibly with antioxidant and anti-platelet properties
Dong quai (*Angelica sinensis*)	Herb (its root is commonly known in Chinese as dong quai) with analgesic, anti-inflammatory, antispasmodic and sedative properties. Also known as 'female ginseng'
Duhuo Jisheng Wan	A classical traditional Chinese medicine combination in tablet form. Widely used to treat joint pain including various form of arthritis

table continues

Eazmov	Ayurvedic herbal preparation containing *Cyperus rotundus, Tinospora cordifolia, Saussurea lappa, Picrorrhiza kurroa* and ginger (*Zingiber officinale*). Produced by Envin Bioceuticals Pvt. Ltd.
Elk velvet antler	Dietary supplement of ground powder produced from the new 'velvet' growth of elks' antlers
Fish oil (omega-3 fatty acids)	Oil from fatty fish such as salmon or mackerel with anti-inflammatory, anticoagulant properties
Flavonoid supplement	See Phytoestrogen
γ-Linolenic acid	Omega-6 fatty acid that exists primarily in plant fats
Garlic (*Allium sativum*)	Perennial plant with antibacterial, antiviral, antifungal, antihypertensive, blood glucose-lowering, antithrombotic, antimutagenic and antiplatelet properties
Geranium (*Pelargonium* spp.)	Perennial flowering plant with antibacterial, antifungal and astringent properties
Gitadyl	A commercial product containing feverfew (*Tanacetum parthenium*), American aspen (*Populus tremuloides*) and milfoil (*Achillea millefolium*); see: http://www.med24.dk
Mangrove (*Rhizophora mangle*)	Bark from the mangrove tree which is purported to have astringent, emmenagogue, expectorant, haemostatic and styptic properties
Moist exposed burn ointment	Oil-based ointment containing sesame oil, β-sitosterol, berberine and other small quantities of plant ingredients
Padma 28	A commercially produced Tibetan herbal formulation; see: http://www.padma-usa.com
Phytodolor	German proprietary medicine containing extracts of aspen (*Populus tremula*), ash (*Fraxinus excelsior*) and European goldenrod (*Solidago virgaurea*); see http://www.steigerwald.de
Phytoestrogens	Phytochemicals with estrogenic, anti-estrogenic, proliferative, antiproliferative, antioxidative and anti-inflammatory properties that can interact with the estrogen receptors in cells. In high enough concentrations, phytoestrogens have many of the properties of natural estrogen for women
Poison ivy (*Rhus toxicodendron* = *Toxicodendron pubescens*)	Woody vine that produces urushiol, a skin irritant which is known for causing an agonising itching rash
Pomegranate (*Punica granatum*)	Fruit-bearing deciduous shrub with astringent, abortive, antioxidant properties
Probiotics	Dietary supplements containing potentially beneficial bacteria. Foods may also contain probiotics in therapeutic amounts, for example yoghurt with live cultures

SECTION FOUR

table continues

Propolis	Antibacterial, antifungal, antiviral, anti-inflammatory, antioxidant, cytotoxic
Qianggu	A capsule made from Chinese herbs, used for fracture healing
Raspberry leaf (*Rubus idaeus*)	Fruit-bearing plant with astringent, vasoconstrictive, anti-inflammatory and estrogenic properties.
Reumalex	A commercial product containing a combination of willow bark, guaiacum resin, black cohosh (*Actaea racemosa*), sarsaparilla (*Smilax* spp.) and poplar bark (*Populus* spp.). Produced by Gerard House, UK
Selenium	Essential trace element with antioxidant properties
Soy protein	Derived from the soya bean plant, a species of legume, native to eastern Asia
Thunder god vine (*Tripterygium wilfordii*)	A species of vine with a long history of use in traditional Chinese medicine
Tiger balm	Commercial product containing, among other ingredients, camphor (*Cinnamomum camphora*), menthol, cajuput oil (*Melaleuca cajuputi*) and clove oil (*Syzygium aromaticum*); see: http://www.tigerbalm.com
Tipi	A mixture of *Withania somnifera*, *Boswellia serrata* and turmeric (*Curcuma longa*)
Toki-shakuyaku-san	Kampo name for Danggui-Shao-Yao-San. See above
Tong luo kai bi	A mixture of traditional Chinese herbs in tablet form for joint pain and arthritis
Xylitol	Naturally occurring sweetener in many berries, fruit, vegetables and mushrooms. Derived from birch, by rendering the structural fibre of the wood, xylan. See: http://www.xylitol.org

Pain syndromes

ABDOMINAL PAIN

SYNONYMS
Stomach ache.

DEFINITION
A symptom in the stomach region. Abdominal pain can arise from the tissues of the abdominal wall that surround the abdominal cavity (i.e. skin, abdominal wall muscles), although the term is generally used to describe pain originating from organs within the abdominal cavity. These organs include the stomach, small intestine, colon, liver, gall bladder and pancreas.

RELATED CONDITIONS
Acute abdominal pain may arise from a number of conditions and may require immediate medical care (e.g. twisted ovarian cyst, ectopic pregnancy, intestinal obstruction, appendicitis, perforated peptic ulcer, perforated diverticulitis, abdominal aortic aneurysm, gall bladder stones, pancreatitis or kidney stones).

CAM USAGE
Herbal medicine is frequently used.

CLINICAL EVIDENCE
ACUPUNCTURE
Two hundred patients undergoing ovum pick-up treatment were assessed in a randomised clinical trial (RCT) and received either electroacupuncture in combination with a paracervical block or conventional medical analgesia plus paracervical block.[1] Directly after the procedure, the acupuncture group reported significantly higher mean and maximum pain scores than the control group. At 30 min thereafter no significant differences between the groups were reported for abdominal pain. For renal colic, an RCT reported that acupuncture is as effective as avafortan injection but with a more rapid analgesic onset.[2] For irritable bowel syndrome-related abdominal pain, a borderline improvement was reported but there was no difference compared with sham acupuncture.[3]

BIOFEEDBACK
In an RCT 64 children and teenagers (mean age 10 years) with diagnosed recurrent abdominal pain were randomly assigned to four interventions: (1) fibre only, (2) fibre and biofeedback-assisted low arousal, (3) fibre, biofeedback and cognitive–behavioural interventions, and (4) fibre, biofeedback, cognitive–behavioural interventions and parental support.[4] All four groups showed improvement in self-reported pain although the active treatment groups showed more improvement than the fibre-only group. A systematic review assessing the evidence for efficacy of biofeedback in the treatment of gastrointestinal problems identified 16 controlled trials of biofeedback for gastrointestinal conditions (Box 5.1).[5] It was concluded that the evidence for effectiveness of biofeedback for gastrointestinal conditions is insufficient. For pelvic floor dyssynergia, an RCT ($n = 110$) reported that five weekly biofeedback sessions produced greater reductions in straining and abdominal pain than polyethylene glycol plus counselling.[6]

HERBAL MEDICINE
A systematic review to evaluate treatments for recurrent abdominal pain in children included one RCT on peppermint (*Mentha piperita*) oil, which reported beneficial effects.[7]

Box 5.1 *Systematic review: biofeedback for gastrointestinal conditions.*[5]

- 16 controlled clinical trials (CCTs) of biofeedback for gastrointestinal problems were identified
- 10 trials had a no-biofeedback control group [constipation and/or encopresis (five), faecal incontinence (three), constipation (one), abdominal pain (one)]
- Of seven trials that provided sufficient data to calculate an effect size, two on faecal incontinence favoured biofeedback; the other five had non-significant results
- **Conclusion**: the evidence is insufficient to support the efficacy of biofeedback for gastrointestinal conditions

A further double-blind RCT in patients with colicky abdominal pain after appendectomy reported no difference for peppermint oil compared with placebo.[8] A review identified eight double-blind RCTs testing 180–200 mg enteric-coated peppermint oil in irritable bowel syndrome and concluded in favour of peppermint oil.[9] The implications for use of herbal medicines for irritable bowel syndrome from a Cochrane review are that, although double-blind RCTs showed a benefit for several herbal preparations that improved the symptoms of irritable bowel syndrome, most of the trials comparing herbal medicines with conventional therapies do not offer convincing evidence to support the use of herbal medicines.[10]

Other trials, which require independent replication, report beneficial effects for fennel (*Foeniculum vulgare*) alone[11] and in a combination preparation,[12] herbal tea,[13] turmeric (*Curcuma longa*) alone[14] and in a combination preparation[15] and wood creosote.[16]

HYPNOTHERAPY

A review of hypnotherapy for irritable bowel syndrome including six CCTs suggested that it improves the cardinal symptoms in the majority of patients.[17] According to the guidelines of the Clinical Psychology Division of the American Psychological Association, hypnotherapy qualifies as being efficacious and specific. A further RCT reported that hypnotherapy in addition to usual management produced greater improvements in pain and overall symptom scores than usual management alone after 3 months,[18] which is supported by another small ($n = 8$) RCT.[19]

MANIPULATION

Two RCTs assessing the effects of chiropractic spinal manipulation for treating infantile colic reported mixed results.[20,21] Whereas one study concluded that spinal manipulation is effective in relieving infantile colic when compared to dimethicone,[21] the other reported that it is no more effective than no treatment for infantile colic.[20] A pilot study of chiropractic for pain in women with primary dysmenorrhoea concluded that it may be a beneficial treatment.[22]

MASSAGE

One RCT evaluated the effectiveness of infant massage compared with that of a crib vibrator in the treatment of infantile colic.[23] Total and colicky crying times were not found to be different in either intervention group. Another RCT examined the effects of adjunctive postoperative massage and vibration therapy on short-term post-surgical pain.[24] It reported that, on the day of surgery, massage was more effective than usual care for affective and sensory pain and better than vibration for affective pain. On post-operative day two, massage was more effective than usual care for distress and better than vibration for sensory pain.

SUPPLEMENTS

A Cochrane review identified four RCTs that assessed the evidence for fibre supplements for abdominal pain relief in patients with irritable bowel syndrome (Box 5.2).[25] It concluded that there is no clear evidence of benefit for such agents. Another RCT reported no difference between a fibre-enriched formula and placebo for reducing crying time in infants with colic.[26]

Data from two RCTs on the effects of *Lactobacillus* spp. on pain in patients with irritable bowel syndrome do not suggest beneficial differences compared with placebo. One study concluded that the administration of *Lactobacillus plantarum* decreased pain in patients with irritable bowel syndrome but there were no differences from use of placebo,[27] and another concluded that *Lactobacillus GG* was not superior to placebo in the treatment of abdominal pain.[28] Two studies,[29,30] one of which is reported as an RCT,[30] concluded that pancreatic extract is not effective compared with placebo for treating abdominal pain caused by chronic pancreatitis.

OTHER THERAPIES

A single quasi-randomised study of reflexology for abdominal pain in irritable bowel syndrome reported no beneficial effects compared with foot massage[31] yet another single trial of reflexology reported effects.[32]

In patients with pain following intestinal surgery, an RCT reported beneficial effects for relaxation and music therapy.[33]

Box 5.2 *Systematic review: bulking agents for the treatment of irritable bowel syndrome*[25]

- 11 RCTs were identified
- Three RCTs ($n = 159$) reported on abdominal pain as a dichotomous outcome
- The pooled relative risk for abdominal pain was 1.22 [95% confidence interval (CI) 0.86 to 1.73]. The test for heterogeneity was significant
- Three RCTs ($n = 128$) reported on abdominal pain as a continuous outcome
- The standardised mean difference was 0.68 (95% CI 0.86 to 2.33). The test for heterogeneity was significant
- There is no clear evidence for use of bulking agents for irritable bowel syndrome

Table 5.1 **Summary of clinical evidence for abdominal pain**

Treatment	Weight of evidence	Direction of evidence	Serious safety concerns
Acupuncture	OO	↗	Yes (see p. 96)
Biofeedback	OO	↗	Yes (see p. 110)
Herbal medicine Peppermint oil	OOO	↗	Yes (see p. 209)
Hypnotherapy	OOO	↑	Yes (see p. 130)
Manipulation	OO	→	Yes (see p. 112)
Massage	OO	→	No (see p. 137)
Supplements Fibre	OOO	→	Yes (see p. 5)
Lactobacillus	OO	↓	Yes (see p. 5)
Pancreatic extract	OO	↓	Yes (see p. 5)

OVERALL RECOMMENDATION

Abdominal pain can be the symptom of serious underlying disease, which may require immediate medical or surgical attention (see above). The best evidence that exists for treating abdominal pain with CAM treatments relates to peppermint oil but even for this option the data are not entirely convincing. However, only a few and usually mild adverse events have been reported using peppermint oil, making it a possible option for treating abdominal pain. Hypnotherapy seems effective for this condition. Encouraging effects have been reported for acupuncture and biofeedback but more data are required.

REFERENCES

1. Humaidan P, Stener-Victorin E. Pain relief during oocyte retrieval with a new short duration electro-acupuncture technique – an alternative to conventional analgesic methods. Hum Reprod 2004;19:1367–1372

2. Lee YH, Lee WC, Chen MT, Huang JK, Chung C, Chang LS. Acupuncture in the treatment of renal colic. J Urol 1992;147:16–18

3. Fireman Z, Segal A, Kopelman Y, Sternberg A, Carasso R. Acupuncture treatment for irritable bowel syndrome. A double-blind controlled study. Digestion 2001;64:100–103

4. Humphreys PA, Gevirtz RN. Treatment of recurrent abdominal pain: components analysis of four treatment protocols. J Pediatr Gastroenterol Nutr 2000;31:47–51

5. Coulter ID, Favreau JT, Hardy ML, Morton SC, Roth EA, Shekelle P. Biofeedback interventions for gastrointestinal conditions: a systematic review. Altern Ther Health Med 2002;8:76–83

6. Chiarioni G, Whitehead WE, Pezza V, Morelli A, Bassotti G. Biofeedback is superior to laxatives for normal transit constipation due to pelvic floor dyssynergia. Gastroenterology 2006;130: 657–664

7. Weydert JA, Ball TM, Davis MF. Systematic review of treatments for recurrent abdominal pain. Pediatrics 2003;111:e1–11

8. Thomas JM, Payne JJ, Carr N, Glick L. Peppermint oil following appendectomy. A (deliberately) small clinical trial. Surg Res Commun 1988;2:285–287

9. Grigoleit HG, Grigoleit P. Peppermint oil in irritable bowel syndrome. Phytomedicine 2005;12:601–606.

10. Liu JP, Yang M, Liu YX, Wei ML, Grimsgaard S. Herbal medicines for treatment of irritable bowel syndrome. The Cochrane Database of Systematic Reviews 2006, Issue 1. Art. No.: CD004116

11. Alexandrovich I, Rakovitskaya O, Kolmo E, Sidorova T, Shushunov S. The effect of fennel (*Foeniculum vulgare*) seed oil emulsion in infantile colic: a randomized, placebo-controlled study. Altern Ther Health Med 2003;9:58–61

12. Savino F, Cresi F, Castagno E, Silvestro L, Oggero R. A randomized double-blind placebo-controlled trial of a standardized extract of *Matricariae recutita, Foeniculum vulgare* and *Melissa officinalis* (ColiMil) in the treatment of breastfed colicky infants. Phytother Res 2005;19:335–340

13. Weizman Z, Alkrinawi S, Goldfarb D, Bitran C. Efficacy of herbal tea preparation in infantile colic. J Pediatr 1993;122:650–652

14. Bundy R, Walker AF, Middleton RW, Booth J. Turmeric extract may improve irritable bowel syndrome symptomatology in otherwise healthy adults: a pilot study. J Altern Complement Med 2004;10:1015–1018

15. Niederau C, Gopfert E. The effect of chelidonium and turmeric root extract on upper abdominal pain due to functional disorders of the biliary system. Results from a placebo-controlled double-blind study. Med Klin (Munich) 1999;94:425–430

16. Kuge T, Shibata T, Willett MS. Multicenter, double-blind, randomized comparison of wood creosote, the principal active ingredient of Seirogan, an herbal antidiarrheal medication, and loperamide in adults with acute nonspecific diarrhea. Clin Ther 2004;26: 1644–1651

17. Tan G, Hammond DC, Joseph G. Hypnosis and irritable bowel syndrome: a review of efficacy and mechanism of action. Am J Clin Hypn 2005;47:161–178

18. Roberts L, Wilson S, Singh S, Roalfe A, Greenfield S. Gut-directed hypnotherapy for irritable bowel syndrome: piloting a primary care-based randomised controlled trial. Br J Gen Pract 2006;56:115–121

SECTION FIVE

19. Barabasz A, Barabasz M. Effects of tailored and manualized hypnotic inductions for complicated irritable bowel syndrome patients. Int J Clin Exp Hypn 2006;54:100–112

20. Olafsdottir E, Forshei S, Fluge G, Markestad T. Randomised controlled trial of infantile colic treated with chiropractic spinal manipulation. Arch Dis Child 2001;84:138–141

21. Wiberg JM, Nordsteen J, Nilsson N. The short-term effect of spinal manipulation in the treatment of infantile colic: a randomized controlled clinical trial with a blinded observer. J Manipulative Physiol Ther 1999;22:517–522

22. Kokjohn K, Schmid DM, Triano JJ, Brennan PC. The effect of spinal manipulation on pain and prostaglandin levels in women with primary dysmenorrhea. J Manipulative Physiol Ther 1992;15:279–285

23. Huhtala V, Lehtonen L, Heinonen R, Korvenranta H. Infant massage compared with crib vibrator in the treatment of colicky infants. Pediatrics 2000;105:E84

24. Taylor AG, Galper DI, Taylor P, Rice LW, Andersen W, Irvin W, Wang XQ, Harrell FE Jr. Effects of adjunctive Swedish massage and vibration therapy on short-term postoperative outcomes: a randomized, controlled trial. J Altern Complement Med 2003;9:77–89

25. Quartero AO, Meineche-Schmidt V, Muris J, Rubin G, de Wit N. Bulking agents, antispasmodic and antidepressant medication for the treatment of irritable bowel syndrome. The Cochrane Database of Systematic Reviews 2005, Issue2. Art. No.: CD003460

26. Treem WR, Hyams JS, Blankschen E, Etienne N, Paule CL, Borschel MW. Evaluation of the effect of a fiber-enriched formula on infant colic. J Pediatr 1991;119:695–701

27. Nobaek S, Johansson ML, Molin G, Ahrne S, Jeppsson B. Alteration of intestinal microflora is associated with reduction in abdominal bloating and pain in patients with irritable bowel syndrome. Am J Gastroenterol 2000;95:1231–1238

28. Bausserman M, Michail S. The use of *Lactobacillus* GG in irritable bowel syndrome in children: a double-blind randomized control trial. J Pediatr 2005;147:197–201

29. Mossner J. Is there a place for pancreatic enzymes in the treatment of pain in chronic pancreatitis? Digestion 1993;54(Suppl. 2):35–39

30. Malesci A, Gaia E, Fioretta A, Bocchia P, Ciravegna G, Cantor P, Vantini I. No effect of long-term treatment with pancreatic extract on recurrent abdominal pain in patients with chronic pancreatitis. Scand J Gastroenterol 1995;30:392–398

31. Tovey P. A single-blind trial of reflexology for irritable bowel syndrome. Br J Gen Pract 2002;52:19–23

32. Bennedbaek O, Viktor J, Carlsen KS, Roed H, Vinding H, Lundbye-Christensen S. Infants with colic. A heterogenous group possible to cure? Treatment by pediatric consultation followed by a study of the effect of zone therapy on incurable colic. Ugeskr Laeger 2001;163:3773–3778

33. Engel JM, Rapoff MA, Pressman AR. Long-term follow-up of relaxation training for pediatric headache disorders. Headache 1992;32:152–156

ANGINA PECTORIS

SYNONYMS/SUBCATEGORIES
Stable and unstable angina.

DEFINITION
Ischaemic pain and tightness in the region of the heart which can radiate into the shoulder, back, arm or jaw. The underlying reason is usually an imbalance of oxygen supply and demand as a result of arteriosclerotic narrowing of the coronary arteries.

RELATED CONDITIONS
Coronary heart disease; risk factors for coronary heart disease (e.g. hypertension, hypercholesterolaemia) are not discussed in this chapter.

CAM USAGE

No reliable prevalence data are available. The use of 'natural' supplements seems popular.

CLINICAL EVIDENCE

ACUPUNCTURE

A Danish research group published several RCTs suggesting that acupuncture reduces angina pectoris better than sham acupuncture and has similarly beneficial effects on cardiac work capacity as well as nitroglycerin consumption.[1-3] These findings were subsequently confirmed in similar studies by Swedish[4-7] and Russian[8] researchers. All of these studies are small and used acupuncture as an adjunct to conventional care. No definitive trial is so far available.

CHELATION THERAPY

A Cochrane review ($n = 5$) generated no conclusive evidence to suggest that chelation therapy is effective for treating ischaemic pain of angina.[9] The methodologically best RCTs fail to show an effect.

HERBAL MEDICINE

The Ayurvedic herbal preparation Abana has been tested in one small ($n = 43$) RCT.[10] Its results suggest that this medication reduces the frequency of angina episodes better than placebo.

A sizable number of Chinese CCTs are available that test various Chinese herbal mixtures as treatments for angina.[11-32] All of them suggest effectiveness but their reliability is difficult to evaluate.

An RCT ($n = 45$) testing pomegranate (*Punica granatum*) extract (240 ml/day intake for 3 months) suggested that this treatment reduces stress-induced ischaemia in patients with coronary heart disease.[33]

An RCT with 58 patients suffering from coronary heart disease compared *Terminalia arjuna* against standard treatments with nitrates.[34] The results suggested that both treatments are similarly effective in treating myocardial ischaemia.

HOMEOPATHY

A CCT ($n = 49$) of the homeopathic remedy pumpan given orally over 15 months in addition to standard care suggested that this treatment improves myocardial ischaemia more than standard treatment alone.[35]

RELAXATION

A systematic review included 27 CCTs of various relaxation techniques used for the adjunctive treatment of coronary heart disease.[36] Their quality was variable but some trials were rigorous. Overall the results demonstrate that relaxation improves exercise tolerance, anxiety and depression and reduces the frequency of ischaemic pain.

SUPPLEMENTS

A systematic review of 10 RCTs found that regular intake of fish oil (omega-3 fatty acids) decreased all-cause mortality but no effect on angina symptoms could be verified.[37]

L-Arginine was not found to improve myocardial ischaemia in an RCT with 25 patients suffering from stable angina.[38]

OTHER THERAPIES

The 'Ornish programme' consists of intensive lifestyle (e.g. smoking cessation) and dietary changes, exercise and stress management. A small RCT ($n = 48$) found that it leads to regression of coronary stenoses if followed for 1–5 years.[39]

SECTION FIVE

OVERALL RECOMMENDATION

Ischaemic pain of coronary heart disease is a serious warning signal. It requires effective medical treatment. Even though there are suggestions that some forms of CAM (e.g. acupuncture and relaxation) might be effective adjuncts to conventional care, it is important to stress that the data are not conclusive. Under no circumstances should angina pectoris be treated solely with CAM.

Table 5.2 **Summary of clinical evidence for angina pectoris**

Treatment	Weight of evidence	Direction of evidence	Serious safety concerns
Acupuncture	OOO	↗	Yes (see p. 96)
Chelation therapy	OO	↘	Yes (see p. 5)
Herbal medicine			
Abana	O	↑	Yes (see p. 5)
Chinese herbal mixtures	OO	↗	Yes (see p. 5)
Pomegranate	O	↑	Yes (see p. 5)
Terminalia arjuna	O	↑	Yes (see p. 5)
Homeopathy	O	↑	No (see p. 124)
Relaxation	OOO	↑	No (see p. 158)
Supplements			
Fish oil	OO	↓	Yes (see p. 5)
L-Arginine	O	↓	No (see p. 5)

REFERENCES

1. Ballegaard S, Jensen G, Pedersen F, Nissen VH. Acupuncture in severe, stable angina pectoris: a randomized trial. Acta Med Scand 1986;220:307–313
2. Ballegaard S, Pedersen F, Pietersen A, Nissen VH, Olsen NV. Effects of acupuncture in moderate, stable angina pectoris: a controlled study. J Intern Med 1990;227:25–30
3. Ballegaard S, Meyer CN, Trojaborg W. Acupuncture in angina pectoris: does acupuncture have a specific effect? J Intern Med 1991;229:357–362
4. Richter A, Herlitz J, Hjalmarson A. Effect of acupuncture in patients with angina pectoris. Eur Heart J 1991;12:175–178
5. Zhou XQ, Liu JX. Metrological analysis for efficacy of acupuncture on angina pectoris. [In Chinese.] Zhongguo Zhong Xi Yi Jie He Za Zhi 1993;13:212–214, 196
6. Liu WP, Xing ZH, Tan HY, Cai CL, Lin ZZ. Efficacy of acupuncture treatment on patients with variant angina pectoris and its effect on the function of vascular endothelial system. [In Chinese.] Chin J Clin Rehab 2004;8:2874–2875
7. Xu FH, Wang JM. Clinical observation on acupuncture combined with medication for intractable angina pectoris. [In Chinese.] Zhongguo Zhen Jiu 2005;25:89–91
8. Zamotrinsky A, Afanasiev S, Karpov RS, Cherniavsky A. Does electroacupuncture reduce severe angina? Coron Artery Dis 1997;8:551–557
9. Villarruz MV, Dans A, Tan F. Chelation therapy for atherosclerotic cardiovascular disease. The Cochrane Database of Systematic Reviews 2002, Issue 4. Art. No.: CD002785
10. Antani JA, Kulkarni RD, Antani NJ. Effect of Abana on ventricular function in ischemic heart disease. Jpn Heart J 1990;31:829–835
11. Cai PY, Xu BT, Shen BY. A clinical study of hehuantang in treating coronary heart disease. [In Chinese.] Zhongguo Zhong Xi Yi Jie He Za Zhi 1996;16:204–206

12. Chen K, Zhou WQ, Gao P. Clinical study on the effect of shuxuening tablet in treatment of coronary heart disease. [In Chinese.] Zhongguo Zhong Xi Yi Jie He Za Zhi 1996;16:24–26

13. Feng P, Qin N, Qin Y. Effect of composite salviae dropping pill on endothelin gene expression in circulating endothelial cells of patients with coronary heart disease. [In Chinese.] Zhongguo Zhong Xi Yi Jie He Za Zhi 1999;19:286–288

14. Hu JX, Jia GX, Yan ZR. Clinical and experimental study of shenshao tongguan pian in treating angina pectoris of coronary heart disease. [In Chinese.] Zhong Xi Yi Jie He Za Zhi 1990;10:596–599, 580

15. Jia Z, Gu F, Xue Y. Effect of tongxinluo capsule in treating variant angina pectoris patients and its influence on endothelial function. [In Chinese.] Zhongguo Zhong Xi Yi Jie He Za Zhi 1999;19:651–652

16. Jin L. Effect of composite salviae dropping pill on function of platelet activation in patients with unstable angina pectoris. [In Chinese.] Zhongguo Zhong Xi Yi Jie He Za Zhi 2000;20:415–417

17. Jiang HW, Qian ZH, Weng WL. Clinical study in treating qi-deficiency and blood-stasis syndrome of angina pectoris with qi xue granule. [In Chinese.] Zhongguo Zhong Xi Yi Jie He Za Zhi 1992;12:663–665, 644

18. Jin M, Qin J, Wu W. Clinical study on "sini" decoction in treating stenocardia for coronary heart disease. [In Chinese.] Zhong Yao Cai 2003;26:71–73

19. Liao JZ, Chen JJ, Wu ZM, Guo WQ, Zhao LY, Qin LM, Wang SR, Zhao YR. Clinical and experimental studies of coronary heart disease treated with yi-qi huo-xue injection. J Tradit Chin Med 1989;9:193–198

20. Li H, Cui L, Zhou W. Clinical observation of the effect of shuxinsu capsule in treating angina pectoris. [In Chinese.] Zhongguo Zhong Xi Yi Jie He Za Zhi 1999; 19:656–659

21. Qiu R, He J. Effects of xin mai tong capsule on vasoregulatory peptides in the patients of coronary heart disease. J Tradit Chin Med 2000;20:251–253

22. Shi YH. Comparative study of composite danshen droplet pills and sordi in treatment of patients with chronic stable angina. [In Chinese.] Zhongguo Zhong Xi Yi Jie He Za Zhi 1997;17:23–25

23. Wang L, Xiong ZY, Wang G. Systematic assessment on randomized controlled trials for treatment of stable angina pectoris by compound salvia pellet. [In Chinese.] Zhongguo Zhong Xi Yi Jie He Za Zhi 2004;24:500–504

24. Wang S, Dai R, Jin C. Clinical observation on artificial shexiang baoxin pill in treating 112 patients of coronary heart disease with angina pectoris. [In Chinese.] Zhongguo Zhong Xi Yi Jie He Za Zhi 1998;18:204–207

25. Wang J, Jing L, Zhong JB, Wang YY, Ma LH, Liu JG. Clinical study on compatibility and dismantlement of Xuefu Zhuyu decoction. [In Chinese.] Zhongguo Zhong Yao Za Zhi 2004;29:803–807

26. Wang SY, Dai RH, Jin C. Clinical observation of shexiang baoxinwan for treatment of coronary heart disease with angina pectoris. [In Chinese.] Zhongguo Zhong Xi Yi Jie He Za Zhi 1996;16:717–720

27. Wang XF, Shi DZ, Tu XH. Clinical observation of wenxin decoction in treating 82 patients with spontaneous angina pectoris. [In Chinese.] Zhongguo Zhong Xi Yi Jie He Za Zhi 1996;16:201–203

28. Wu HL, Wang X, Li XM, Luo WJ, Deng TT. Trial study on DENG Tie-tao's coronary heart disease capsules in improving patients' quality of life. [In Chinese.] Chin J Integr Med 2005;11:173–178

29. Xu GC, Gao RL, Wu YL. Clinical study on tongxinluo capsule in treatment of patients with angina pectoris caused by coronary heart disease. [In Chinese.] Zhongguo Zhong Xi Yi Jie He Za Zhi 1997;17:414–416

30. Ye H, Du J, Shen D, Shi S, Huang T, Hong Z, Mao YS, Li FJ, Zhou LN. Effect of shexiang baoxin pill on the function of vascular endothelium in patients with diabetes mellitus type 2 complicated with angina pectoris. [In Chinese.] Zhongguo Zhong Xi Yi Jie He Za Zhi 2004;24:1077–1079

31. Zhang Q, Peng JH, Zhang XN. A clinical study of Safflower Yellow injection in treating coronary heart disease angina pectoris with Xin-blood stagnation syndrome. [In Chinese.] Chin J Integr Med 2005;11:222–225

32. Zhang XL. Preliminary study of rose shu-xin oral liquid in the treatment of angina pectoris in coronary heart disease. [In Chinese.] Zhongguo Zhong Xi Yi Jie He Za Zhi 1992;12:414–416, 389

33. Sumner MD, Elliott-Eller M, Weidner G, Daubenmier JJ, Chew MH, Marlin R, Raisin CJ, Ornish D. Effects of pomegranate juice consumption on myocardial perfusion in patients with coronary heart disease. Am J Cardiol 2005;96:810–814

34. Bharani A, Ganguli A, Mathur LK, Jamra Y, Raman PG. Efficacy of Terminalia arjuna in chronic stable angina: a double-blind, placebo-controlled, crossover study comparing Terminalia arjuna with isosorbide mononitrate. Indian Heart J 2002;54:170–175

35. Parshina SS, Golovacheva TV, Afanas'eva TN, Panchenko OV, Baldina AA, Starostina NV, Lial'chenko IF, Egorova LP. Results of the use of pumpan preparation in the treatment of severe forms of angina pectoris. [In Russian.] Ter Arkh 2000;72:36–41

36. van Dixhoorn J, White A. Relaxation therapy for rehabilitation and prevention in ischaemic heart disease: a systematic review and meta-analysis. Eur J Cardiovasc Prev Rehabil 2005;12:193–202

37. Yzebe D, Lievre M. Fish oils in the care of coronary heart disease patients: a meta-analysis of randomized controlled trials. Fundam Clin Pharmacol 2004;18:581–592

38. Bednarz B, Wolk R, Chamiec T, Herbaczynska-Cedro K, Winek D, Ceremuzynski L. Effects of oral L-arginine supplementation on exercise-induced QT dispersion and exercise tolerance in stable angina pectoris. Int J Cardiol 2000;75:205–210

39. Ornish D, Scherwitz LW, Billings JH, Brown SE, Gould KL, Merritt TA, Sparler S, Armstrong WT, Ports TA, Kirkeeide RL, Hogeboom C, Brand RJ. Intensive lifestyle changes for reversal of coronary heart disease. JAMA 1998;280:2001–2007; erratum in: JAMA 1999;281:1380

BACK PAIN

SYNONYMS/SUBCATEGORIES

Mechanical back pain, idiopathic back pain, non-specific back pain, low back pain, back ache, lumbago, sciatica.

DEFINITION

Pain, muscle tension or stiffness below the costal margin with many (often undefined) causes. Acute means less than 12 weeks.

RELATED CONDITIONS

Back pain with specific causes, i.e. specific back pain (e.g. caused by ankylosing spondylitis, vertebral canal stenosis, etc.); can be differentiated from non-specific back pain where no cause can be identified. The latter type is much more common.

CAM USAGE

Many surveys demonstrate that back pain is the most frequent indication for which patients try CAM.[1] The most commonly employed CAM treatments include acupuncture, herbal remedies, massage therapy and spinal manipulation (chiropractic or osteopathy). In our survey of professional CAM organisations the following additional treatments were recommended for back pain: Bowen technique, magnet therapy, reflexology and yoga.[2]

CLINICAL EVIDENCE

ACUPUNCTURE/ACUPRESSURE

In the past, systematic reviews have generated contradictory conclusions. Two new meta-analyses generated overall positive results (Box 5.3).[3,4] A more recent, large ($n = 298$) RCT compared acupuncture with 'minimal acupuncture' as a placebo or a waiting list control group.[5] Its results show no difference between acupuncture and placebo but both of these approaches generated more pain relief than no treatment at all. One RCT suggested that the beneficial effects of acupuncture last for 2 years after the initial treatment but this requires independent confirmation.[6] An RCT ($n = 129$) of acupressure versus physical therapy showed greater pain reduction with the former intervention when applied regularly for 1 month.[7]

Box 5.3 *Meta-analysis: acupuncture for back pain*[3]

- Thirty-three RCTs were included, of which 22 were meta-analysed
- The methodological quality was variable but for some studies it was good
- For short-term relief of chronic pain the standardised mean difference was 0.54 (95% CI 0.35 to 0.73) compared to sham treatment
- For acute pain, the data were inconclusive
- **Conclusion**: acupuncture is effective for chronic low back pain

Box 5.4 *Systematic review: exercise for chronic back pain*[10]

- Forty-three RCTs were included
- Methodological quality was variable
- Overall results were positive
- High-dose exercise programmes were superior to low-dose
- **Conclusion**: exercise may improve pain and function in chronic back pain

Box 5.5 *Systematic review: Harpagophytum procumbens for low back pain*[13]

- Four RCTs were included
- Methodological quality was good on average
- There is moderate evidence that 100 mg harpagoside/day is effective for back pain
- **Conclusion**: this remedy is an effective symptomatic treatment for low back pain

ALEXANDER TECHNIQUE

A systematic review included one CCT with back pain sufferers and showed encouraging results for this approach.[8]

EXERCISE

Systematic reviews of therapeutic exercise have drawn positive conclusions (Box 5.4).[9,10] It seems important that the treatment is individually designed, includes stretching and strengthening, and is supervised.[11]

HERBAL MEDICINE

Several herbal remedies have shown promising results in alleviating musculoskeletal pain.[12] The one that has been most thoroughly investigated for back pain specifically is devil's claw (*Harpagophytum procumbens*). A systematic review (Box 5.5) of devil's claw included four RCTs on back pain and concluded that this remedy is an effective symptomatic treatment.[13]

HYDROTHERAPY/BALNEOTHERAPY

Systematic reviews assessing balneotherapy identified encouraging evidence for this approach as a treatment of low back pain.[14,15]

MASSAGE

A Cochrane review (Box 5.6) included eight RCTs and arrived at a cautiously positive conclusion.[16]

Box 5.6 *Systematic review: massage for back pain*[16]

- Eight RCTs were included
- Five RCTs were of high methodological quality
- Various comparator interventions were used
- Results were not uniform
- **Conclusion:** massage might be beneficial

Box 5.7 *Meta-analysis: spinal manipulation/mobilisation for low-back pain*[18]

- Thirty-nine RCTs were included
- Methodological quality was variable
- Acute low back pain: spinal manipulation therapy was superior to sham, ineffective or harmful interventions, but not to general practitioner care, analgesics, physical therapy, exercise or back school
- For chronic low back pain, results were similar
- **Conclusion:** there is no evidence that spinal manipulation therapy is superior to other treatments

PROLOTHERAPY

A systematic review included four RCTs of prolotherapy for back pain.[17] The results show positive effects on pain and function in two instances, while the two other RCTs failed to confirm this.

SPINAL MANIPULATION

A Cochrane review of all types of manipulation and mobilisation failed to show that these approaches are superior to other treatment options (Box 5.7).[18] More recent RCTs demonstrated positive effects of spinal manipulation on back pain but not on disability[19] and suggested that chiropractic care is associated with higher costs without producing better clinical outcomes.[20] A large ($n = 681$) RCT with long-term follow-up tested the effects of chiropractic with or without physical therapy.[21] The differences in outcomes between medical and chiropractic care were 'not clinically meaningful'. An RCT with 252 patients suffering from osteoarthritic back pain suggested that chiropractic care with heat is more effective in reducing pain than heat alone.[22] An RCT ($n = 102$) of chiropractic spinal manipulation for acute sciatica suggested that manipulation generates greater pain relief than sham manipulation.[23]

WATER INJECTIONS

Sterile water injections have been used for a number of pain syndromes. Two placebo-controlled RCTs suggested that they are effective in alleviating back pain of various causes.[24,25]

YOGA

Several studies have suggested effectiveness.[26] Two good quality RCTs ($n = 60$ and $n = 101$) demonstrated that 16 or 12 weeks of regular yoga exercises improve back pain more than control treatments such as conventional exercise, education or a self-help book.[27,28]

OTHER THERAPIES

A combination of back school, relaxation and qigong yielded promising preliminary results[29] and there is preliminary evidence for breath therapy,[30] meditation,[31] hypnotherapy[32] and imagery.[33] For music therapy, the results of two RCTs are contradictory.[34,35]

OVERALL RECOMMENDATION

The CAM treatments for back pain with the most promising risk–benefit profile are probably acupuncture, exercise, devil's claw and massage. Perhaps, with the exception of therapeutic exercise, none of these therapies are completely risk free, but serious complications are rare. The effect sizes of CAM modalities for low back pain are invariably small to moderate, yet this also applies to all conventional treatments of back pain.[36] The bottom line therefore is that the above options are worthy of consideration. The most important advice to back pain sufferers remains to keep up normal activity as much as possible and to realise that having back problems is not a disease.

Table 5.3 **Summary of clinical evidence for back pain**

Treatment	Weight of evidence	Direction of evidence	Serious safety concerns
Acupuncture/acupressure	OOO	↗	Yes (see p. 96)
Alexander technique	O	↗	No (see p. 102)
Exercise	OOO	↗	Yes (see p. 5)
Herbal medicine Devil's claw	OOO	↗	Yes (see p. 190)
Hydro-/balneotherapy	OOO	↗	No (see p. 126)
Massage	OOO	↗	No (see p. 137)
Prolotherapy	OO	→	Yes (see p. 5)
Spinal manipulation	OOO	↗	Yes (see p. 112)
Water injections	O	↗	Yes (see p. 5)
Yoga	OO	↗	Yes (see p. 169)

REFERENCES

1. Eisenberg DM, David RB, Ettner SL, Appel S, Wilkey S, Van Rompay M, Kessler RC. Trends in alternative medicine use in the United States, 1990–1997. JAMA 1998;280:1569–1575
2. Long L, Huntley A, Ernst E. Which complementary and alternative therapies benefit which conditions? A survey of the opinions of 223 professional organizations. Complement Ther Med 2001;9:178–185
3. Manheimer E, White A, Berman B, Forys K, Ernst E. Meta-analysis: acupuncture for low back pain. Ann Intern Med 2005;142:651–663
4. Furlan AD, van Tulder M, Cherkin D, Tsukayama H, Lao L, Koes B, Berman B. Acupuncture and dry-needling for low back pain: an updated systematic review within the framework of the Cochrane collaboration. Spine 2005;30:944–963
5. Brinkhaus B, Witt CM, Jena S, Linde K, Streng A, Wagenpfeil S, Irnich D, Walther HU, Melchart D, Willich SN. Acupuncture in patients with chronic low back pain: a randomized controlled trial. Arch Intern Med 2006;166:450–457
6. Thomas KJ, MacPherson H, Ratcliffe J, Thorpe L, Brazier J, Campbell M, Fitter M, Roman M, Walters S, Nicholl JP. Longer term clinical and economic benefits of offering acupuncture care to patients with chronic low back pain. Health Technol Assess 2005;9:1–109
7. Hsieh LL, Kuo CH, Lee LH, Yen AM, Chien KL, Chen TH. Treatment of low back pain by acupressure and physical therapy: randomised controlled trial. BMJ 2006;332:696–700
8. Ernst E, Canter PH. The Alexander technique: a systematic review of controlled clinical trials. Forsch Komplementarmed Klass Naturheilkd 2003;10:325–329
9. Brox JI, Hagen KB, Juel NG, Storheim K. Is exercise therapy and manipulation effective in low back pain? [In Norwegian.] Tidsskr Nor Laegeforen 1999;119:2042–2050

10. Hayden JA, van Tulder MW, Tomlinson G. Systematic review: strategies for using exercise therapy to improve outcomes in chronic low back pain. Ann Intern Med 2005;142:776–785

11. Hayden JA, van Tulder MW, Malmivaara AV, Koes BW. Meta-analysis: exercise therapy for non-specific low back pain. Ann Intern Med 2005;142:765–775

12. Ernst E, Chrubasik S. Phyto-antiinflammatories. A systematic review of randomized, placebo-controlled, double-blind trials. Rheum Dis Clin North Am 2000;26:13–27

13. Gagnier JJ, Chrubasik S, Manheimer E. *Harpagophytum procumbens* for osteoarthritis and low back pain: a systematic review. BMC Complement Altern Med 2004;4:13

14. Nasermoaddeli A, Kagamimori S. Balneotherapy in medicine: a review. Environ Health Prev Med 2005;10:171–179

15. Pittler MH, Karagülle MZ, Karagülle M, Ernst E. Balneotherapy and spa therapy for treating chronic low back pain: meta-analysis of randomised controlled trials. Rheumatology (Oxford) 2006;45:880–884

16. Furlan A D, Brosseau L, Imamura M, Irvin E. Massage for low-back pain: a systematic review within the framework of the Cochrane Collaboration Back Review Group. Spine 2002;27:1896–1910

17. Rabago D, Best TM, Beamsley M, Patterson J. A systematic review of prolotherapy for chronic musculoskeletal pain. Clin J Sport Med 2005;15:376–380

18. Assendelft WJJ, Morton SC, Yu Emily I, Suttorp MJ, Shekelle PG. Spinal manipulative therapy for low back pain. The Cochrane Database of Systematic Reviews 2004, Issue 1. Art No: CD000447

19. Geisser ME, Wiggert EA, Haig AJ, Colwell MO. A randomized, controlled trial of manual therapy and specific adjuvant exercise for chronic low back pain. Clin J Pain 2005;21:463–470

20. Kominski GF, Heslin KC, Morgenstern H, Hurwitz EL, Harber PI. Economic evaluation of four treatments for low-back pain: results from a randomized controlled trial. Med Care 2005;43:428–435

21. Hurwitz EL, Morgenstern H, Kominski GF, Yu F, Chiang LM. A randomized trial of chiropractic and medical care for patients with low back pain: eighteen-month follow-up outcomes from the UCLA low back pain study. Spine 2006;31:611–621

22. Beyerman KL, Palmerino MB, Zohn LE, Kane GM, Foster KA. Efficacy of treating low back pain and dysfunction secondary to osteoarthritis: chiropractic care compared with moist heat alone. J Manipulative Physiol Ther 2006;29:107–114

23. Santilli V, Beghi E, Finucci S. Chiropractic manipulation in the treatment of acute back pain and sciatica with disc protrusion: a randomized double-blind clinical trial of active and simulated spinal manipulations. Spine J 2006;6:131–137

24. Labrecque M, Nouwen A, Bergeron M, Rancourt J. A randomized controlled trial of non-pharmacologic approaches for relief of low back pain during labor. J Fam Pract 1999;48:259–263

25. Trolle B, Moller M, Kronborg H, Thomsen S. The effect of sterile water blocks on low back labor pain. Am J Obstet Gynecol 1991;164:1277–1281

26. Nespor K. Psychosomatics of back pain and the use of yoga. Int J Psychosom 1989;36:72–78

27. Williams KA, Petronis J, Smith D, Goodrich D, Wu J, Ravi N, Doyle EJ Jr, Gregory Juckett R, Munoz Kolar M, Gross R, Steinberg L. Effect of Iyengar yoga therapy for chronic low back pain. Pain 2005;115:107–117

28. Sherman KJ, Cherkin DC, Erro J, Miglioretti DL, Deyo RA. Comparing yoga, exercise, and a self-care book for chronic low back pain: a randomized, controlled trial. Ann Intern Med 2005; 143:849–856

29. Berman BM, Sing BB. Chronic low back pain: an outcome analysis of a mind–body intervention. Complement Ther Med 1997;5:29–35

30. Mehling WE, Hamel KA, Acree M, Byl N, Hecht FM. Randomized, controlled trial of breath therapy for patients with chronic low-back pain. Altern Ther Health Med 2005;11:44–52

31. Carson JW, Keefe FJ, Lynch TR, Carson KM, Goli V, Fras AM, Thorp SR. Loving-kindness meditation for chronic low back pain: results from a pilot trial. J Holist Nurs 2005;23:287–304

32. McCauley JD, Thelen MH, Frank RG, Willard RR, Callen KE. Hypnosis compared to relaxation in the outpatient management of chronic low back pain. Arch Phys Med Rehab 1983;64:548–552

33. Basler HD, Jakle C, Kroner-Herwig B. Incorporation of cognitive-behavioral treatment into the medical care of chronic low back patients: a controlled randomized study in German pain treatment centers. Patient Educ Couns 1997;31:113–124

34. Kullich W, Bernatzky G, Hesse HP, Wendtner F, Likar R, Klein G. Music therapy-effect on pain, sleep and quality of life in low back pain. [In German.] Wien Med Wochenschr. 2003;153:217–221

35. Guetin S, Coudeyre E, Picot MC, Ginies P, Graber-Duvernay B, Ratsimba D, Vanbiervliet W, Blayac JP, Herisson C. Effect of music therapy among hospitalized patients with chronic low back pain: a controlled, randomized trial. [In French.] Ann Readapt Med Phys 2005;48:217–224

36. Van Tulder MW, Koes BW, Bouter LM. Conservative treatment of acute and chronic non-specific low back pain: a systematic review of the most common interventions. Spine 1997;22:2128–2156

BURN PAIN

SUBCATEGORIES

Thermal burns, electrical burns, chemical burns, scalds, cold burns.

DEFINITION

Burns are bodily injuries resulting from exposure to heat, caustics, electricity or some forms of radiation. Superficial burns comprise a spectrum of injury severity depending on the depth of the wound and the proportion of the body affected. Burn depth is classified as erythema (first-degree) involving the epidermis only, superficial partial thickness (second-degree) involving the epidermis and upper dermis, deep partial thickness (second-degree) involving the epidermis and dermis, and full thickness (third-degree) involving the epidermis, dermis and damage to appendages. The extent of the injury is usually expressed as a percentage of the total body surface area which is burnt.

CAM USAGE

Topically, dressings containing herbal and non-herbal preparations for burn wound management are available. To reduce anxiety and pain, relaxation therapies have been used particularly during dressing change and debridement.

CLINICAL EVIDENCE

HYPNOTHERAPY

An RCT ($n = 44$) reported decreased degrees of pain and anxiety caused by burns physiotherapy in patients receiving hypnotherapy compared with controls not receiving hypnotherapy.[1] In an RCT of 61 patients with severe burns, the pain scores of patients receiving either hypnosis or a control intervention consisting of attention, information and brief relaxation instructions did not differ when all patients were considered; however, a subset of patients with high levels of baseline pain reported less pain after receiving hypnosis.[2] In an RCT of 30 severely burned patients, both hypnosis and a stress-reducing strategy reduced pain and increased patient satisfaction compared to baseline.[3] Hypnotherapy alone reduced anxiety but not pain and pain control during dressing changes compared to the stress-reducing strategy. A small RCT of 32 severely burned patients receiving hypnosis, lorazepam, hypnosis with lorazepam or placebo in addition to opioids found no differences between groups in burn pain control (see Table 5.4).[4]

MASSAGE

In an RCT ($n = 28$), massage therapy before debridement sessions was reported to reduce pain and state of anxiety compared to standard treatment.[5] Massage therapy with cocoa butter during the remodelling phase of wound healing was found to reduce pain, itching and anxiety compared to standard treatment in a small RCT of 20 patients with burn injuries.[6]

MUSIC THERAPY

The effects of music-based imagery and music alternate engagement in the management of pain and anxiety during debridement were tested in an RCT ($n = 25$) using a repeated measure design with patients serving as their own controls.[7] It found a reduction of self-reported pain in patients receiving music therapy. A small RCT found no difference between the music and no music group for pain or anxiety during the rehabilitation of patients with burns.[8]

SUPPLEMENTS

A systematic review of the use of honey (Box 5.8) as a wound dressing including six RCTs concluded that, although the results from individual studies were positive, the poor methodological quality prevented any firm conclusions being reached.[9]

A non-randomised unblinded trial comparing a propolis skin cream with silver sulfadiazine reported beneficial effects of propolis on the healing of partial-thickness burn wounds.[10]

Box 5.8 *Systematic review: honey as wound dressing in burns*[9]

- Six trials were located, all were performed by the same researcher and were of low quality (Jadad score = 1)
- Controls were potato peelings and amniotic membrane as well as conventional treatments
- Two of the studies involved superficial burns, three were partial-thickness burns, one comprised moderate to severe burns that included full-thickness injury, and one was infected post-operative wounds
- Five studies reported positive outcomes on healing time and infection rates
- One trial was negative, in which tangential excision was better than honey
- **Conclusion**: confidence in a conclusion that honey is a useful treatment for superficial wounds or burns is low yet there is biological plausibility

Table 5.4 **Controlled clinical trials of hypnotherapy for burn pain**

Reference	Sample size	Interventions (regimen)	Result	Comment
Harandi[1]	44	(A) Hypnotherapy, 4× (B) No hypnotherapy	A better than B	Procedural pain related to physiotherapy
Patterson[2]	61	(A) Hypnosis (B) Attention, information, brief relaxation	A equal to B	A better than B in a subgroup of patients with high levels of baseline pain
Frenay[3]	30	(A) Hypnotherapy (B) Stress-reducing strategy	A equal to B in pain, pain control and satisfaction, A superior to B in anxiety scores	A and B improved compared to baseline
Everett[4]	32	(A) Hypnosis (B) Lorazepam (C) Hypnosis and lorazepam (D) Placebo	No differences between groups	All groups improved compared to baseline

OTHER THERAPIES

An RCT of moist exposed burn ointment in 115 patients with partial-thickness burns found it equal to conventional treatment in general and superior in relieving pain during the first week after burns.[11]

In a single-blind RCT ($n = 99$) patients receiving therapeutic touch reported greater reduction in pain and anxiety than those receiving sham therapeutic touch.[12]

OVERALL RECOMMENDATION

There is some evidence that hypnotherapy might be a useful adjunct to standard pain control with opioid analgesics and anxiolytic drugs in burned patients. There is not sufficient evidence to recommend any other intervention.

Table 5.5 **Summary of clinical evidence for burn pain**

Treatment	Weight of evidence	Direction of evidence	Serious safety concerns
Hypnotherapy	OO	↗	Yes (see p. 130)
Massage	O	↗	No (see p. 137)
Music	O	→	No (see p. 142)
Supplements			
Honey	OOO	↗	Yes (see p. 5)
Propolis	O	↗	Yes (see p. 5)

REFERENCES

1. Harandi AA, Esfandani A, Shakibaei F. The effect of hypnotherapy on procedural pain and state anxiety related to physiotherapy in women hospitalized in a burn unit. Contemp Hypn 2004;21:28–34
2. Patterson DR, Ptacek JT. Baseline pain as a moderator of hypnotic analgesia for burn injury treatment. J Consult Clin Psychol 1997;65:60–67
3. Frenay MC, Faymonville ME, Devlieger S, Albert A, Vanderkelen A. Psychological approaches during dressing changes of burned patients: a prospective randomised study comparing hypnosis against stress reducing strategy. Burns 2001;27:793–799
4. Everett JJ, Patterson DR, Burns GL, Montgomery B, Heimbach D. Adjunctive interventions for burn pain control: comparison of hypnosis and ativan: the 1993 Clinical Research Award. J Burn Care Rehabil 1993;14:676–683
5. Field T, Peck M, Krugman S, Tuchel T, Schanberg S, Kuhn C, Burman I. Burn injuries benefit from massage therapy. J Burn Care Rehabil;19:241–244
6. Field T, Peck M, Scd, Hernandez-Reif M, Krugman S, Burman I, Ozment-Schenck L. Postburn itching, pain, and psychological symptoms are reduced with massage therapy. J Burn Care Rehabil 2000;21:189–193
7. Fratianne RB, Prensner JD, Huston MJ, Super DM, Yowler CJ, Standley JM. The effect of music-based imagery and musical alternate engagement on the burn debridement process. J Burn Care Rehabil 2001;22:47–53
8. Ferguson SL, Voll KV. Burn pain and anxiety: the use of music relaxation during rehabilitation. J Burn Care Rehabil 2004;25:8–14
9. Moore OA, Smith LA, Campbell F, Seers K, McQuay HJ, Moore RA. Systematic review of the use of honey as a wound dressing. BMC Complement Altern Med 2001;1:2
10. Gregory SR, Piccolo N, Piccolo MT, Piccolo MS, Heggers JP. Comparison of propolis skin cream to silver sulfadiazine: a naturopathic alternative to antibiotics in treatment of minor burns. J Altern Complement Med 2002;8:77–83

11. Ang E, Lee ST, Gan CS, Chan YH, Cheung YB, Machin D. Pain control in a randomized, controlled, clinical trial comparing moist exposed burn ointment and conventional methods in patients with partial-thickness burns. J Burn Care Rehabil 2003;24:289–296

12. Turner JG, Clark AJ, Gauthier DK, Williams M. The effect of therapeutic touch on pain and anxiety in burn patients. J Adv Nurs 1998;28:10–20

CANCER PAIN

SYNONYMS/SUBCATEGORIES

Pain associated with malignant tumours or neoplasms.

DEFINITION

General term used to describe any type of pain associated with malignant neoplasm. Acute pain can be caused by diagnostic or therapeutic interventions for cancer. Chronic cancer pain can be caused by therapy or by the direct effects of the malignancy.

RELATED CONDITIONS

Biopsy pain, breakthrough pain, chemotherapy-associated or radiotherapy-associated pain, diffuse bone pain, mucositis, neuralgia, neuropathy, perioperative pain and procedural pain.

CAM USAGE

Cancer patients are understandably desperate to try any treatment that offers hope; therefore, many of them try some form of CAM. A systematic review of 26 surveys from 13 countries found an average prevalence of CAM use of 31%.[1] Some CAM therapies are promoted as 'cures', some are used for palliative care, e.g. for pain management, and some are promoted for cancer prevention. Claims to cure cancer, lower the tumour burden or prolong the life of cancer patients are rife within CAM. For none of these therapies is the evidence convincingly positive.[2] It is also not likely that 'alternative cancer cures' alleviate cancer pain effectively.

However, many CAM modalities have the potential to increase well-being, e.g. by reducing pain. Thus, they are often used in addition to conventional treatments in palliative and supportive care for cancer patients.

CLINICAL EVIDENCE

ACUPUNCTURE

A systematic review of six clinical trials testing the effectiveness of acupuncture to control cancer pain found no compelling evidence for this indication[3] (Box 5.9). This was confirmed by other reviewers who concluded that the analgesic effects of acupuncture are promising but not convincing and need further study.[4] A subsequent RCT did, however, produce promising results in terms of pain control in cancer patients.[5] Encouraging data suggest that acupuncture alleviates nausea and vomiting[6] as well as radiation-induced xerostomia[7] and reduces vasomotor symptoms in men receiving hormone therapy for prostate cancer.[8]

AROMATHERAPY AND MASSAGE

A Cochrane review[9] found that aromatherapy and/or massage have positive short-term effects on the well-being of cancer patients. The questions of whether essential oils are important for this effect and whether prominent analgesic effects are associated with these techniques remain unanswered (Box 5.10).

EXERCISE

A substantial body of evidence suggests that regular physical exercise will reduce the severity of treatment-related symptoms such as fatigue and nausea and possibly pain.[10,11]

Box 5.9 *Systematic review: acupuncture for cancer pain*[3]

- Two RCTs and four uncontrolled clinical trials
- Methodological quality was, on average, poor
- Best studies fail to show positive effects
- **Conclusion:** effectiveness not proven

Box 5.10 *Systematic review: aromatherapy/massage for cancer*[9]

- Eight RCTs including 357 patients
- Methodological quality was variable
- Most consistent effect was short-term anxiolytic effect
- **Conclusion:** short-term benefits on psychological well-being

HERBAL MEDICINE

Aloe vera gel was tested against placebo in an RCT ($n = 58$) for control of radiation-induced mucositis.[12] The results failed to demonstrate any beneficial effects. In a similar RCT of *A. vera*, no decrease in skin reaction was noted with low-dose radiotherapy[13] but, with high-dose radiotherapy (>2700 cGy), skin reactions occurred on average 2 weeks later compared with placebo.

Calendula officinalis cream was compared to trolamine cream in an RCT ($n = 254$) testing their usefulness in preventing radiation-induced dermatitis in breast cancer patients.[14] The occurrence of grade 2 dermatitis was 41% with *Calendula* and 63% with trolamine.

Ginkgo (*Ginkgo biloba*) reduced limb heaviness and pain in an RCT including 48 patients with upper extremity lymphoedema after breast cancer treatment.[15]

HOMEOPATHY

A systematic review including six RCTs found no convincing evidence that homeopathic remedies have analgesic effects in cancer patients.[16]

HYPNOTHERAPY

Several RCTs have suggested the usefulness of hypnotherapy in palliative cancer care. It was effective in controlling pain and nausea/vomiting.[17,18] However, the evidence for hypnotherapy to control procedural pain in children with cancer is inconclusive, not least because of the methodological limitations of the trial data.[19,20] One RCT suggested its ineffectiveness in reducing anxiety in cancer patients receiving radiotherapy.[21] A systematic review of all types of clinical investigations found encouraging evidence that hypnotherapy can alleviate cancer pain[22] but, because of the often poor methodology of the primary data, this evidence was not deemed conclusive.

MASSAGE

A systematic review found encouraging evidence for massage as a method to control cancer pain.[23]

MUSIC THERAPY

An RCT ($n = 60$) suggested that procedural pain and anxiety are not influenced by music therapy compared to simple distraction.[24]

REFLEXOLOGY

A small, sham-controlled RCT ($n = 12$) generated no convincing evidence that reflexology improves quality of life or pain of cancer patients.[25] A less rigorously controlled CCT with 23 breast and lung cancer patients suggested that reflexology reduces anxiety and pain.[26]

RELAXATION

The effectiveness of several relaxation therapies has been tested repeatedly. In one RCT ($n = 56$) the programme consisted of breathing exercises, muscle relaxation and imagery. This regimen was superior to no intervention in controlling the pain of cancer patients.[27] A three-armed RCT ($n = 60$) found no evidence that pain is reduced by either imagery or relaxation in cancer patients after colorectal resections.[28]

In another RCT, 96 women with advanced breast cancer were randomised to receive either regular relaxation training and imagery or standard care only. The experimental group experienced better quality of life than the control group.[29] Other relaxation therapies supported by similar data from RCTs or CCTs include a comprehensive coping strategy programme with imagery,[30] mindfulness meditation,[31–33] stress management training,[34] autogenic training,[35] progressive muscle relaxation training[36–39] and qigong.[40] Whether these techniques have direct analgesic effects remains, however, uncertain.

SUPPLEMENTS

A systematic review of cannabinoids in supportive cancer care included nine RCTs. The authors concluded that cannabinoids are not superior to codeine in controlling cancer pain. As cannabinoids cause central nervous system depression, their introduction into routine care was deemed 'undesirable'.[41]

OVERALL RECOMMENDATION

CAM has an important role in palliative/supportive cancer care, and some treatments, such as exercise or hypnotherapy, have been shown to be potentially useful contributors to pain

Table 5.6 **Summary of clinical evidence for cancer pain**

Treatment	Weight of evidence	Direction of evidence	Serious safety concerns
Acupuncture (pain)	OO	→	Yes (see p. 96)
Aromatherapy/massage	OO	→	Yes (see p. 103/137)
Exercise	OOO	↗	Yes (see p. 5)
Herbal medicine			
Aloe vera gel	OO	→	Yes (see p. 5)
Calendula	O	↑	Yes (see p. 5)
Ginkgo	O	↗	Yes (see p. 5)
Homeopathy	OO	↘	No (see p. 124)
Hypnotherapy	OOO	↗	Yes (see p. 130)
Massage	OO	↗	No (see p. 137)
Music therapy	O	↗	No (see p. 142)
Reflexology	O	↗	No (see p. 155)
Relaxation	OO	→	No (see p. 158)
Supplements			
Cannabinoids	OOO	→	Yes (see p. 179)

control. This area clearly deserves more research; in particular, we need to know which treatments are in any way superior to conventional methods of pain management.

REFERENCES

1. Ernst E, Cassileth BR. The prevalence of complementary/alternative medicine in cancer. A systematic review. Cancer 1998;83:777–782
2. Ernst E, Pittler M, Wider B, Boddy K. The desktop guide to complementary and alternative medicine, 2nd edn. Edinburgh: Mosby; 2006
3. Lee H, Schmidt K, Ernst E. Acupuncture for the relief of cancer-related pain – a systematic review. Eur J Pain 2005;9:437–441
4. Cohen AJ, Menter A, Hale L. Acupuncture: role in comprehensive cancer care – a primer for the oncologist and review of the literature. Integr Cancer Ther 2005;4:131–143
5. Nguyen J. Analgesic effects of auricular acupuncture for cancer pain: a randomized blinded, controlled trial. Acupunct Moxibustion 2005;4:144–146
6. Ernst E, Pittler M, Wider B, Boddy K. The desktop guide to complementary and alternative medicine, 2nd edn. Edinburgh: Mosby; 2006:214–224
7. Rydholm N, Strang P. Acupuncture for patients in hospital-based home care suffering from xerostomia. J Palliat Care 1999;15:20–23
8. Hammar M, Frisk J, Grimas O. Acupuncture treatment of vasomotor symptoms in men with prostatic carcinoma: a pilot study. J Urol 1999;161:853–857
9. Fellowes D, Barnes K, Wilkinson S. Aromatherapy and massage for symptom relief in patients with cancer. The Cochrane Database of Systematic Reviews 2004, Issue 3. Art No.: CD002287
10. Dimeo F. Welche Rolle spielt körperliche Aktivität in der Prävention, Therapie und Rehabilitation von neoplastischen Erkrankungen? Deutsche Zeitschr Sportmed 2004;55:177–182
11. Adamsen L, Quist M, Midtgaard J, Andersen C, Moller T, Knutsen L, Tveteras A, Rorth M. The effect of a multidimensional exercise intervention on physical capacity, well-being and quality of life in cancer patients undergoing chemotherapy. Support Care Cancer 2006;14:116–127
12. Su CK, Mehta V, Ravikumar L, Shah R, Pinto H, Halpern J, Koong A, Goffinet D, Le QT. Phase II double-blind randomized study comparing aloe vera versus placebo to prevent radiation-related mucositis in patients with head-and-neck neoplasms. Int J Radiat Oncol Biol Phys 2004;60:171–177
13. Olsen SL, Raub W Jr, Bradley C, Johnson M, Macias JL, Love V, Markoe A. The effect of aloe vera gel/mild soap versus mild soap alone in preventing skin reactions in patients undergoing radiation therapy. Oncol Nurs Forum 2001;28:543–547
14. Pommier P, Gomez F, Sunyach MP, D'Hombres A, Carrie C, Montbarbon X. Phase III randomized trial of *Calendula officinalis* compared with trolamine for the prevention of acute dermatitis during irradiation for breast cancer. J Clin Oncol 2004;22:1447–1453
15. Cluzan RV, Pecking AP, Mathiex-Fortunet H, Leger Picherit E. Efficacy of BN165 (Ginkor Fort) in breast cancer related upper limb lymphedema: a preliminary study. Lymphology 2004;37:47–52
16. Milazzo S, Russell N, Ernst E. Efficacy of homeopathic therapy in cancer treatment. Eur J Cancer 2006;42:282–289
17. Syrjala KL, Cummings C, Donaldson GW. Hypnosis or cognitive behavioral training for the reduction of pain and nausea during cancer treatment: a controlled clinical trial. Pain 1992;50:237–238
18. Elkins G, Cheung A, Marcus J, Palamara L, Rajab MH. Hypnosis to reduce pain in cancer survivors with advanced disease: a prospective study. J Cancer Integr Med 2004;2:167–172
19. Wild MR, Espie C. The efficacy of hypnosis in the reduction of procedural pain and distress in pediatric oncology: a systematic review. J Dev Behav Pediatr 2004;25:207–213
20. Richardson J, Smith JE, McCall G, Pilkington K. Hypnosis for procedure-related pain and distress in pediatric cancer patients: a systematic review of effectiveness and methodology related to hypnosis interventions. J Pain Symptom Manage 2006;31:70–84
21. Stalpers LJ, da Costa HC, Merbis MA, Fortuin AA, Muller MJ, van Dam FS. Hypnotherapy in radiotherapy patients: a randomized trial. Int J Radiat Oncol Biol Phys 2005;61:499–506
22. Rajasekaran M, Edmonds PM, Higginson IL. Systematic review of hypnotherapy for treating symptoms in terminally ill adult cancer patients. Palliat Med 2005;19:418–426
23. Corbin L. Safety and efficacy of massage therapy for patients with cancer. Cancer Control 2005;12:158–164

24. Kwekkeboom KL. Music versus distraction for procedural pain and anxiety in patients with cancer. Oncol Nurs Forum 2003;30:433–440

25. Hodgson H. Does reflexology impact on cancer patients' quality of life? Nurs Stand 2000;14:33–38

26. Stephenson NL, Weinrich SP, Tavakoli AS. The effects of foot reflexology on anxiety and pain in patients with breast and lung cancer. Oncol Nurs Forum 2000;27:67–72

27. Sloman R, Brown P, Aldana E, Chee E. The use of relaxation for the promotion of comfort and pain relief in persons with advanced cancer. Contemporary Nurse 1994;3:6–12

28. Haase O, Schwenk W, Hermann C, Muller JM. Guided imagery and relaxation in conventional colorectal resections: a randomized, controlled, partially blinded trial. Dis Colon Rectum 2005;48:1955–1963

29. Walker LG, Walker MB, Ogston K, Heys SD, Ah-See AK, Miller ID, Hutcheon AW, Sarkar TK, Eremin O. Psychological, clinical and pathological effects of relaxation training and guided imagery during primary chemotherapy. Br J Cancer 1999;80:262–268

30. Gaston-Johansson F, Fall-Dickson JM, Nanda J, Ohly KV, Stillman S, Krumm S, Kennedy MJ. The effectiveness of the comprehensive coping strategy program on clinical outcomes in breast cancer autologous bone marrow transplantation. Cancer Nurs 2000;23:277–285

31. Speca M, Carlson LE, Goodey E, Angen M. A randomized, wait-list controlled clinical trial: the effect of a mindfulness meditation-based stress reduction program on mood and symptoms of stress in cancer outpatients. Psychosom Med 2000;62:613–622

32. Carlson LE, Ursuliak Z, Goodey E, Angen M, Speca M. The effects of a mindfulness meditation-based stress reduction program on mood and symptoms of stress in cancer outpatients: 6-month follow-up. Support Care Cancer 2001;9:112–123

33. Shapiro SL, Bootzin RR, Figueredo AJ, Lopez AM, Schwartz GE. The efficacy of mindfulness-based stress reduction in the treatment of sleep disturbance in women with breast cancer: an exploratory study. J Psychosom Res 2003;54:85–91

34. Jacobsen PB, Meade CD, Stein KD, Chirikos TN, Small BJ, Ruckdeschel JC. Efficacy and costs of two forms of stress management training for cancer patients undergoing chemotherapy. J Clin Oncol 2002;20:2851–2862

35. Hidderley M, Holt M. A pilot randomized trial assessing the effects of autogenic training in early stage cancer patients in relation to psychological status and immune system responses. Eur J Oncol Nurs 2004;8:61–65

36. Baider L, Peretz T, Hadani PE, Koch U. Psychological intervention in cancer patients: a randomized study. Gen Hosp Psychiatry 2001;23:272–277

37. Molassiotis A, Yung HP, Yam BM, Chan FY, Mok TS. The effectiveness of progressive muscle relaxation training in managing chemotherapy-induced nausea and vomiting in Chinese breast cancer patients: a randomised controlled trial. Support Care Cancer 2002; 10:237–246

38. Sloman R. Relaxation and imagery for anxiety and depression control in community patients with advanced cancer. Cancer Nurs 2002;25:432–435

39. Cheung YL, Molassiotis A, Chang AM. The effect of progressive muscle relaxation training on anxiety and quality of life after stoma surgery in colorectal cancer patients. Psychooncology 2003;12:254–266

40. Lee TI, Chen HH, Yeh ML. Effects of chan-chuang qigong on improving symptom and psychological distress in chemotherapy patients. Am J Chin Med 2006;34:37–46

41. Campbell FA, Tramer MR, Carroll D, Reynolds DJ, Moore RA, McQuay HJ. Are cannabinoids an effective and safe treatment option in the management of pain? A qualitative systematic review. BMJ 2001;323:13–16

CARPAL TUNNEL SYNDROME

SYNONYM

Median nerve dysfunction.

DEFINITION

Carpal tunnel syndrome is a neuropathy caused by compression of the median nerve within the carpal tunnel. Classical symptoms of carpal tunnel syndrome include numbness, tingling,

Box 5.11 *Cochrane review: non-surgical treatments for carpal tunnel syndrome*[1]

- Randomised or quasi-randomised studies of participants with the diagnosis of carpal tunnel syndrome who had not previously undergone surgical release
- Twenty-one trials involving 884 patients were included
- **Conclusion:** 'Current evidence shows significant short-term benefit from oral steroids, splinting, ultrasound, yoga and carpal bone mobilisation. Other non-surgical treatments do not produce significant benefit'

burning or pain in at least two of the three digits supplied by the median nerve (i.e. the thumb, index and middle fingers). Injury or trauma to the area, including repetitive movement of the wrists caused by sports such as handball or use of tools, especially vibrating tools, can cause carpal tunnel syndrome.

RELATED CONDITIONS
Arthritis, bursitis.

CAM USAGE
Herbal medicine, homeopathy and manipulative treatments are popular.

CLINICAL EVIDENCE
Non-surgical treatments have been evaluated in a Cochrane review (Box 5.11).[1]

ACUPUNCTURE
A Cochrane review identified one RCT.[1] This trial evaluated the short-term effects of laser acupuncture on paraesthesiae and night pain compared with placebo laser acupuncture. No differences in paraesthesiae or night pain were demonstrated between laser acupuncture and placebo over a 3-week treatment period. It was concluded that the limited evidence suggests that laser acupuncture does not improve short-term paraesthesiae and night pain in patients with carpal tunnel syndrome.

CHIROPRACTIC
A systematic review aimed to critically evaluate the evidence for or against the effectiveness of chiropractic manipulation for non-spinal conditions.[2] It identified one RCT and concluded that claims that this approach is effective for pain reduction in carpal tunnel syndrome are not based on data from rigorous clinical trials.

HOMEOPATHY
Two RCTs (*n* = 99) compared homeopathic arnica with placebo.[3,4] One trial reported significant pain reduction compared with baseline in favour of homeopathic arnica,[3] whereas the other reported no intergroup differences for pain and bruising after hand surgery.[4] Thus, there is no convincing evidence that homeopathic arnica is effective for pain reduction in carpal tunnel syndrome.

MAGNETS
A Cochrane review identified one RCT evaluating the short-term effect of applying a magnetic device over the carpal tunnel (for 45 minutes) on pain compared with a placebo device.[1] No significant effect in favour of magnet therapy was demonstrated immediately following treatment or 2 weeks after.

SECTION FIVE

MOBILISATION

A Cochrane review identified one RCT.[1] This trial evaluated the short-term effect of mobilisation on pain, hand function, wrist motion and need for surgery compared with no treatment. No significant effect in favour of mobilisation was demonstrated for improving symptoms, pain, hand function, active wrist motion or need for surgery after 3 weeks of treatment. It was concluded that limited evidence suggests that neurodynamic mobilisation does not improve such signs and symptoms in the short term or reduce the likelihood of surgery.

VITAMIN B6

A Cochrane review identified two RCTs ($n = 50$).[1] The medium-term effects of oral vitamin B6 (pyridoxine) were compared with placebo. No significant effect of vitamin B6 was demonstrated for improvement in symptoms and nocturnal discomfort after 10–12 weeks of treatment. However, a significant effect was demonstrated for movement discomfort after 12 weeks of intervention. Therefore, limited evidence exists that 12 weeks of vitamin B6 treatment improves movement discomfort.

YOGA

A Cochrane review identified one RCT.[1] It evaluated the short-term effects of yoga on a pain visual analogue scale when compared to wrist splinting. A significant improvement of pain was demonstrated after 8 weeks of treatment. It was concluded that there is limited evidence that yoga results in superior short-term pain relief compared to wrist splinting.

OTHER THERAPIES

A small ($n = 16$) RCT of massage reported reduced pain and increased grip strength and concluded that 'symptoms can be relieved by a daily regimen of massage therapy.'[5] In an RCT ($n = 21$) testing therapeutic touch for changes in median motor nerve distal latencies, pain scores and relaxation scores did not differ compared with sham therapeutic touch.[6]

OVERALL RECOMMENDATION

There is no convincing evidence that any complementary therapy reduces pain caused by carpal tunnel syndrome. Encouraging evidence from single RCTs exists but it requires independent replication.

Table 5.7 **Summary of clinical evidence for carpal tunnel syndrome**

Treatment	Weight of evidence	Direction of evidence	Serious safety concerns
Acupuncture (laser)	OO	↘	Yes (see p. 96)
Chiropractic	OO	↘	Yes (see p. 112)
Exercise	OO	↘	Yes (see p. 5)
Homeopathic arnica	OO	↘	No (see p. 176)
Magnets	O	↘	Yes (see p. 164)
Mobilisation	O	↘	Yes (see p. 112)
Vitamin B6	OO	↗	Yes (see p. 5)
Yoga	O	↗	Yes (see p. 169)

REFERENCES

1. O'Connor D, Marshall S, Massy-Westropp N. Non-surgical treatment (other than steroid injection) for carpal tunnel syndrome. The Cochrane Database of Systematic Reviews 2003, Issue 1. Art. No.: CD003219
2. Ernst E. Chiropractic manipulation for non-spinal pain – a systematic review. NZ Med J 2003;116:U539
3. Jeffrey SL, Belcher HJ. Use of Arnica to relieve pain after carpal-tunnel release surgery. Altern Ther Health Med 2002;8:66–68
4. Stevinson C, Devaraj VS, Fountain-Barber A, Hawkins S, Ernst E. Homeopathic arnica for prevention of pain and bruising: randomized placebo-controlled trial in hand surgery. J R Soc Med 2003;96:60–65
5. Field T, Diego M, Cullen C, Hartshorn K, Gruskin A, Hernandez-Reif M, Sunshine W. Carpal tunnel syndrome symptoms are lessened following massage therapy. J Bodywork Movement Ther 2004;8:9–14
6. Blankfield RP, Sulzmann C, Fradley LG, Tapolyai AA, Zyzanski SJ. Therapeutic touch in the treatment of carpal tunnel syndrome. J Am Board Fam Pract 2001;14:335–342

COMPLEX REGIONAL PAIN SYNDROME

SYNONYMS/SUBCATEGORIES

Reflex sympathetic dystrophy, causalgia.

DEFINITION

Regional progressive pain syndromes usually occur after relatively minor injury often resulting in impaired motor functions. Type I (reflex sympathetic dystrophy) develops after an initiating noxious event and is characterised by oedema, skin blood flow abnormalities and abnormal sudomotor activity. Type II develops after nerve injury. Pain is not necessarily limited to the territory of the injured nerve. Otherwise, symptoms are similar to type I.

CAM USAGE

No definitive data available, likely to be high.

CLINICAL EVIDENCE

ACUPUNCTURE

A small ($n = 14$) RCT suggested that acupuncture is better than sham acupuncture in reducing the pain of reflex sympathetic dystrophy.[1]

AUTOGENIC TRAINING

An RCT ($n = 18$) tested the effectiveness of autogenic training plus standard treatment compared to standard therapy alone.[2] There were improvements in both groups of patients suffering from reflex sympathetic dystrophy but no differences between groups in terms of pain relief.

IMAGERY

A small ($n = 13$) crossover RCT of imagery for reflex sympathetic dystrophy suggested effectiveness of this approach in terms of pain control compared to no-treatment controls.[3]

MASSAGE

An RCT ($n = 35$) compared lymph drainage plus exercise with exercise alone.[4] Its results suggest better pain control in the former group.

SECTION FIVE

QIGONG

An RCT ($n = 26$) suggested that, compared to sham therapy, qigong was more effective in reducing the pain of late-stage complex regional pain syndrome.[5]

OVERALL RECOMMENDATION

Complex regional pain syndromes are notoriously difficult to treat with any type of intervention. Even though for some CAM treatments encouraging results have emerged, these require independent replication before recommendations can be issued.

Table 5.8 **Summary of clinical evidence for complex regional pain syndrome**

Treatment	Weight of evidence	Direction of evidence	Serious safety concerns
Acupuncture	O	↑	Yes (see p. 96)
Autogenic training	O	↗	Yes (see p. 106)
Imagery	O	↑	No (see p. 132)
Massage	O	↑	No (see p. 137)
Qigong	O	↑	No (see p. 152)

REFERENCES

1. Ernst E, Resch KL, Fialka V, Ritter-Dittrich D, Alcamioglu Y, Chen O, Leitha T, Kluger R. Traditional acupuncture for reflex sympathetic dystrophy: a randomised, sham-controlled, double-blind trial. Acupunct Med 1995;2:78

2. Fialka V, Korpan M, Saradeth T, Paternostro-Slugo T, Hexel O, Frischenschlager O, Ernst E. Autogenic training for reflex sympathetic dystrophy: a pilot study. Complement Ther Med 1996;4: 103–105

3. Moseley GL. Graded motor imagery is effective for long-standing complex regional pain syndrome: a randomised controlled trial. Pain 2004;108:192–198

4. Uher EM, Vacariu G, Schneider B, Fialka V. Comparison of manual lymph drainage with physical therapy in complex regional pain syndrome, type I. A comparative randomized controlled therapy study. [In German.] Wien Klin Wochenschr 2000;112:133–137

5. Wu WH, Bandilla E, Ciccone DS, Yang J, Cheng SC, Carner N, Wu Y, Shen R. Effects of qigong on late-stage complex regional pain syndrome. Altern Ther Health Med 1999;5:45–54

DENTAL PAIN

SYNONYMS

Toothache.

DEFINITION

Pain that is most commonly caused by a dental cavity or by conditions affecting the gum. Dental pain can also be caused by conditions that do not originate from a tooth or the jaw such as trigeminal neuralgia.

RELATED CONDITIONS

Facial pain.

Box 5.12 *Systematic review: acupuncture for dental pain*[2]

- Of 11 RCTs all but four were positive
- Most trials used acupuncture in a clinical situation; five studies related to experimental set-ups where dental pain was induced in volunteers
- Methodological quality ranged between zero and three points (Jadad)
- **Conclusion**: acupuncture can alleviate dental pain and future investigations should define the optimal acupuncture technique and its relative efficacy compared with conventional methods of analgesia

CAM USAGE
Acupuncture, biofeedback, relaxation.[1]

CLINICAL EVIDENCE
ACUPUNCTURE
A systematic review identified 11 RCTs that assessed acupuncture for dental pain (Box 5.12).[2] Seven of these RCTs were sham-controlled and patient and/or observer blind. Of these all but four were positive and the review concluded that the data suggest that acupuncture can be effective in alleviating dental pain. A subsequent double-blind, placebo-controlled RCT ($n = 39$) tested acupuncture in treating post-operative oral surgery pain.[3] Pain-free post-operative time was significantly longer in the acupuncture group than in the placebo group, as was the time until moderate pain. A pilot RCT tested whether acupuncture can reduce the induction time of a local anaesthetic and suggested that the onset time of local anaesthesia is reduced if segmentally administered acupuncture is given before the regional inferior dental block.[4]

OTHER THERAPIES
A pilot study evaluated the effect of propolis in subjects with dentinal hypersensitivity.[5] Some positive effects were noted after 4 weeks of treatment on subjective reporting of pain.

OVERALL RECOMMENDATION
The data suggest that acupuncture is effective in alleviating dental pain in a number of settings such as following surgery or during dental operations. Its relative effectiveness compared with conventional methods of analgesia is unclear. There are no data from rigorous clinical trials for any other CAM intervention for dental pain.

Table 5.9 **Summary of clinical evidence for dental pain**

Treatment	Weight of evidence	Direction of evidence	Serious safety concerns
Acupuncture	OOO	↑	Yes (see p. 96)

REFERENCES
1. Myers CD, White BA, Heft MW. A review of complementary and alternative medicine use for treating chronic facial pain. J Am Dent Assoc 2002;133:1189–1196
2. Ernst E, Pittler MH. The effectiveness of acupuncture in treating acute dental pain: a systematic review. Br Dent J 1998;184:443–447

SECTION FIVE

3. Lao L, Bergman S, Hamilton GR, Langenberg P, Berman B. Evaluation of acupuncture for pain control after oral surgery: a placebo-controlled trial. Arch Otolaryngol Head Neck Surg 1999;125:567–572

4. Rosted P, Bundgaard M. Can acupuncture reduce the induction time of a local anaesthetic? A pilot study. Acupunct Med 2003;21:92–99

5. Mahmoud AS, Almas K, Dahlan AA. The effect of propolis on dentinal hypersensitivity and level of satisfaction among patients from a university hospital Riyadh, Saudi Arabia. Indian J Dent Res 1999;10:130–137

DEPRESSION

This chapter differs from other chapters included in this section in that depression is not painful per se. However, more than 75% of depressive patients seen in primary care report pain,[1] and 69% of patients later diagnosed with depression initially presented with somatic symptoms.[2] Therefore, the associations between pain and depression (and vice versa) are of sufficient importance to merit a chapter specifically on depression.

SYNONYMS/SUBCATEGORIES

Depressive disorder, depressive illness, dysthymic disorder, neurotic depression, psychotic depression.

DEFINITION

Persistent low mood, loss of interest and enjoyment and reduced energy. Mild to moderate depression is characterised by depressive symptoms and some functional impairment. Severe depression is characterised by additional agitation or psychomotor retardation with marked somatic symptoms.

CAM USAGE

Depression is one of the most common reasons for using CAM. The most popular therapies include exercise, herbal medicine, relaxation and spiritual healing.[3,4]

CLINICAL EVIDENCE

ACUPUNCTURE

A systematic review[5] of six RCTs demonstrated that the evidence for the effectiveness of acupuncture in depression was inconclusive (Box 5.13). More recent CCTs have invariably reported encouraging results.[6–9]

AUTOGENIC TRAINING

A systematic review of all clinical trials of autogenic training (for any condition) found encouraging evidence for its effectiveness in depression.[10]

EXERCISE

A large body of positive evidence exists for the antidepressant effects of exercise. The majority of studies are not of high quality, but over a dozen RCTs collectively provide convincing evidence of efficacy in clinically depressed patients. Two meta-analyses have found effects. One included 80 studies of any design with all types of participants.[11] The other was restricted to controlled trials with clinically depressed patients (Box 5.14).[12] Both aerobic and non-aerobic forms of exercise were effective. Three RCTs have suggested that aerobic exercise may be as effective as psychological or pharmacological treatment (Table 5.10).[13–15] One RCT suggested that exercise improves the mood even in cases of major

SECTION FIVE

Box 5.13 *Systematic review: acupuncture for depression*[5]

- Six RCTs were found with a total of 509 patients
- Only three of these were of good methodological quality
- The results were inconsistent
- **Conclusion**: the evidence from RCTs is insufficient for firm recommendations

Box 5.14 *Meta-analysis: exercise for depression*[12]

- Thirty controlled trials including 2158 patients
- Depression as primary disorder or secondary to other psychiatric disorder
- Comparison groups were mainly waiting lists or psychotherapy
- Trial quality ranged from good to poor
- Significant effect of exercise (mean effect size −0.72; standard error 0.10)
- **Conclusion**: all types of exercise appear to have similar effects

Table 5.10 **RCTs of exercise compared with psychiatric treatment for depression**

Reference	Sample size	Interventions (regimen)	Result	Comment
Klein[13]	74	(A) Running [2 × for 45 min/week for 12 weeks] (B) Meditation/relaxation (C) Group psychotherapy	A no different to B or C	Improvements maintained at 9 months
Freemont[14]	49	(A) Running [3 × 20 min/ week for 10 weeks] (B) Cognitive therapy (C) Combination of A and B	A no different to B or C	Improvements maintained at 4 months
Blumenthal[15]	156	(A) Walking/jogging [3 × 45 min/week for 16 weeks] (B) Sertraline [200 mg/day] (C) Combination of A and B	A no different to B or C; less relapse in A after 6 months	Patients were all ⩾50 years

depression.[16] A further RCT suggested beneficial effects of combining exercise with light exposure.[17]

HERBAL MEDICINE

Ginkgo (*Ginkgo biloba*) was tested against placebo in a small RCT with 27 patients suffering from 'winter depression'.[18] The results failed to demonstrate effectiveness. Lavender (*Lavandula angustifolia*) was compared to imipramine in a small RCT with 45 moderately depressed patients.[19] Depressive symptoms improved similarly in both groups, and the authors concluded that lavender 'may be of therapeutic benefit'.

Saffron (*Crocus sativus*) generated similar improvements as imipramine in a small RCT with 30 patients suffering from mild to moderate depression.[20]

Box 5.15 *Meta-analysis: St John's wort for depression*[21]

- Thirty RCTs were included
- Mainly but not exclusively for mild to moderate depression
- Trial quality generally good
- Placebo-controlled trials with a total of 2129 patients favoured St John's wort [relative risk (RR) = 0.66, 95% CI 0.57 to 0.78, numbers needed to treat = 42)
- Five compared with other antidepressants (n = 2231, RR = 0.96, 95% CI 0.85 to 1.08)
- Favourable side effects profile
- **Conclusion**: St John's wort is effective for mild to moderate depression

There is compelling evidence from numerous meta-analyses for the efficacy of St John's wort (*Hypericum perforatum*) in mild to moderate depression. A recent meta-analysis (Box 5.15), which also includes the more recent negative RCTs,[21] comes to a positive conclusion for mild to moderate depression. This overall encouraging finding was modified[22] and it was noted that the effect size was inversely related to the sample size in placebo-controlled RCTs. Newer RCTs and those originating from countries other than Germany tended to generate smaller response rates. Some RCTs also suggest that St John's wort is as effective as synthetic antidepressants[23] and also works for major depression.[24]

HOMEOPATHY

A systematic review included two RCTs and found no convincing evidence that homeopathy represents an effective approach to the treatment of depression.[25]

HYPNOTHERAPY

A systematic review found one RCT and 26 other types of investigations.[26] It concluded that the value of hypnotherapy for treating depression is uncertain.

IMAGERY

A review of 46 studies of imagery (regardless of indication) found 'preliminary evidence for the effectiveness of imagery in the management of depression'.[27]

MAGNETS

An RCT tested exposure to a magnetic field (15 microTesla) against sham therapy in 24 patients on antidepressants. The results suggest that magnetic therapy has a positive additional symptomatic effect.[28]

MASSAGE

Massage was more effective in improving symptoms of depression and anxiety, night-time sleep and cortisol levels than watching relaxing videos in an RCT (n = 72) involving children and adolescent inpatients with depression and adjustment disorder.[29] A further recent RCT confirmed these positive findings[30] and a meta-analysis of all RCTs of massage therapy (regardless of indication) concluded that 'reductions of trait anxiety and depression were massage therapy's largest effects'.[31]

MINDFULNESS-BASED STRESS REDUCTION

A systematic review of all clinical studies of this approach (regardless of indication) found encouraging evidence that mindfulness-based stress reduction reduces depression.[32]

Table 5.11 **RCTs of relaxation therapy for depression**

Reference	Sample size	Interventions (regimen)	Result	Comment
Reynolds[38]	30	(A) Relaxation training [10 × 50 min over 5 weeks] (B) Cognitive–behavioural therapy (C) Waiting list	A no different to B; both superior to C	Patients were adolescents; improvements maintained at 5-week follow-up
Broota[39]	30	(A) Progressive muscle relaxation [1 × 20 min/day for 3 days] (B) Yoga and autosuggestion (C) Discussion	A no different to B; both superior to C	Patients all on medication
Murphy[40]	37	(A) Relaxation training [1–2 × 50 min/week for 12 weeks] (B) Cognitive–behavioural therapy (C) Desipramine [150–300 mg]	A no different to B; both superior to C	Substantial non-compliance in medication group

MUSIC THERAPY

An RCT of music therapy in depressed elderly patients ($n = 30$) found superior results with a music-based intervention compared with no treatment.[33] The intervention involved various therapeutic modalities. Other RCTs involving depressed adolescent females who listened to rock music while control groups received massage[34] or simply relaxed[35] reported changes to physiological and biochemical parameters but not to mood or behaviour. An RCT ($n = 65$) suggested that music therapy reduced pain and depression in patients hospitalised with chronic back pain[36] or in patients suffering from moderate to severe burns.[37]

RELAXATION

Three small RCTs of relaxation for depression have suggested that relaxation training is superior to no treatment and potentially similar to cognitive–behavioural therapy (Table 5.11).[38–40] Clearly, non-specific effects are difficult to control for with this therapy. Nonetheless, the evidence can be considered encouraging. Relaxation training also seems to be effective for depression secondary to somatic disease[41] or organ transplantation.[42]

SUPPLEMENTS

Fish oil (omega-3 fatty acids) was assessed in a systematic review including four RCTs.[43] It concluded that the evidence is encouraging but not fully convincing.

Encouraging evidence was also found in a systematic review of S-adenosylmethionine.[44]

Zinc was tested against placebo in an RCT with 14 severely depressed and medically treated patients.[45] The results suggest that 12 weeks of zinc supplementation (25 mg/day) has beneficial effects on the symptoms of depression.

YOGA

A systematic review of five RCTs found encouraging evidence for yoga as a treatment for depression but cautioned that the evidence, because of methodological flaws in the primary data, was not conclusive.[46]

OTHER THERAPIES

In a small non-randomised trial ($n = 20$) with male inpatients, adjunctive aromatherapy enabled the dose of antidepressants to be reduced compared with patients receiving the usual care.[47]

An RCT ($n = 35$) suggested that patients undergoing stem cell transplantation experienced less depression after having been trained to do regular breathing exercises.[48] Single sessions of dance and movement therapy produced promising results in two small trials with inpatients when compared with no intervention.[49,50]

Reiki was compared with distant Reiki healing and with no treatment at all in an RCT involving 46 patients.[51] The results suggest that both Reiki interventions reduced depressive symptoms.

OVERALL RECOMMENDATIONS

No complementary treatment is more effective than conventional pharmacological or psychological interventions. Exercise and St John's wort, however, seem to be equivalent to conventional treatment and certainly have fewer adverse effects. Other approaches for which research is encouraging include autogenic training, massage, relaxation and yoga. As these options are considered relatively safe they may benefit some individuals.

Table 5.12 **Summary of clinical evidence for depression**

Treatment	Weight of evidence	Direction of evidence	Serious safety concerns
Acupuncture	OOO	↗	Yes (see p. 96)
Autogenic training	OO	↗	Yes (see p. 106)
Exercise	OOO	↑	Yes (see p. 5)
Herbal medicine			
Ginkgo	O	↓	Yes (see p. 5)
Lavender	O	↗	Yes (see p. 204)
Saffron	O	↗	Yes (see p. 5)
St John's wort	OOO	↑	Yes (see p. 5)
Homeopathy	OO	→	No (see p. 124)
Hypnotherapy	OO	→	Yes (see p. 130)
Imagery	O	↑	No (see p. 132)
Magnets	O	↗	No (see p. 164)
Massage	OO	↑	No (see p. 137)
Mindfulness-based stress reduction	O	↗	No (see p. 5)
Music therapy	OOO	↗	No (see p. 142)
Relaxation	OOO	↑	No (see p. 158)
Supplements			
Fish oil	OO	↗	Yes (see p. 5)
S-adenosylmethionine	OO	↗	No (see p. 212)
Zinc	O	↑	No (see p. 5)
Yoga	OO	↗	Yes (see p. 169)

REFERENCES

1. Simon GE, VonKorff M, Piccinelli M, Fullerton C, Ormel J. An international study of the relation between somatic symptoms and depression. N Engl J Med 1999;341:1329–1335
2. Kirmayer LJ, Robbins JM, Dworkind M, Yaffe MJ. Somatization and the recognition of depression and anxiety in primary care. Am J Psychiatry 1993;150:734–741
3. Astin JA. Why patients use alternative medicine. JAMA 1998;279:1548–1553
4. Eisenberg DM, Davis RB, Ettner SL, Appel S, Wilkey S, Rompay MV, Kessler RC. Trends in alternative medicine use in the United States, 1990–1997. JAMA 1998;280:1569–1575
5. Mukaino Y, Park J, White A, Ernst E. Effectiveness of acupuncture for depression: a systematic review. Acupunct Med 2005;23:70–76
6. Fan L, Fu WB, Meng CR, Zhu XP, Mi JP, Li WX, Wen X. Effect of acupuncture at routine acupoint and non-acupoint on depressive neurosis evaluated with Hamilton depression scale. [In Chinese.] Chin J Clin Rehab 2005;9:14–16
7. He D, Hostmark AT, Veiersted KB, Medbo JI. Effect of intensive acupuncture on pain-related social and psychological variables for women with chronic neck and shoulder pain – an RCT with six month and three year follow up. Acupunct Med 2005;23:52–61
8. Hou Q, Yan L, Fu L, Du YH. Tiaoshen shugan acupuncture versus routine acupuncture for intervention of depression and anxiety. [In Chinese.] Clin J Clin Rehab 2005;9:11–13
9. Quah-Smith JI, Tang WM, Russell J. Laser acupuncture for mild to moderate depression in a primary care setting — a randomised controlled trial. Acupunct Med 2005;23:103–111
10. Stetter F, Kupper S. Autogenic training: a meta-analysis of clinical outcome studies. Appl Psychophysiol Biofeedback 2002;27:45–98
11. North TC, McCullagh P, Vu Tran Z. Effect of exercise on depression. Ex Sport Sci Rev 1990; 18:379–415
12. Craft LL, Landers DM. The effect of exercise on clinical depression and depression resulting from mental illness: a meta-analysis. J Sport Exercise Psychol 1998;20:339–357
13. Klein MH, Greist JH, Gurman AS, Neimeyer RA, Lesser DP, Bushnell NJ, Smith, RE. A comparative outcome study of group psychotherapy vs exercise treatments for depression. Int J Ment Health 1985;13:148–177
14. Freemont J, Craighead LW. Aerobic exercise and cognitive therapy in the treatment of dysphoric moods. Cognitive Ther Res 1987;11:241–251
15. Blumenthal JA, Babyak MA, Moore KA, Craighead WE, Herman S, Khatri P, Waugh R, Napolitano MA, Forman LM, Appelbaum M, Doraiswamy PM, Krishnan KR. Effects of exercise training on older patients with major depression. Arch Intern Med 1999;159: 2349–2356
16. Bartholomew JB, Morrison D, Ciccolo JT. Effects of acute exercise on mood and well-being in patients with major depressive disorder. Med Sci Sports Exerc 2005;37:2032–2037
17. Leppamaki S, Haukka J, Lonnqvist J, Partonen T. Drop-out and mood improvement: a randomized controlled trial with light exposure and physical exercise. BMC Psychiatry 2004;4:22
18. Lingaerde O, Foreland AR, Magnusson A. Can winter depression be prevented by *Ginkgo biloba* extract? A placebo-controlled trial. Acta Psychiatr Scand 1999;1000:62–66
19. Akhondzadeh S, Kashani L, Fotouhi A, Jarvandi S, Mobaseri M, Moin M, Khani M, Jamshidi AH, Baghalian K, Taghizadeh M. Comparison of *Lavandula angustifolia* Mill. Tincture and imipramine in the treatment of mild to moderate depression: a double-blind, randomized trial. Prog Neuropsychopharmacol Biol Psychiatry 2003;27:123–127
20. Akhondzadeh S, Fallah-Pour H, Afkham K, Jamshidi AH, Khalighi-Cigaroudi F. Comparison of *Crocus sativus* L. and imipramine in the treatment of mild to moderate depression: a double-blind randomized trial. BMC Complement Altern Med 2004;4:12
21. Roder C, Schaefer M, Leucht S. Meta-analysis of effectiveness and tolerability of treatment of mild to moderate depression with St John's wort. [In German.] Fortschr Neurol Psychiatr 2004;72:330–343
22. Linde K, Mulrow C, Berner M, Egger M. St John's wort for depression. The Cochrane Database of Systematic Reviews 2005, Issue 2. Art No.: CD000448
23. Gastpar M, Singer A, Zeller K. Comparative efficacy and safety of a once-daily dosage of *Hypericum* extract STW3-VI and citalopram in patients with moderate depression: a double-blind, randomised, multicentre, placebo-controlled study. Pharmacopsychiatry 2006;39:66–75
24. Fava M, Alpert J, Nierenberg AA, Mischoulon D, Otto MW, Zajecka J, Murck H, Rosenbaum JF. A double-blind, randomized trial of St John's wort, fluoxetine, and placebo in major depressive disorder. J Clin Psychopharmacol 2005;25:441–447

25. Pilkington K, Kirkwood G, Rampes H, Fisher P, Richardson J. Homeopathy for depression: a systematic review of the research evidence. Homeopathy 2005;94:153–163

26. Rajasekaran M, Edmonds PM, Higginson IL. Systematic review of hypnotherapy for treating symptoms in terminally ill adult cancer patients. Palliat Med 2005;19:418–426

27. Eller LS. Guided imagery interventions for symptom management. Ann Rev Nurs Res 1999; 17:57–84

28. Sieron A, Hese RT, Sobis J, Ciesla G. Estimation of therapeutical efficacy of weak variable magnetic fields with low value of induction in patients with depression. [In Polish.] Psychiatr Pol 2004;38:217–225

29. Field T, Morrow C, Valdeon C, Larson S, Kuhn C, Schanberg S. Massage reduces anxiety in child and adolescent psychiatric patients. J Am Acad Child Adolesc Psychiatr 1992;31:125–131

30. Muller-Oerlinghausen B, Berg C, Scherer P, Mackert A, Moestl HP, Wolf J. Effects of slow-stroke massage as complementary treatment of depressed hospitalized patients. [In German.] Dtsch Med Wochenschr 2004;129:1363–1368

31. Moyer CA, Rounds J, Hannum JW. A meta-analysis of massage therapy research. Psychol Bull 2004;130:3–18

32. Grossman P, Niemann L, Schmidt S, Walach H. Mindfulness-based stress reduction and health benefits. A meta-analysis. J Psychosom Res 2004;57:35–43

33. Hanser SB. Thompson LW. Effects of music therapy strategy on depressed older adults. J Gerontol 1994;49:265–269

34. Jones NA, Field T. Massage and music therapies attenuate frontal EEG asymmetry in depressed adolescents. Adolescence 1999;34:529–534

35. Field T, Martinez A, Nawrocki T, Pickens J, Fox NA, Schanberg S. Music shifts frontal EEG in depressed adolescents. Adolescence 1998;33:109–116

36. Guetin S, Coudeyre E, Picot MC, Ginies P, Graber-Duvernay B, Ratsimba D, Vanbiervliet W, Blayac JP, Herisson C. Effect of music therapy among hospitalized patients with chronic low backpain: a controlled, randomized trial. [In French.] Ann Readapt Med Phys 2005;48:217–224

37. Wang D, Wu XP, Sun CZ, Song ZJ, Xu YX, Xia XI, He YD, Wang CM, Sun XL. Effect of music therapy plus selective serotonin reuptake inhibitors on emotion and burn wound healing in burn patients. [In Chinese.] Chin J Evid Based Med 2006;6:90–93

38. Reynolds WM, Coats KI. A comparison of cognitive-behavioral therapy and relaxation training for the treatment of depression in adolescents. J Consult Clin Psychol 1986;54: 653–660

39. Broota A, Dhir R. Efficacy of two relaxation techniques in depression. J Pers Clin Stud 1990;6:83–90

40. Murphy GE, Carney RM, Knesevich MA, Wetzel RD, Whitworth P. Cognitive behavior therapy, relaxation training, and tricyclic antidepressant medication in the treatment of depression. Psychol Rep 1995;77:403–420

41. Bu XM, Wang X, Cao LJ, Zhu GC. Effect of comprehensive relaxation training on anxiety and depression in patients with hepatic carcinoma. Chin J Clin Rehab 2005;9: 16–17

42. Kreitzer MJ, Gross CR, Ye X, Russas V, Treesak C. Longitudinal impact of mindfulness meditation on illness burden in solid-organ transplant recipients. Prog Transplant 2005;15:166–172

43. Sontrop J, Campbell MK. Omega-3 polyunsaturated fatty acids and depression: a review of the evidence and a methodological critique. Prev Med 2006;42:4–13

44. Jorm AF, Christensen H, Griffiths KM, Rodgers B. Effectiveness of complementary and self-help treatments for depression. Med J Aust 2002;176:S84-S96

45. Nowak G, Siwek M, Dudek D, Zieba A, Pilc A. Effect of zinc supplementation on antidepressant therapy in unipolar depression: a preliminary placebo-controlled study. Pol J Pharmacol 2003;55:1143–1147

46. Pilkington K, Kirkwood G, Rampes H, Richardson J. Yoga for depression: the research evidence. J Affect Disord 2005;89:13–24

47. Komori T, Fujiwara R, Tanida M, Nomura J, Yokoyama MM. Effects of citrus fragrance on immune function and depressive states. Neuroimmunomodulation 1995;2:174–180

48. Kim SD, Kim HS. Effects of a relaxation breathing exercise on anxiety, depression, and leukocytes in hemopoietic stem cell transplantation patients. Cancer Nurs 2005;28: 79–83

49. Brooks D, Stark A. The effect of dance/movement therapy on affect: a pilot study. Am J Dance Ther 1989;11:101–112

50. Stewart NJ, McMullen LM, Rubin LD. Movement therapy with depressed inpatients: a randomized multiple single-case design. Arch Psychiatr Nurs 1994;8:22–29

51. Shore AG. Long-term effects of energetic healing on symptoms of psychological depression and self-perceived stress. Altern Ther Health Med 2004;10:42–48

DYSMENORRHOEA

SYNONYMS/SUBCATEGORIES

Menstrual pain, pelvic pain; primary and secondary dysmenorrhoea.

DEFINITION

Dysmenorrhoea is painful menstrual cramps of uterine origin. It is commonly divided into primary dysmenorrhoea (pain without organic pathology) and secondary dysmenorrhoea (pelvic pain associated with an identifiable pathological condition, such as endometriosis or ovarian cysts). The initial onset of primary dysmenorrhoea is usually shortly after menarche (6–12 months), when ovulatory cycles are established. Pain duration is commonly 8–72 hours and is usually associated with the onset of menstrual flow. Secondary dysmenorrhoea can occur at any time after menarche, but may arise as a new symptom during a woman's fourth and fifth decades, after the onset of an underlying causative condition.

RELATED CONDITIONS

Premenstrual syndrome, menopausal symptoms.

CAM USAGE

Acupuncture and herbal and non-herbal supplements are commonly used by patients with dysmenorrhoea.

CLINICAL EVIDENCE

ACUPUNCTURE

A systematic review of acupuncture or acupressure for women's reproductive health included four RCTs of dysmenorrhoea.[1] It concluded that acupressure ($n = 2$) is superior to standard care and equal to ibuprofen. Greater pain relief was reported for acupuncture ($n = 2$) compared to sham acupuncture, usual care and 'control' visitation but methodological limitations render the results not convincing. A subsequent controlled trial of 57 women with primary dysmenorrhoea reported decreased medication use in patients receiving real acupuncture compared to sham acupuncture.[2]

EXERCISE

Four RCTs including 492 patients reported that exercise (aerobic training, daily Golub exercises, Billig exercises, Mosher exercises) reduced the symptoms of dysmenorrhoea.[3]

HERBAL MEDICINE

The Chinese herbal formula Danggui-Shao-Yao-San was suggested to reduce pain in a double-blind, placebo-controlled trial of 40 women with dysmenorrhoea.[3]

Toki-shakuyaku-san, a Japanese combination of six herbs, was shown in one double-blind trial ($n = 40$) to be more effective for pain relief than placebo, and less additional pain medication was taken by the treatment group.[4]

MAGNETS

In a double-blind postal questionnaire RCT of 65 women with primary dysmenorrhoea a static magnet with a field strength of 2700 gauss was reported to reduce pain compared to a placebo magnet of only 140 gauss.[5] Results of an RCT of 23 women with primary dysmenorrhoea suggested that a magnetic device of 800–1299 gauss was superior to a non-magnetic device in reducing pain.[6]

SPINAL MANIPULATION

A Cochrane review of five RCTs concluded that there is no evidence to suggest that spinal manipulation is effective in the treatment of primary and secondary dysmenorrhoea (Box 5.16).[7]

SUPPLEMENTS

A systematic review included seven controlled trials of dietary supplements (Box 5.17).[4] Encouraging results were found for magnesium ($n = 3$) but it is unclear what dose or regimen of treatments to use because there were variations between the included trials. The review concluded that, based on the results of one large ($n = 556$) placebo-controlled RCT, vitamin B1 taken at 100 mg daily was an effective treatment for dysmenorrhoea.

Box 5.16 *Systematic review: spinal manipulation for primary and secondary dysmenorrhoea*[7]

- Five RCTs were included
- Four RCTs ($n = 206$) of high-velocity, low-amplitude manipulation found it no more effective than sham manipulation, although it was possibly more effective than no treatment
- One small RCT ($n = 30$) of Toftness technique reported it to be more effective than sham treatment but no strong conclusions could be made because of the small size of the trial and other methodological considerations
- No greater risk of adverse effects was found with spinal manipulation than with sham manipulation

Box 5.17 *Systematic review: herbal and dietary therapies for primary and secondary dysmenorrhoea*[4]

- Seven controlled trials were included
- Three small double-blind trials ($n = 97$) found magnesium more effective than placebo for pain relief and the need for additional medication was less
- One small double-blind RCT with four groups compared magnesium, vitamin B6, a combination of vitamin B6 and magnesium and placebo. It found no difference between the magnesium and placebo groups, the magnesium and vitamin B6 groups, the magnesium or the magnesium/vitamin B6 combination groups but found vitamin B6 to be superior to placebo
- One large double-blind RCT ($n = 556$) showed vitamin B1 to be more effective than placebo in reducing pain
- One open RCT ($n = 50$) comparing a combination of vitamin E (taken daily) and ibuprofen (taken during menses) versus ibuprofen (taken during menses) alone showed no difference in pain relief between the two treatments
- One double-blind RCT showed fish oil (omega-3 fatty acids) to be more effective than placebo for pain relief
- Toki-shakuyaku-san, a Japanese combination of six herbs, was shown in one double-blind RCT ($n = 40$) to be more effective for pain relief than placebo, and less additional pain medication was taken by the treatment group

A further systematic review reports encouraging results for vitamin E ($n = 2$), fish oil ($n = 1$), and fish oil in combination with vitamin B1 ($n = 1$) in reducing the severity of pain in women with dysmenorrhoea.[3]

A double-blind, placebo-controlled RCT reported that the dietary supplement Karinat, containing β-carotene, α-tocopherol, ascorbic acid and garlic powder, reduced the severity of dysmenorrhoea, mastalgia and premenstrual syndrome.[8]

TRANSCUTANEOUS ELECTRICAL NERVE STIMULATION

A Cochrane review located seven RCTs of transcutaneous electrical nerve stimulation (TENS) for primary dysmenorrhoea and found that high-frequency TENS was more effective for pain relief than placebo TENS and that low-frequency TENS was not more effective in reducing pain than placebo.[9]

OVERALL RECOMMENDATION

The evidence for TENS and exercise in treating dysmenorrhoea is positive and encouraging results exist for acupuncture/acupressure and vitamin E. These therapies are associated with few risks and can be useful, particularly in patients who are unable to use analgesics. The evidence for spinal manipulation is negative and there is no convincing evidence for any other intervention.

Table 5.13 **Summary of clinical evidence for dysmenorrhoea**

Treatment	Weight of evidence	Direction of evidence	Serious safety concerns
Acupuncture/acupressure	OO	↗	Yes (see p. 96)
Exercise	OO	↑	Yes (see p. 5)
Herbal medicine			
Danggui-Shao-Yao-San	O	↗	Yes (see p. 5)
Toki-shakuyaku-san	O	↗	Yes (see p. 5)
Magnets	O	↑	No (see p. 164)
Spinal manipulation	OO	↓	Yes (see p. 112)
Supplements			
Fish oil	O	↑	Yes (see p. 5)
Karinat	O	↗	Yes (see p. 5)
Magnesium	OO	↗	No (see p. 5)
Vitamin B1	O	↑	Yes (see p. 5)
Vitamin E	OO	↗	Yes (see p. 5)
TENS	OOO	↗	Yes (see p. 5)

TENS, transcutaneous electrical nerve stimulation.

SECTION FIVE

REFERENCES

1. White AR. A review of controlled trials of acupuncture for women's reproductive health care. J Fam Plann Reprod Health Care 2003;29:233–236
2. Habek D, Cerkez Habek J, Bobic-Vukovic M, Vujic B. Efficacy of acupuncture for the treatment of primary dysmenorrhea. Gynakol Geburtshilfliche Rundsch 2003;43:250–253
3. Fugh-Berman A, Kronenberg F. Complementary and alternative medicine (CAM) in reproductive-age women: a review of randomized controlled trials. Reprod Toxicol 2003;17:137–152
4. Proctor ML, Murphy PA. Herbal and dietary therapies for primary and secondary dysmenorrhoea. The Cochrane Database of Systematic Reviews 2001, Issue 2. Art. No.: CD002124

5. Eccles NK. A randomized, double-blinded, placebo-controlled pilot study to investigate the effectiveness of a static magnet to relieve dysmenorrhea. J Altern Complement Med 2005;11:681–687

6. Kim KS, Lee YJ. The effect of magnetic application for primary dysmenorrhoea. [In Korean.] Kanhohak Tamgu 1994;3:148–173

7. Proctor ML, Hing W, Johnson TC, Murphy PA. Spinal manipulation for primary and secondary dysmenorrhoea. The Cochrane Database of Systematic Reviews 2001, Issue 4. Art. No.: CD002119

8. Bespalov VG, Barash NIu, Ivanova OA, Krzhivitskii PI, Semiglazov VF, Aleksandrov VA, Sobenin NA, Orekhov AN. Study of an antioxidant dietary supplement "Karinat" in patients with benign breast disease. [In Russian.] Vopr Onkol 2004;50:467–472

9. Proctor ML, Smith CA, Farquhar CM, Stones RW. Transcutaneous electrical nerve stimulation and acupuncture for primary dysmenorrhoea. The Cochrane Database of Systematic Reviews 2002, Issue 1. Art. No.: CD002123

FIBROMYALGIA

SYNONYMS

Fibromyalgia syndrome, tension myalgia.

DEFINITION

A painful disorder, more common in women, in which diffuse pain, stiffness, fatigue, functional impairment and disrupted sleep are associated with the presence of bilateral tender points.

CAM USAGE

Many fibromyalgia patients try some form of CAM. One survey found that 91% had used CAM.[1] CAM therapies frequently employed include massage, dietary therapies, vitamins and herbs, relaxation and imagery, spirituality/prayer, acupressure, acupuncture, biofeedback and meditation.[2]

CLINICAL EVIDENCE

Three systematic reviews of CCTs of all types of CAM treatments[3–5] and one of various non-pharmacological approaches[6] are available. These articles emphasise the often poor methodological quality of research in this area.

ACUPUNCTURE

One good-quality RCT of acupuncture with 70 patients found that 25% of them improved markedly, 50% had satisfactory relief of symptoms and 25% had no benefit.[7] This study was the principal evidence in a systematic review[8] (Box 5.18) which reached a positive overall conclusion. Two subsequent RCTs ($n = 114$ and $n = 100$) both found real acupuncture to be no better than sham acupuncture in relieving fibromyalgia pain.[9,10] A recent study shows that acupuncture increases microcirculatory blood flow over tender points in fibromyalgia patients, thus reducing pain.[11] A further CCT compared acupuncture with connective tissue massage and found the former to be more clinically effective than the latter.[12]

BALNEOTHERAPY

One small study ($n = 39$) implied that balneotherapy with plain fresh-water baths reduces pain and the addition of valerian to the water may improve other outcomes such as well-being and sleep.[13] Similarly, encouraging results emerged from two RCTs[14,15] and one CCT[16] of balneotherapy without the addition of herbal extracts. A recent RCT of spa therapy (thalassotherapy combined with exercise and group education) showed that, compared to treatment as usual, it temporarily improves the symptoms of fibromyalgia[17] and a further RCT suggested that the effects were long-lasting.[18]

Box 5.18 *Systematic review: acupuncture for fibromyalgia*[8]

- Three RCTs and four cohort studies involving 300 subjects
- Quality of studies ranged from poor to adequate
- A single high-quality RCT suggested that acupuncture is more effective than placebo for relieving pain and morning stiffness
- Long-term effects remain unknown
- **Conclusion**: based on a single high-quality study the evidence suggests that real acupuncture is more effective than sham acupuncture; further robust data on effectiveness are required

Box 5.19 *Systematic review: exercise for treating fibromyalgia syndrome*[21]

- Seventeen RCTs involving 724 patients
- Quality was variable but seven studies were rigorous
- All high-quality studies of aerobic exercise showed greater improvements compared to controls
- For other forms of exercise, the evidence is less conclusive
- Poor reporting was a common weakness
- **Conclusion**: aerobic exercise training has beneficial effects on physical capacity and symptoms

BIOFEEDBACK

Although several RCTs have suggested that fibromyalgia patients can benefit from various mind–body therapies, appropriate attention controls have rarely been used. In one study, 12 patients received 15 sessions of either biofeedback or sham biofeedback over 5 weeks.[19] Persistent improvements in tender points, pain intensity and morning stiffness were found. In an RCT involving 119 subjects, biofeedback with relaxation was compared to exercise, a combination of biofeedback and exercise, and attention control.[20] Biofeedback was superior to the control group only in terms of tender points and enhanced self-efficacy of function.

EXERCISE

A Cochrane review[21] (Box 5.19) produced good evidence for aerobic exercise to increase physical capacity and alleviate symptoms of patients suffering from fibromyalgia. This was recently confirmed in a further systematic review evaluating the health benefits of exercise for any indication.[22] A subsequent RCT with 79 female fibromyalgia patients showed that a home-based exercise programme is an effective, low-cost approach for reducing pain and improving function.[23] A further RCT suggests that group exercise can be usefully combined with pain and stress management and education.[24]

HOMEOPATHY

In one RCT, 30 patients receiving homeopathic *Rhus toxicodendron* experienced greater reduction in tender points, pain and sleep disturbance, but global assessment was not different.[25] Another RCT ($n = 62$) also found good symptomatic improvements when comparing individualised homeopathy with placebo in a double-blind fashion.[26]

MASSAGE

Connective tissue massage was compared with no treatment or attention control in an RCT involving 52 patients.[27] The treated group experienced greater relief of pain and depression

Box 5.20 *Systematic review: mind–body therapies for fibromyalgia*[29]

- Thirteen CCTs involving 802 patients were included
- Quality was variable, but seven trials were rigorous
- Mind–body therapies improved self-efficacy (strong evidence), quality of life (limited evidence) and pain (limited evidence)
- Whether mind–body therapies are superior to physiotherapy, psychotherapy or education is not clear
- **Conclusion**: exercise is more effective than mind–body therapies

and improvement in quality of life. A small ($n = 37$) CCT compared regular Swedish massage for 4 weeks with standard care and suggested modest symptomatic effects which, however, were not substantiated at the 28-week follow-up.[28]

MIND–BODY THERAPIES

A systematic review[29] found encouraging results for mind–body therapies such as meditation, hypnotherapy, relaxation, etc. (Box 5.20). A subsequent RCT confirmed positive effects of imagery on pain[30] while another RCT showed no effect of imagery on pain compared to standard care.[31] A further RCT suggested that mindfulness meditation plus qigong was more helpful than education plus support.[32]

SUPPLEMENTS

Forty-five patients treated with topical capsaicin reported less tenderness and a significant increase in grip strength, but no difference in pain scores compared with placebo.[33]

Of four placebo-controlled RCTs of S-adenosyl-L-methionine (SAM-e), three suggested positive effects on pain. The negative RCT, however, was the one rated to have the highest methodological quality.[3]

OTHER THERAPIES

A small ($n = 19$) RCT found that, although treatment with chiropractic manipulation and soft tissue massage was associated with improvements in many parameters such as spinal pain and mobility, the changes were not superior to no treatment in terms of the physical symptoms.[34] Outcome measures specific to fibromyalgia were not used.

A small ($n = 30$) RCT of cognitive–behavioural therapy versus self monitoring suggested that this approach improves the ability of adolescent fibromyalgia patients to cope with pain.[35]

Compared to an educational program, regular Feldenkrais treatment was followed by only minor functional improvements, which were not maintained over time.[36]

An RCT in which 40 patients with fibromyalgia were randomised to receive either hypnotherapy or physical therapy for 12 weeks found improvements in several measures including pain ratings, sleep disturbance and somatic and psychological discomfort scores, though not physicians' global assessments.[37]

Low-dose laser therapy was not found to provide any greater relief of pain than placebo laser in a crossover study involving 60 patients.[38]

Two RCTs suggested that, compared to placebo, magnet therapy may decrease pain in patients with fibromyalgia.[39,40]

A single trial suggested that music therapy was associated with reduced pain and disability in chronic pain patients, including those with fibromyalgia, compared with untreated controls, but there was no change in anxiety or depression.[41]

A small ($n = 24$) RCT with four parallel groups suggested that osteopathic spinal manipulation effectively reduced the pain of fibromyalgia.[42]

Encouraging evidence from one RCT ($n = 128$) also exists for internal qigong.[43]

An RCT comparing a vegetarian diet with amitriptyline therapy suggested a modest analgesic effect after dieting which, however, was much smaller than that observed with drug treatment.[44]

OVERALL RECOMMENDATION

Many CAM approaches have been tested but in only a few cases are there sufficient data. Several treatments have shown considerable promise. The most convincing evidence exists for exercise and biofeedback. It is unlikely that any complementary therapy alone has greater impact on fibromyalgia symptoms than conventional therapies. Combinations of therapies are often used for fibromyalgia. For example, the judicious use of oral medications to alleviate pain and insomnia can be usefully combined with biofeedback or (supervised) exercise and perhaps acupuncture.

Table 5.14 **Summary of clinical evidence for fibromyalgia**

Treatment	Weight of evidence	Direction of evidence	Serious safety concerns
Acupuncture	OOO	→	Yes (see p. 96)
Balneotherapy	OO	↑	Yes (see p. 126)
Biofeedback	OO	↑	No (see p. 110)
Exercise	OOO	↑	Yes (see p. 5)
Homeopathy	O	↗	No (see p. 124)
Massage	O	↑	No (see p. 137)
Mind–body therapies	OO	↗	No (see p. 5)
Supplements			
Capsaicin	O	↗	Yes (see p. 5)
S-adenosyl-L-methionine	OO	↗	No (see p. 212)

REFERENCES

1. Pioro-Boisset M, Esdaile JM, Fitzcharles M-A. Alternative medicine use in fibromyalgia syndrome. Arthritis Care Res 1996;9:13–17
2. Nicassio PM, Schuman C, Kim J, Cordova A, Weisman MH. Psychosocial factors associated with complementary treatment use in fibromyalgia. J Rheumatol 1997;24:2008–2013
3. Holdcraft LC, Assefi N, Buchwald D. Complementary and alternative medicine in fibromyalgia and related syndromes. Best Pract Res Clin Rheumatol 2003;17:667–683
4. Ko GD, Whitmore S, Gottfried B, Hum A, Rahman M, Traitses G, Loong S, Steward K, Berbrayer D, Jokic M. Fibromyalgia/chronic pain syndrome: an alternative medicine perspective. Crit Rev Phys Rehabil Med 2005;17:1–30
5. Sarac AJ, Gur A. Complementary and alternative medical therapies in fibromyalgia. Curr Pharm Des 2006;12:47–57
6. Sim J, Adams N. Systematic review of randomized controlled trials of nonpharmacological interventions for fibromyalgia. Clin J Pain 2002;18:324–336
7. Deluze C, Bosia L, Zirbs A, Chantraine A, Vischer TL. Electroacupuncture in fibromyalgia: results of a controlled trial. Br Med J 1992;305:1249–1252

8. Berman BM, Ezzo J, Hadhazy V, Swyers JP. Is acupuncture effective in the treatment of fibromyalgia? J Fam Pract 1999;48:213–218

9. Harris RE, Tian X, Williams DA, Tian TX, Cupps TR, Petzke F, Groner KH, Biswas P, Gracely RH, Clauw DJ. Treatment of fibromyalgia with formula acupuncture: investigation of needle placement, needle stimulation, and treatment frequency. J Altern Complement Med 2005;11:663–671

10. Assefi NP, Sherman KJ, Jacobsen C, Goldberg J, Smith WR, Buchwald D. A randomized clinical trial of acupuncture compared with sham acupuncture in fibromyalgia. Ann Intern Med 2005; 143:10–19.

11. Sprott H, Jeschonneck M, Grohmann G, Hein G. Änderung der Durchblutung über den tender points bei Fibromyalgie-Patienten nach einer Akupunkturtherapie (gemessen mit der Laser-Doppler-Flowmetrie). Wien Klin Wochenschr 2000;112:580–586

12. Uhlemann C, Schreiber TU, Smolenski UC, Loth D. Randomisierte Studie zur Akupunktur und Bindegewebmassage als Therapieoption bei Patienten mit Fibromyalgiesyndrom (FMS). Phys Med Rehab Kuror 2001;11:153

13. Ammer K, Melnizky P. Medicinal baths for treatment of generalized fibromyalgia. [In German.] Forsch Komplementärmed 1999;6:80–85

14. Neumann L, Sukenik S, Bolotin A, Abu-Shakra M, Amir M, Flusser D, Buskila D. The effect of balneotherapy at the Dead Sea on the quality of life of patients with fibromyalgia syndrome. Clin Rheumatol 2001;20:15–19

15. Vitorino DF, Carvalho LB, Prado GF. Hydrotherapy and conventional physiotherapy improve total sleep time and quality of life of fibromyalgia patients: randomized clinical trial. Sleep Med 2006; 7:293–296.

16. Evcik D, Kizilay B, Gokcen E. The effects of balneotherapy on fibromyalgia patients. Rheumatol Int 2002;22:56–59

17. Zijlstra TR, van de Laar MA, Bernelot Moens HJ, Taal E, Zakraoui L, Rasker JJ. Spa treatment for primary fibromyalgia syndrome: a combination of thalassotherapy, exercise and patient education improves symptoms and quality of life. Rheumatology (Oxford) 2005;44:539–546

18. Donmez A, Karagulle MZ, Tercan N, Dinler M, Issever H, Karagulle M, Turan M. Spa therapy in fibromyalgia: a randomised controlled clinic study. Rheumatol Int 2005;26:168–172

19. Ferraccioli G, Gherilli L, Scita F, Nolli M, Mozzani M, Fontana S, Scorsonelli M, Tridenti A, De Risio C. EMG-biofeedback training in fibromyalgia syndrome. J Rheumatol 1987; 14:820–825

20. Buckelew SP, Conway R, Parker J, Deuser WE, Read J, Witty TE, Hewett JE, Minor M, Johnson JC, Van Male L, McIntosh MJ, Nigh M, Kay DR. Biofeedback/relaxation training and exercise interventions for fibromyalgia: a prospective trial. Arthritis Care Res 1998;11:196–209

21. Busch A, Schachter CL, Peloso PM, Bombardier C. Exercise for treating fibromyalgia syndrome. The Cochrane Database of Systematic Reviews 2002, Issue 2. Art. No.: CD003786

22. Karmisholt K, Gotzsche PC. Physical activity for secondary prevention of disease. Systematic reviews of randomised clinical trials. Dan Med Bull 2005;52:90–94

23. Da Costa D, Abrahamowicz M, Lowensteyn I, Bernatsky S, Dritsa M, Fitzcharles MA, Dobkin PL. A randomized clinical trial of an individualized home-based exercise programme for women with fibromyalgia. Rheumatology (Oxford) 2005;44:1422–1427

24. Lemstra M, Olszynski WP. The effectiveness of multidisciplinary rehabilitation in the treatment of fibromyalgia: a randomized controlled trial. Clin J Pain 2005;21: 166–174

25. Fisher P, Greenwood A, Huskisson EC, Turner P, Belon P. Effect of homeopathic treatment on fibrositis (primary fibromyalgia). Br Med J 1989;299:365–366

26. Bell IR, Lewis DA, Brooks AJ, Schwartz GE, Lewis SE, Walsh BT, Baldwin CM. Improved clinical status in fibromyalgia patients treated with individualized homeopathic remedies versus placebo. Rheumatology (Oxford) 2004;43:577–582

27. Brattberg G. Connective tissue massage in the treatment of fibromyalgia. Eur J Pain 1999; 3:235–245

28. Alnigenis MNY, Bradly JD, Wallick J, Emsley CL. Massage therapy in the management of fibromyalgia: a pilot study. J Musculoskeletal Pain 2001;9:55–68

29. Hadhazy VA, Ezzo J, Creamer P, Berman BM. Mind-body therapies for the treatment of fibromyalgia. A systematic review. J Rheumatol 2000;27:2911–2918

30. Fors EA, Sexton H, Gotestam KG. The effect of guided imagery and amitriptyline on daily fibromyalgia pain: a prospective, randomized, controlled trial. J Psychiatr Res 2002;36:179–187

31. Menzies V, Taylor AG, Bourguignon C. Effects of guided imagery on outcomes of pain, functional status, and self-efficacy in persons diagnosed with fibromyalgia. J Altern Complement Med 2006;12:23–30

32. Astin JA, Berman BM, Bausell B, Lee WL, Hochberg M, Forys KL. The efficacy of mindfulness meditation plus Qigong movement therapy in the treatment of fibromyalgia: a randomized controlled trial. J Rheumatol 2003;30:2088–2089

33. McCarty DJ, Csuka M, McCarthy G, Trotter D. Treatment of pain due to fibromyalgia with topical capsaicin: a pilot study. Semin Arthritis Rheum 1994;23(Suppl. 3):41–47

34. Blunt KL, Rajwani MH, Guerriero RC. The effectiveness of chiropractic management of fibromyalgia patients: a pilot study. J Manip Physiol Ther 1997;20:389–399

35. Kashikar-Zuck S, Swain NF, Jones BA, Graham TB. Efficacy of cognitive-behavioral intervention for juvenile primary fibromyalgia syndrome. J Rheumatol 2005;32:1594–1602

36. Aspegren Kendall S, Ekselius L, Gerdle B, Sörén B, Bengtsson A. Feldenkrais intervention in fibromyalgia patients: a pilot study. J Musculoskelet Pain 2001;9:25–35

37. Haanen HCM, Hoenderdos HTW, Romunde LKJ, Hop WC, Mallee C, Terwiel JP, Hekster GB. Controlled trial of hypnotherapy in the treatment of refractory fibromyalgia. J Rheumatol 1991;18:72–75

38. Waylonis GW, Wilke S, O'Toole D, Waylonis DA, Waylonis DB. Chronic myofascial pain: management by low-output helium-neon laser therapy. Arch Phys Med Rehabil 1998; 69: 1017–1020

39. Alfano P, Taylor AG, Foresman PA, Dunkl PR, McConnell GG, Conaway MR, Gillies GT. Static magnetic fields for treatment of fibromyalgia: a randomized controlled trial. J Altern Complement Med 2001;7:53–64

40. Colbert AP, Markov MS, Banerji M, Pilla A. Magnetic mattress pad use in patients with fibromyalgia: a randomized, double-blind pilot study. J Back Musculoskel Rehab 1999;13:19–31

41. Müller-Busch HC, Hoffmann P. Aktive Musiktherapie bei chronischen Schmerzen. Schmerz 1997;11:91–100

42. Gamber RG, Shores JH, Russo DP, Jimenez C, Rubin BR. Osteopathic manipulative treatment in conjunction with medication relieves pain associated with fibromyalgia syndrome: results of a randomized clinical pilot project. J Am Osteopath Ass 2002;102:321–325

43. Astin JA, Berman BM, Bausell B, Lee WL, Hochberg M, Forys KL. The efficacy of mindfulness meditation plus Qigong movement therapy in the treatment of fibromyalgia: a randomized controlled trial. J Rheumatol 2003;30:2257–2262

44. Azad KA, Alam MN, Haq SA, Nahar S, Chowdury MA, Ali SM, Ullah AK. Vegetarian diet in the treatment of fibromyalgia. Bangladesh Med Res Counc Bull 2000;26:41–47

HEADACHE

SYNONYMS/SUBCATEGORIES

Tension headache, chronic or episodic tension-type headache, cephalodynia, cephalalgia, cephalea, cerebralgia, encephalalgia, encephalodynia, cervicogenic headache (formerly muscle tension headache). For migraine see p. 298.

DEFINITION

The 1988 International Headache Society criteria for chronic tension-type headache are headaches on 15 or more days a month (180 days/year) for at least 6 months; pain that is bilateral, pressing or tightening in quality, of mild or moderate intensity, which does not prohibit activities and is not aggravated by routine physical activity; presence of no more than one additional clinical feature (nausea, photophobia or phonophobia) and no vomiting. Episodic tension-type headache can last for 30 minutes to 7 days and occurs for fewer than 180 days a year.

CAM USAGE

Thirty-two per cent of Americans with headache have used CAM in the previous 12 months, most frequently relaxation and chiropractic.[1] Many other therapies are also popular, especially herbal medicine, homeopathy, acupuncture and reflexology.

CLINICAL EVIDENCE

A Cochrane review[2] found encouraging evidence for spinal manipulation, therapeutic touch, electrotherapy and transcutaneous electrical nerve stimulation (TENS) for treating tension-type headaches. It also noted that spinal manipulation and exercise are promising for cervico-genic headache.

ACUPUNCTURE

Three good-quality studies were included in a systematic review.[3] It concluded that acupuncture might have a role to play in idiopathic headache but the current evidence was insufficient to make firm recommendations. Since then, results of RCTs have been mixed. Three placebo-controlled RCTs ($n = 69$, $n = 37$ and $n = 50$) suggested positive effects of acupuncture on pain or quality of life.[4–6] Another RCT also generated positive results but the majority of patients suffered from migraine.[7] Four further RCTs ($n = 39$, $n = 50$, $n = 30$ and $n = 270$) showed no effects compared to sham acupuncture.[8–11] A recent systematic review of six RCTs (only five were of high quality) concluded that there is only limited evidence in favour of acupuncture for tension-type headache.[12]

AUTOGENIC TRAINING

In one study, 146 patients with tension headache were randomised to autogenic training, hypnotherapy or waiting list control.[13] Autogenic training (but not hypnotherapy) was better than waiting list for symptom control.

BIOFEEDBACK

A systematic review[14] (Box 5.21) concluded that both relaxation and biofeedback (either on its own or in combination with relaxation) were superior to no treatment and to placebo therapy. Subsequent RCTs[15–17] (Table 5.15) tested biofeedback in adolescents and adults, mainly in comparison with relaxation. The majority found that biofeedback was more effective. One study demonstrated that the clinical improvements correlated with changes in self-efficacy but not in electromyography (EMG) or electroencephalogram activity.[18] Another study found that patients who have a preference for highly structured practice respond better when they are given explicit guidelines than when they are left to their own devices.[19]

Box 5.21 *Meta-analysis: biofeedback and relaxation for headache*[14]

- All prospective investigations, including uncontrolled studies
- Seventy-eight studies were included in the review, involving 2866 patients
- Mean (SD) effect size from 29 studies of EMG biofeedback was 47% (26%)
- Mean (SD) effect size from 38 studies of relaxation was 36% (20%)
- For comparison, mean (SD) effect size from pharmacological treatment was 39% (23%) and for placebo treatment was 20% (38%)
- **Conclusion**: biofeedback is likely to be an effective option for headache

Table 5.15 **Parallel-arm RCTs of biofeedback for headache**

Reference	Sample size	Interventions (regimen)	Result	Comment
Arena[15]	26	(A) Frontal EMG biofeedback [12 sessions] (B) Trapezius EMG biofeedback [12 sessions] (C) Relaxation [seven sessions]	B better than A or C at 3 months	
Bussone[16]	35	(A) Biofeedback relaxation [10 sessions in 5 weeks] (B) Relaxation placebo	A better than B at 1 year	Adolescents
Kroner-Herwig[17]	50	(A) Biofeedback [12 30-minute sessions in 6 weeks] (B) Relaxation [six 1-hour sessions in 6 weeks] (C) Untreated control	No difference between A and B. Both better than C for some outcomes	Children; parental involvement had no influence

EXERCISE

A small ($n = 53$) RCT suggested that workplace physical exercise reduced headaches during a 4-week period.[20]

HERBAL MEDICINE

In an RCT involving 41 adults with a history of tension headache, 164 acute headache episodes were treated with either peppermint (*Mentha piperita*) oil or placebo oil locally and either paracetamol (acetaminophen) or placebo tablet orally.[21] Peppermint oil was superior to placebo and not different from the analgesic drug in reducing headache.

The use of tiger balm was supported in one multicentre RCT in which 57 patients were given either tiger balm to apply locally, placebo balm or standard analgesic medication.[22] Tiger balm and medication were both more effective than placebo at reducing the headache intensity, though the success of subject blinding is questionable because tiger balm produces local warmth.

HOMEOPATHY

One rigorous RCT with 98 subjects included patients with tension-type headache as well as those with migraine and found no benefit from 12 weeks of individualised homeopathy compared with placebo.[23] The results were similar after 1 year of follow-up.[24]

HYPNOTHERAPY

Like other forms of therapy involving regular relaxation, self-hypnosis appears to be more effective than waiting list control.[25] However, it is not clear whether it is superior to other forms of relaxation. Several trials have compared different combinations of therapies including hypnotherapy with various control interventions.[13,26] Subjects who are highly hypnotisable tend to show a greater reduction of headaches than those who are less easily hypnotised.[13]

Box 5.22 *Systematic review: spinal manipulation for tension-type headache*[30]

- Four RCTs were included
- Three studies were of chiropractic, one of osteopathic techniques
- Overall methodological quality was poor
- Best evidence synthesis generated no convincing evidence for spinal manipulation
- Few adverse events were reported
- **Conclusion**: the evidence is insufficient

RELAXATION

A systematic review[14] of biofeedback and relaxation (Box 5.21) concluded that relaxation is effective, with a mean effect size of 36%. In children and adolescents, RCTs indicate that relaxation has a positive effect on tension headache, though the size of the effect is often modest. More than two-thirds of the children in one study ($n = 26$) recorded at least 50% improvement at follow-up after 6 months, compared with only a quarter of controls.[27] Follow-up over an average of 4 years found that continuing to practice relaxation maintained some of the improvements.[28] Most studies have compared relaxation with no treatment. One exception is a trial among 202 adolescents in which relaxation was compared with placebo relaxation (sitting quietly, thinking of an episode from their life) and no difference was found.[29] Relaxation techniques could therefore be of benefit predominantly through non-specific effects.

SPINAL MANIPULATION

The most recent and authoritative systematic review[30] of spinal manipulation found that, because of the small number and poor quality of the primary data, it is not possible to draw valid conclusions about the effectiveness of this approach (Box 5.22). An independent research group reached similar conclusions regarding both spinal manipulation and mobilisation.[31]

OTHER THERAPIES

Cranial electrotherapy, applies a high-frequency, low-intensity current transcranially. It was found to be more effective in treating acute headache than placebo in a multicentre RCT of 100 patients, reducing headache scores by 35% after 20 minutes compared with 18% in the placebo group.[32]

Imagery was used as an adjunct to standard medical treatment in an RCT of 260 adults with chronic tension headache with or without migraine.[33] The intervention group received an imagery tape to listen to every day for 1 month and controls received standard medical treatment alone. Imagery was superior in global assessment and some quality of life measures.

Neither classic massage (one RCT) nor connective tissue massage (one RCT) are supported by convincing evidence in the treatment of tension-type headache.[31]

In one double-dummy RCT involving 32 patients, reflexology was compared with flunarizin. Improvements in headache severity were twice as great with reflexology, but the difference was not significant and several methodological flaws of this trial prevent any firm conclusions.[34]

Non-contact therapeutic touch was more effective than a sham intervention in the treatment of acute headache in an RCT of reasonable quality that involved 90 subjects. However, the difference was no longer apparent after 4 hours.[35]

Recent RCTs generated encouraging results for percutaneous electrical nerve stimulation,[36] impulse magnetic-field therapy[37] and the Trager approach[38] as treatments for various types of headache. Preliminary data from a CCT suggest that yoga is effective in relieving headache.[39]

OVERALL RECOMMENDATION

The evidence is not convincing that any particular CAM therapy is more effective than placebo in preventing tension headaches. However, in the absence of genuinely safe and effective conventional preventive measures, patients may benefit from treatments involving relaxation. Relaxation in various forms, including muscular and mental relaxation, hypnotherapy and autogenic training, is simple, relatively safe and beneficial compared with no treatment. The addition of biofeedback may increase the benefit compared with simple relaxation alone. In the treatment of acute headache, preliminary evidence supports the use of tiger balm or peppermint oil locally, and possibly electrotherapy. It seems unlikely, however, that these options are superior to conventional treatments.

Table 5.16 **Summary of clinical evidence for headache**

Treatment	Weight of evidence	Direction of evidence	Serious safety concerns
Acupuncture	OO	→	Yes (see p. 96)
Autogenic training	O	↗	Yes (see p. 106)
Biofeedback	OOO	↗	No (see p. 110)
Herbal medicine			
Peppermint oil (local)	O	↑	Yes (see p. 209)
Tiger balm (local)	O	↗	Yes (see p. 5)
Homeopathy	O	↓	No (see p. 124)
Hypnotherapy	OO	↗	Yes (see p. 130)
Relaxation	OO	↗	No (see p. 158)
Spinal manipulation	OO	→	Yes (see p. 112)

REFERENCES

1. Eisenberg DM, Davis R, Ettner SL, Appel S, Wilkey S, Rompay MV. Trends in alternative medicine use in the United States, 1990–1997. JAMA 1998;280:1569–1575
2. Bronfort G, Nilsson N, Haas M, Evans R, Goldsmith CH, Assendelft WJJ, Bouter LM. Non-invasive treatments for chronic/recurrent headache. The Cochrane Database of Systematic Reviews 2004, Issue 3. Art No.: CD001878
3. Melchart D, Linde K, Fischer P, Berman B, White A, Vickers A, Allais G. Acupuncture for idiopathic headache. The Cochrane Database of Systematic Reviews 2001, Issue 1. Art No.: CD001218
4. Karst M, Reinhard M, Thum P, Wiese B, Rollnik J, Fink M. Needle acupuncture in tension-type headache: a randomized, placebo-controlled study. Cephalalgia 2001;21:637–642
5. Xue CC, Dong L, Polus B, English RA, Zheng Z, Da Costa C, Li CG, Story DF. Electroacupuncture for tension-type headache on distal acupoints only: a randomized, controlled, crossover trial. Headache 2004;44:333–341
6. Ebneshahidi NS, Heshmatipour M, Moghaddami A, Eghtesadi-Araghi P. The effects of laser acupuncture on chronic tension headache – a randomised controlled trial. Acupunct Med 2005; 23:13–18
7. Vickers AJ, Rees RW, Zollman CE, McCarney R, Smith CM, Ellis N, Fisher P, Van Haselen R. Acupuncture for chronic headache in primary care: large, pragmatic, randomised trial. BMJ 2004;328:744
8. Karst M, Rollnik JD, Fink M, Reinhard M, Piepenbrock S. Pressure pain threshold and needle acupuncture in chronic tension-type headache – a double-blind placebo-controlled study. Pain 2000;88:199–203
9. White AR, Resch KL, Chan JC, Norris CD, Modi SK, Patel JN, Ernst E. Acupuncture for episodic tension-type headache: a multicentre randomized controlled trial. Cephalalgia 2000;20:632–637

10. Karakurum B, Karaalin O, Coskun O, Dora B, Ucler S, Inan L. The 'dry-needle technique': intramuscular stimulation in tension-type headache. Cephalalgia 2001;21:813–817

11. Melchart D, Streng A, Hoppe A, Brinkhaus B, Witt C, Wagenpfeil S, Pfaffenrath V, Hammes M, Hummelsberger J, Irnich D, Weidenhammer W, Willich SN, Linde K. Acupuncture in patients with tension-type headache: randomised controlled trial. BMJ 2005;331:376–382

12. Jedel E, Carlsson J. Acupuncture in the management of tension-type headache. Phys Ther Rev 2005;10:131–139

13. Ter Kuile MM, Spinhoven P, Linssen ACG, Zitman FG, Van Dyck R, Rooijmans HGM. Autogenic training and cognitive self-hypnosis for the treatment of recurrent headaches in three different subject groups. Pain 1994;58:331–340

14. Bogaards MC, ter Kuile MM. Treatment of recurrent tension headache: a meta-analytic review. Clin J Pain 1994;10:174–190

15. Arena JG, Bruno GM, Hannah SL, Meador KJ. A comparison of frontal electromyographic biofeedback training, trapezius electromyographic biofeedback training, and progressive muscle relaxation therapy in the treatment of tension headache. Headache 1995;35:411–419

16. Bussone G, Grazzi L, D'Amico D, Leone M, Andraski F. Biofeedback-assisted relaxation training for young adolescents with tension-type headache: a controlled study. Cephalalgia 1998;18:463–467

17. Kroner-Herwig B, Mohn U, Pothmann R. Comparison of biofeedback and relaxation in the treatment of pediatric headache and the influence of parent involvement on outcome. Appl Psychophysiol Biofeedback 1998;23:143–157

18. Rokicki LA, Holroyd KA, France CR, Lipchik GL, France JL, Kvaal SA. Change mechanisms associated with combined relaxation/EMG biofeedback training for chronic tension headache. Applied Psychophysiol Biofeedback 1997;22:21–41

19. Hart JD. Predicting differential response to EMG biofeedback and relaxation training: the role of cognitive structure. J Clin Psychol 1984;40:453–457

20. Sjögren T, Nissinen KJ, Jarvenpaa SK, Ojanen MT, Vanharanta H, Malkia EA. Effects of a workplace physical exercise intervention on the intensity of headache and neck and shoulder symptoms and upper extremity muscular strength of office workers: a cluster randomized controlled crossover trial. Pain;116:119–128

21. Gobel H, Fresenius J, Heinze A, Dworschak M, Soyka D. Effectiveness of Oleum menthae piperitae and paracetamol in therapy of headache of the tension type. Nervenarzt 1996; 67:672–681

22. Schattner P, Randerson D. Tiger Balm as a treatment of tension headache. A clinical trial in general practice. Aust Fam Physician 1996;25:216,218,220 passim

23. Walach H, Haeusler W, Lower T, Mussbach D, Schamell U, Springer W, Stritzl G, Gaus W, Haag G. Classical homeopathic treatment of chronic headaches. Cephalalgia 1997;17:119–126

24. Walach H, Lowes T, Mussbach D, Schamell U, Springer W, Stritzl G, Haag G. The long-term effects of homeopathic treatment of chronic headaches: one year follow-up and single case time series analysis. Br Homeopath J 2001;90:61–62

25. Melis PM, Rooimans W, Spierings EL, Hoogduin CA. Treatment of chronic tension-type headache with hypnotherapy: a single-blind time controlled study. Headache 1991;31:686–689

26. Reich BA. Non-invasive treatment of vascular and muscle contraction headache: a comparative longitudinal clinical study. Headache 1989;29:34–41

27. Larsson B, Melin L. Chronic headaches in adolescents: treatment in a school setting with relaxation training as compared with information-contact and self-registration. Pain 1986;25:325–336

28. Engel JM, Rapoff MA, Pressman AR. Long-term follow-up of relaxation training for pediatric headache disorders. Headache 1992;32:152–156

29. Passchier J, Van Den Bree MB, Emmen HH, Osterhaus SO, Orlebeke JF, Verhage F. Relaxation training in school classes does not reduce headache complaints. Headache 1990;30:660–664

30. Lenssinck ML, Damen L, Verhagen AP, Berger MY, Passchier J, Koes BW. The effectiveness of physiotherapy and manipulation in patients with tension-type headache: a systematic review. Pain 2004;112:381–388

31. Fernandez-de-Las-Penas C, Alonso-Blanco C, Cuadrado ML, Miangolarra JC, Barriga FJ, Pareja JA. Are manual therapies effective in reducing pain from tension-type headache?: a systematic review. Clin J Pain 2006;22:278–285

32. Solomon S, Elkind A, Freitag F, Gallagher RM, Moore K, Swerdlow B, Malkin S. Safety and effectiveness of cranial electrotherapy in the treatment of tension headache. Headache 1989;29: 445–450

33. Mannix LK, Chandurkar RS, Rybicki LA, Tusek DL, Solomon GD. Effect of guided imagery on quality of life for patients with chronic tension-type headache. Headache 1999;39:326–334

34. Lafuente A, Noguera M, Puy C, Molins A, Titus F, Sanz F. Effekt der Reflexzonenbehandlung am Fuß bezüglich der prophylaktischen Behandlung mit Funarizin bei an Cephalea-Kopfschmerzen leidenden Patienten. Erfahrungsheilkunde 1990;39:713–715

35. Keller E, Bzdek VM. Effects of therapeutic touch on tension headache pain. Nurs Res 1986;35: 101–106

36. Ahmed HE, White PF, Craig WF, Hamza MA, Ghoname E, Gajraj NM. Use of percutaneous electrical nerve stimulation (PENS) in the short-term management of headache. Headache 2000;40: 311–315

37. Pelka RB, Jaenicke C, Gruenwald J. Impulse magnetic-field therapy for migraine and other headaches: a double-blind, placebo-controlled study. Adv Ther 2001;18:101–109

38. Foster KA, Liskin J, Cen S, Abbott A, Armisen V, Globe D, Knox L, Mitchell M, Shtir C, Azen S. The Trager approach in the treatment of chronic headache: a pilot study. Altern Ther Health Med 2004;10:40–46

39. Michalsen A, Grossman P, Acil A, Langhorst J, Ludtke R, Esch T, Stefano GB, Dobos GJ. Rapid stress reduction and anxiolysis among distressed women as a consequence of a three-month intensive yoga program. Med Sci Monit 2005;11:CR555–561

LABOUR PAIN

SYNONYMS

Childbirth, parturition; parodynia.

DEFINITION

Labour is the act of giving birth to a baby. Labour pains are rhythmical uterine contractions, which under normal conditions increase in intensity, frequency and duration, resulting in vaginal delivery of the infant.

CAM USAGE

Hypnosis, acupuncture and some herbal medicines (particularly raspberry leaves) are commonly used.

CLINICAL EVIDENCE

Several systematic reviews of complementary therapies for pain management during labour have been published.[1–4]

ACUPUNCTURE

A systematic review of acupuncture for labour pain management (Box 5.23) concluded that the evidence for acupuncture as an adjunct to conventional pain control during labour is encouraging but not convincing because of the paucity of trial data.[5]

The effects of acupressure during labour were assessed in two RCTs. One ($n = 127$), which compared acupressure at LI4 and BL67 with light skin stroking, no treatment or conversation, only indicated decreased labour pain in the acupressure group but found no effects on uterine contractions.[6] The other RCT ($n = 75$) found SP6 acupressure compared with SP6 touch control to be more effective in reducing pain and shortening labour.[7]

Box 5.23 *Systematic review: acupuncture for pain management in labour.*[5]

- Three trials including 496 parturients
- All trials were of good quality
- Two RCTs compared adjunctive acupuncture with usual care and reported a reduction of meperidine and/or epidural analgesia use
- One placebo-controlled RCT showed differences in both subjective and objective outcome measures of pain
- No adverse events were reported in any of the trials
- **Conclusion**: the evidence for acupuncture is promising but, because of the paucity of trial data, not convincing

AROMATHERAPY

A systematic review included one double-blind RCT in which 22 multiparous women with a singleton pregnancy took baths with essential oils of ginger or lemongrass.[3] There were no differences between groups regarding analgesic consumption or outcome of delivery.

BIOFEEDBACK

Biofeedback for pain relief during labour was tested in two small RCTs; one found it to lower pain and shorten labour compared with controls[8] while the other found no difference between effectively trained EMG, ineffectively trained skin-conductance groups and standard antenatal classes.[9]

HERBAL MEDICINE

The Chinese herbal medicine mixture Chanlibao was suggested to accelerate the second stage of labour when compared to oxytocin and no intervention in an RCT ($n = 161$).[10]

In a double-blind, placebo-controlled RCT ($n = 192$), raspberry leaf (*Rubus idaeus*) tablets were found to shorten the second but not the first stage of labour and no differences were found in birth outcome.[11]

HYPNOTHERAPY

A systematic review of hypnotherapy (Box 5.24) for labour pain relief included four randomised and two non-randomised trials and found that fewer parturients receiving hypnosis required analgesia.[12] A subsequent large RCT ($n = 520$) reported fewer complications at birth in women receiving prenatal hypnosis compared with attention only or no contact.[13]

INTRACUTANEOUS STERILE WATER INJECTIONS

Four RCTs compared low back pain in labouring women receiving intracutaneous sterile water injections with controls receiving a saline placebo[14–16] or TENS, movement, massage and baths.[17] All four found sterile water injections to be effective in decreasing severe low back pain within minutes although no decrease in the request for other pain medication was reported in three studies assessing pain relief consumption.

MASSAGE

A systematic review included two RCTs.[3] One included 28 women receiving massage in addition to coaching in breathing or coaching in breathing alone; in the other ($n = 60$) the women underwent massage or attention control. Both trials found that massage provides pain relief and psychological support during labour. A further RCT ($n = 40$) reported nurse- and self-administered massage in combination with breathing techniques to be effective in reducing the perception of pain.[18]

Box 5.24 *Meta-analysis: hypnosis for pain management in labour*[12]

- Four RCTs of 224 women and two non-randomised CTs were included
- Meta-analysis of three RCTs showed that fewer parturients receiving hypnosis required analgesia (RR 0.51, CI 95% 0.28 to 0.95); one RCT was rated poor on quality assessment
- Of the two non-randomised CTs included, one showed lower pain ratings and the other had reduced opioid and pharmacological analgesia requirements with hypnosis
- **Conclusion**: hypnosis alone or in combination with other anaesthetic techniques may offer advantages over conventional analgesia alone

Box 5.25 *Meta-analysis: immersion in water during labour and birth*[22]

- Eight RCTs ($n = 2939$) comparing any kind of bath tub or pool use with no immersion during pregnancy, labour or birth
- Reduction in the use of epidural/spinal/paracervical analgesia/anaesthesia among women allocated to water immersion during the first stage of labour (odds ratio 0.84, 95% CI 0.71 to 0.99, $n = 4$)
- Less pain reported by women who used water immersion during the first stage of labour (odds ratio 0.23, 95% CI 0.08 to 0.63, $n = 1$)
- Labour duration, operative delivery rates or neonatal well-being were not adversely affected and did not differ between groups
- **Conclusion**: there is evidence that water immersion during the first stage of labour reduces the use of analgesia and reported maternal pain without increasing adverse outcomes; further research is needed to assess the effect of immersion in water on neonatal and maternal morbidity

MUSIC THERAPY

Music therapy was assessed in an RCT of 110 labouring women; less pain sensation and less distress were reported in the music group and there was also a delayed increase of affective pain for 1 hour.[19] One small RCT ($n = 30$) compared the effect of standard antenatal psychoprophylactic childbirth instruction combined with music with standard psychoprophylaxis alone and found no difference in the frequency of analgesia use between the two groups.[20] Music did not have an effect on analogued labour pain using nulliparous volunteers in two small trials when compared to no-treatment controls or various forms of imagery.[21]

WATER IMMERSION

A systematic review[22] of eight RCTs (Box 5.25) comparing any kind of bath tub or pool use with no immersion during pregnancy, labour or birth found that water immersion during the first stage of labour reduced both the use of analgesia and reported maternal pain without increasing adverse outcomes such as operative delivery rates or neonatal well-being. A subsequent RCT reported similar findings.[23]

OTHER THERAPIES

In an RCT, 53 women in the seventh month of pregnancy received either nine weekly sessions of respiratory autogenic training ($n = 23$) or a traditional psychoprophylactic course ($n = 30$) for childbirth preparation.[3] The respiratory autogenic training participants tended to report less pain during labour than the traditional psychoprophylactic course women, but the difference only reached statistical significance after removing the influence of the unbalanced initial anxiety level in the two groups.

OVERALL RECOMMENDATION

Labour pain is arguably one of the most severe forms of pain that many women will experience during their lives. Pain management during childbirth has always been controversial and the possible effects of anesthaesia on progress of labour and on the neonate continue to concern health-care professionals and patients. Epidural anaesthesia, the current gold standard for pain relief during childbirth, is not acceptable for all women and many are drawn to non-pharmacological interventions. Patients should, however, always be advised of safety issues associated with complementary therapies. Particularly during pregnancy, the precautionary principle that a treatment is not considered risk free unless evidence suggests otherwise should be applied.

Hypnosis and water immersion, as well as intracutaneous sterile water injections and massage, seem to be effective in reducing pain during labour and are not associated with serious safety concerns. The evidence for acupuncture is encouraging but further research is required. There is not enough evidence for any other complementary therapy to make any firm recommendations.

Table 5.17 **Summary of clinical evidence for labour**

Treatment	Weight of evidence	Direction of evidence	Serious safety concerns
Acupuncture	OO	↗	Yes (see p. 96)
Acupressure	OO	↗	Yes (see p. 96)
Aromatherapy	O	→	Yes (see p. 103)
Biofeedback	O	→	No (see p. 110)
Herbal medicine			
Chanlibao	O	↗	Yes (see p. 5)
Raspberry leaf	O	↗	Yes (see p. 5)
Hypnotherapy	OOO	↑	Yes (see p. 130)
Intracutaneous sterile water injections	OO	↗	Yes (see p. 5)
Massage	OO	↑	No (see p. 137)
Music	OO	↘	No (see p. 142)
Water immersion	OOO	↑	No (see p. 5)

REFERENCES

1. Anderson FWJ, Johnson CT. Complementary and alternative medicine in obstetrics. Int J Gynecol Obstet 2005;91:116–124
2. Simkin P, Bolding A. Update on nonpharmacologic approaches to relieve labor pain and prevent suffering. J Midwifery Womens Health 2004;49:489–504
3. Huntley AL, Coon JT, Ernst E. Complementary and alternative medicine for labor pain: a systematic review. Am J Obstet Gynecol 2004;191:36–44
4. Smith CA, Collins CT, Cyna AM, Crowther CA. Complementary and alternative therapies for pain management in labour. The Cochrane Database of Systematic Reviews 2003, Issue 2. Art. No.: CD003521

5. Lee H, Ernst E. Acupuncture for labor pain management: a systematic review. Am J Obstet Gynecol 2004;191:1573–1579

6. Chung UL, Hung LC, Kuo SC, Huang CL. Effects of LI4 and BL67 acupressure on labor pain and uterine contractions in the first stage of labor. J Nurs Res 2003;11: 251–260

7. Lee MK, Chang SB, Kang DH. Effects of SP6 acupressure on labor pain and length of delivery time in women during labor. J Altern Complement Med 2004;10:959–965

8. Duchene P. Effects of biofeedback on childbirth pain. J Pain Symptom Manage 1989;4: 117–123

9. St James-Roberts I, Chamberlain G, Haran FJ, Hutchinson CM. Use of electromyographic and skin-conductance biofeedback relaxation training of facilitated childbirth in primiparae. J Psychosom Res 1982;26:455–462

10. Qiu H, Zhu H, Ouyang W, Wang Z, Sun H. Clinical effects and mechanism of chanlibao in accelerating second stage of labor. J Tongji Med Univ 1999;19:141–144

11. Simpson M, Parsons M, Greenwood J, Wade K. Raspberry leaf in pregnancy: its safety and efficacy in labor. J Midwifery Womens Health 2001;46:51–59

12. Cyna AM, McAuliffe GL, Andrew MI. Hypnosis for pain relief in labour and childbirth: a systematic review. Br J Anaesth 2004;93:505–511

13. Mehl-Madrona LE. Hypnosis to facilitate uncomplicated birth. Am J Clin Hypn 2004; 46:299–312

14. Martensson L, Wallin G. Labour pain treated with cutaneous injections of sterile water: a randomised controlled trial. Br J Obstet Gynaecol 1999;106:633–637

15. Ader L, Hansson B, Wallin G. Parturition pain treated by intracutaneous injections of sterile water. Pain 1990;41:133–138

16. Trolle B, Moller M, Kronborg H, Thomsen S. The effect of sterile water blocks on low back labor pain. Am J Obstet Gynecol 1991;164:1277–1281

17. Labrecque M, Nouwen A, Bergeron M, Rancourt JF. A randomized controlled trial of nonpharmacologic approaches for relief of low back pain during labor. J Fam Pract 1999; 48:259–263

18. Yildirim G, Sahin NH. The effect of breathing and skin stimulation techniques on labour pain perception of Turkish women. Pain Res Manag 2004;9:183–187

19. Phumdoung S, Good M. Music reduces sensation and distress of labor pain. Pain Manag Nurs 2003;4:54–61

20. Durham L, Collins M. The effect of music as a conditioning aid in prepared childbirth education. J Obstet Gynecol Neonatal Nurs 1986;15:268–270

21. Geden EA, Lower M, Beattie S, Beck N. Effects of music and imagery on physiologic and self-report of analogued labor pain. Nurs Res 1989;38:37–41

22. Cluett ER, Nikodem VC, McCandlish RE, Burns EE. Immersion in water in pregnancy, labour and birth. The Cochrane Database of Systematic Reviews 2004, Issue 1. Art. No.: CD000111

23. Cluett ER, Pickering RM, Getliffe K, St George Saunders NJ. Randomised controlled trial of labouring in water compared with standard of augmentation for management of dystocia in first stage of labour. BMJ 2004;328:314

MASTALGIA

SYNONYMS/SUBCATEGORIES

Mastodynia, idiopathic breast pain.

DEFINITION

Mastalgia can be differentiated into cyclical mastalgia (worse before a menstrual period) or non-cyclical mastalgia (unrelated to the menstrual cycle). Cyclical pain is often bilateral, usually most severe in the upper outer quadrants of the breast, and may be referred to the medial aspect of the upper arm. Non-cyclical pain may be caused by true breast pain or chest wall pain located over the costal cartilages.

CAM USAGE

Oral and topical applications of herbal medicines, particularly evening primrose oil.

CLINICAL EVIDENCE

HERBAL MEDICINE

A solution containing a chaste tree (*Vitex agnus-castus*) extract was shown to have a small effect in treating cyclical mastalgia in a placebo-controlled RCT of 97 women.[1] Another RCT compared chaste tree fruits to bromocriptine in the treatment of hyperprolactinaemia and cyclical mastalgia and found that pain scores decreased in all groups with no differences between groups.[2] A placebo-controlled, double-blind RCT ($n = 120$) found a chaste tree-containing preparation to be superior in treating premenstrual mastalgia.[3] A systematic safety review reported only mild and reversible adverse events following treatment with chaste tree.[4]

In a double-blind RCT, 120 women with severe chronic mastalgia received fish oil and control oil, evening primrose oil (*Oenothera biennis*) and control oil, fish oil and evening primrose oil, or both control oils.[5] All groups showed a decrease in pain but neither evening primrose oil nor fish oil had any clear benefit over control.

In a double-blind RCT, 555 women with moderate to severe mastalgia receiving gamolenic acid from evening primrose and antioxidants, placebo fatty acids and antioxidants, gamolenic acid and placebo antioxidants or placebo fatty acids and placebo antioxidants reported improvement in all groups with no differences between groups.[6] An open, non-randomised trial reported evening primrose oil to be less effective than topical non-steroidal anti-inflammatory drugs (NSAIDs) in the treatment of 50 women with mastalgia.[7]

A systematic review of red clover (*Trifolium pratense*) included 11 RCTs.[8] Five studies tested the effects of red clover isoflavones on vasomotor symptoms in menopausal women and were suitable for inclusion in a meta-analysis. Data were limited regarding the effects on cyclical mastalgia.

SUPPLEMENTS

A double-blind, placebo-controlled RCT reported that the dietary supplement Karinat, which contains β-carotene, α-tocopherol, ascorbic acid and garlic powder, reduces the severity of mastalgia, premenstrual syndrome and dysmenorrhoea.[9]

Encouraging results for phytoestrogens (40 or 80 mg of isoflavones) in reducing cyclical mastalgia were found in a small double-blind, placebo-controlled RCT ($n = 18$).[10]

A small double-blind RCT ($n = 20$) comparing soy protein with flavoured cow's milk suggested that the ingestion of soy protein improved breast pain yet compliance was poor, which makes the interpretation of results difficult.[11]

OVERALL RECOMMENDATION

There is some encouraging evidence for chaste tree in reducing the symptoms of mastalgia. It is associated with only mild adverse events and might be worth considering in patients with cyclical mastalgia. Evening primrose oil does not have any effects beyond those of placebo and no convincing evidence is available for any other complementary therapies.

Table 5.18 **Summary of clinical evidence for mastalgia**

Treatment	Weight of evidence	Direction of evidence	Serious safety concerns
Herbal medicine			
Chaste tree	OO	↑	Yes (see p. 5)
Evening primrose	OO	↘	Yes (see p. 191)
Red clover	OO	→	Yes (see p. 211)
Supplements			
Karinat	O	↗	Yes (see p. 5)
Phytooestrogens	O	↗	Yes (see p. 5)
Soy protein	O	→	Yes (see p. 5)

REFERENCES

1. Halaska M, Beles P, Gorkow C, Sieder C. Treatment of cyclical mastalgia with a solution containing a *Vitex agnus-castus* extract: results of a placebo-controlled double-blind study. Breast 1999;8:175–181

2. Kilicdag EB, Tarim E, Bagis T, Erkanli S, Aslan E, Ozsahin K, Kuscu E. Fructus agni-casti and bromocriptine for treatment of hyperprolactinemia and mastalgia. Int J Gynaecol Obstet 2004;85:292–293

3. Wuttke W, Splitt G, Gorkow C, Sieder C. Behandlung zyklusabhängiger Brustschmerzen mit einem Agnus-castus-haltigen Arzneimittel. Geburtshilfe Frauenheilkunde 1997:57:1–14

4. Daniele C, Thompson Coon J, Pittler MH, Ernst E. *Vitex agnus castus*: a systematic review of adverse events. Drug Saf 2005;28:319–332

5. Blommers J, de Lange-De Klerk ES, Kuik DJ, Bezemer PD, Meijer S. Evening primrose oil and fish oil for severe chronic mastalgia: a randomized, double-blind, controlled trial. Am J Obstet Gynecol 2002;187:1389–1394

6. Goyal A, Mansel RE; Efamast Study Group. A randomized multicenter study of gamolenic acid (Efamast) with and without antioxidant vitamins and minerals in the management of mastalgia. Breast J 2005;11:41–47

7. Qureshi S, Sultan N. Topical nonsteroidal anti-inflammatory drugs versus oil of evening primrose in the treatment of mastalgia. Surgeon 2005;3:7–10

8. Thompson Coon J, Pittler MH, Ernst E. *Trifolium pratense* isoflavones in the treatment of menopausal hot flushes. A systematic review and meta-analysis of randomized trials. Phytomedicine 2007;14:153–159

9. Bespalov VG, Barash NIu, Ivanova OA, Krzhivitskii PI, Semiglazov VF, Aleksandrov VA, Sobenin NA, Orekhov AN. Study of an antioxidant dietary supplement "Karinat" in patients with benign breast disease. [In Russian.] Vopr Onkol 2004;50:467–472

10. Ingram DM, Hickling C, West L, Mahe LJ, Dunbar PM. A double-blind randomized controlled trial of isoflavones in the treatment of cyclical mastalgia. Breast 2002;11:170–174

11. McFadyen IJ, Chetty U, Setchell KD, Zimmer-Nechemias L, Stanley E, Miller WR. A randomized double blind-cross over trial of soya protein for the treatment of cyclical breast pain. Breast 2000;9:271–276

MIGRAINE

SYNONYMS

Vascular headache, bilious headache, sick headache, blind headache, hemicrania. May also be named according to associated symptom, e.g. hemiplegic, ophthalmoplegic and ophthalmic nerve migraines. For headache see p. 285.

DEFINITION

Migraine is a primary headache disorder manifesting as recurring headaches usually lasting for 4–72 hours and involving pain of moderate to severe intensity, often with nausea, sometimes vomiting, and/or sensitivity to light, sound and other sensory stimuli.

CAM USAGE

Patients with this chronic complaint are very likely to seek help from CAM, the commonest forms being herbal medicine, spinal manipulation, acupuncture, homeopathy and reflexology.[1]

CLINICAL EVIDENCE

The available evidence relates mostly to prevention of migraine rather than treatment of an acute headache. Several overviews are available.[2–4]

ACUPUNCTURE

A systematic review[5] (Box 5.26) concluded cautiously in favour of acupuncture for prevention of migraine. However, the generally modest quality of studies prevented a firm conclusion.

SECTION FIVE

Box 5.26 *Systematic review: acupuncture for migraine*[5]

- Twenty-six RCTs involving 1151 patients with idiopathic headache (16 RCTs of migraine)
- Quality of studies was variable and often poor
- Sixteen sham-controlled RCTs showed efficacy of acupuncture
- **Conclusion**: the existing evidence supports the value of acupuncture

Since then, the trial data have generated mixed results. In one RCT, 160 patients received either acupuncture or oral flunarizine.[6] After 2 and 4 months of treatment, the frequency of headaches was lower in the acupuncture group, while at 6 months there was no longer a difference. An RCT involving 179 patients in the early stages of acute migraine suggested that acupuncture reduces the number of patients who develop a full migraine within 48 hours compared with placebo; the effect was similar to sumatriptan.[7] A large ($n = 302$) three-armed RCT found that acupuncture is not better than sham acupuncture for migraine prevention but both were better than waiting list control.[8] Similar results emerged from another German RCT with three parallel groups ($n = 794$) receiving acupuncture, sham acupuncture or standard medical prevention. The authors concluded that outcomes (number of migraine days) do not differ between patients treated with sham acupuncture, true acupuncture or standard therapy.[9] Comparing TENS, low-dose laser therapy and acupuncture for 4 months, acupuncture proved to be best for migraine prevention.[10] When 401 patients with chronic headache, predominantly migraine, were randomised to either receive advice to consult an acupuncturist or have the usual treatment, acupuncture led to a persistent reduction in headache scores.[11] A small RCT ($n = 28$) found no differences in the prevention of menstrually-related migraine between real and sham acupuncture.[12]

BIOFEEDBACK AND RELAXATION

A meta-analysis suggests that these therapies generate benefits for adults with migraine[13] (Box 5.27) but the conclusions must be cautious because appropriate controls are difficult to arrange. Moreover, the review included any type of prospective study. More recent RCTs show positive results for a multidisciplinary approach, including stress-management,[14] as well as for thermal biofeedback[15] and for a complex relaxation programme.[16] They also suggest biofeedback-assisted breathing exercises to have an effect similar to that of propranolol.[17] A 1995 National Institutes of Health Technology Assessment Panel found moderate evidence in support of the hypothesis that biofeedback is more effective than either relaxation or no treatment in relieving migraine headache.[18] The evidence was less clear when biofeedback was compared with placebo. Seven RCTs show that therapist-assisted relaxation training is an effective treatment for adolescents suffering from migraine.[19] Prospective studies in paediatric migraine[20] suggest the effectiveness of biofeedback, either alone or in combination with relaxation, with a similar effect to propranolol, though the result is not supported by the evidence from controlled studies (Box 5.28).

DIET

Of 88 children with severe, frequent migraine, 93% improved on a low-allergen diet. The role of foods in provoking migraine was established by double-blind challenge in 40 of the children.[21] Confirmation of the role of food allergy in causing migraine was provided by a study of 43 adults with migraine who were skin tested for allergies.[22] Those who were positive were more likely to respond to dietary manipulation than those who were negative. Migraines were provoked in several cases (71%) by blinded food challenge but not by placebo. Clearly, if

Box 5.27 *Meta-analysis: biofeedback/relaxation for migraine (adults)*[13]

- Thirty-five prospective trials of relaxation and/or biofeedback (sample sizes not quoted)
- Simultaneous analysis of 25 trials of propranolol for comparison
- Overall, effect size similar to propranolol: 43% reduction in headache activity (improvement as a percentage of baseline symptoms)
- Effect size for those who received placebo medication was 14% and for untreated group 0%
- **Conclusion**: evidence provides substantial support for effectiveness of relaxation/biofeedback and for propranolol

Box 5.28 *Meta-analysis: biofeedback/relaxation for migraine (children)*[20]

- Twenty-nine prospective investigations of behavioural interventions, mainly biofeedback and/or relaxation, involving 471 subjects
- Investigations of drug therapy ($n = 556$) used for comparison
- Effect sizes (measured in standard deviations): biofeedback, 2.6; relaxation, 1.0; biofeedback combined with relaxation, 3.1; placebo, 0.6; waiting list, 0.6; propranolol, 2.8; ergotamine, 1.6; clonidine, 1.5
- Further analysis restricted to controlled trials found no differences compared to various control interventions
- **Conclusion**: cautiously positive; lack of good-quality studies

Box 5.29 *Systematic review: feverfew for migraine*[25]

- Five RCTs including 343 subjects
- Results favoured feverfew over placebo for migraine prevention but had limitations, in particular the short duration
- No major safety problems emerged
- **Conclusion**: the evidence is insufficient

trigger foods such as chocolate, cheese, shellfish or red wine are identified, these should be avoided. No rigorous studies of other nutritional approaches are available.

HERBAL MEDICINE

Butterbur (*Petasites hybridus*) was compared to placebo in a 12-week RCT with 60 migraineurs.[23] The frequency of migraines proved to be lower in the verum group. A reanalysis of these data showed that the responder rate with butterbur was 45%, while that of the placebo group was 15%.[24]

A systematic review[25] of feverfew (*Tanacetum parthenium*) (Box 5.29) found three positive studies but there were weaknesses in most of these and the evidence was not considered to be conclusive in favour of feverfew. The most recent RCT ($n = 170$) suggested that feverfew reduces migraine frequency by more than 50%.[26]

Encouraging results were also reported for a Chinese patent medicine (shutianning granule)[27] and for a combination of soy isoflavones, dong quai and black cohosh (for menstrual migraine).[28]

Box 5.30 *Systematic review: homeopathy for migraine*[29]

- Four RCTs including 294 subjects
- One study also included patients with other forms of chronic headache
- One RCT, the lowest quality, found improvement in frequency, duration and intensity of migraines
- The remaining three RCTs were negative for attack frequency, severity and intensity, although, in one, the neurologist's assessment favoured homeopathy
- **Conclusion**: homeopathy is not superior to placebo

Box 5.31 *Systematic reviews: spinal manipulation for migraine*[31,32]

- Eight RCTs including patients with various forms of headache
- Three RCTs on migraine including a total of 430 patients
- Quality was satisfactory to moderate
- **Conclusion**: overall these studies imply effectiveness

HOMEOPATHY

A systematic review[29] of homeopathy for chronic headache, mainly migraine (Box 5.30), suggested that this therapy is not superior to placebo. More recently, a double-blind, placebo-controlled RCT ($n = 73$) of individualised homeopathy showed a trend in favour of homeopathy in migraine prevention.[30]

SPINAL MANIPULATION

Two systematic reviews of spinal manipulation for various forms of headache are available.[31,32] They include three RCTs on migraine patients. Their results suggest the effectiveness of this treatment for migraine. (Box 5.31)

SUPPLEMENTS

A small placebo-controlled RCT ($n = 42$) suggested that co-enzyme Q10 (3×100 mg/ day) is effective in reducing the number of migraines of chronic migraine sufferers.[33]

Two RCTs ($n = 27$ and $n = 196$) tested the effects of fish oil (omega-3 fatty acid) in migraine prevention. In the smaller study[34] no effect was found, yet a slight reduction (by 1.1 episodes per 4 months) was noted in the larger trial.[35]

OTHER THERAPIES

No benefits were demonstrated in an RCT of hyperbaric oxygen therapy.[36] A double-blind, placebo-controlled RCT of impulse magnetic-field therapy generated encouraging results,[37] but they require independent replication.

In an RCT involving 20 subjects with mixed migraine and tension headache over 4 months, yoga in addition to standard medication produced a reduction in headache activity in contrast to standard medication alone.[38]

OVERALL RECOMMENDATION

Reasonable choices for prevention of migraine are acupuncture, biofeedback (either alone or with relaxation) or exclusion diets (in suitable patients). For acupuncture, the evidence is encouraging but not fully convincing. Some herbal remedies, such as feverfew or butterbur, may also be beneficial. The results with co-enzyme Q10 are encouraging but require independent confirmation. Compared to conventional treatments, these CAM therapies seem similarly effective in the prevention of migraine episodes. It should be noted, however, that simply increasing the daily water intake has been shown to reduce the total number of hours and intensity of migraine episodes.[39] None of the CAM therapies is associated with major risks and thus may be preferable to long-term use of conventional preventive drugs. The role of CAM therapies in the treatment of acute migraine episodes has not been investigated or compared with modern medications such as triptans.

Table 5.19 **Summary of clinical evidence for migraine**

Treatment	Weight of evidence	Direction of evidence	Serious safety concerns
Acupuncture	OOO	↗	Yes (see p. 96)
Biofeedback	OOO	↑	No (see p. 110)
Diet	OO	↑	No (see p. 5)
Herbal medicine			
Butterbur	O	↑	Yes (see p. 5)
Feverfew	OO	↗	Yes (see p. 194)
Homeopathy	OO	↘	No (see p. 124)
Relaxation	OOO	↑	No (see p. 158)
Spinal manipulation	OO	↗	Yes (see p. 112)
Supplements			
Co-enzyme Q10	O	↑	Yes (see p. 5)
Fish oil	O	↗	Yes (see p. 5)

REFERENCES

1. Eisenberg DM, Davis R, Ettner SL, Appel S, Wilkey S, Rompay MV. Trends in alternative medicine use in the United States, 1990–1997. JAMA 1998;280:1569–1575
2. Tepper SJ. Alternative medicine in migraine: is it ever a good alternative? Headache Pain Diagn Chall Curr Ther 2005;16:69–74
3. Biondi DM. Physical treatments for headache: a structured review. Headache 2005;45:738–746
4. Sandor PS, Dydak U, Schoenen J, Kollias SS, Hess K, Boesiger P, Agosti RM. MR-spectroscopic imaging during visual stimulation in subgroups of migraine with aura. Cephalalgia 2005;25:507–518
5. Melchart D, Linde K, Fischer P, Berman B, White A, Vickers A, Allais G. Acupuncture for idiopathic headache. The Cochrane Database of Systematic Reviews 2001, Issue 1. Art No.: CD001218
6. Allais G, De Lorenzo C, Quirico PE, Airola G, Tolardo G, Mana O, Benedetto C. Acupuncture in the prophylactic treatment of migraine without aura: a comparison with flunarizine. Headache 2002;42:855–861
7. Melchart D, Thormaehlen J, Hager S, Liao J, Linde K, Weidenhammer W. Acupuncture versus placebo versus sumatriptan for early treatment of acute migraine attacks – a randomized controlled trial. J Intern Med 2003;253:181–188
8. Linde K, Streng A, Jurgens S, Hoppe A, Brinkhaus B, Witt C, Wagenpfeil S, Pfaffenrath V, Hammes MG, Weidenhammer W, Willich SN, Melchart D. Acupuncture for patients with migraine: a randomized controlled trial. JAMA 2005;293:2118–2125
9. Diener HC, Kronfeld K, Boewing G, Lungenhausen M, Maier C, Molsberger A, Tegenthoff M, Trampisch HJ, Zenz M, Meinert R; GERAC Migraine Study Group. Efficacy of acupuncture for the prophylaxis of migraine: a multicentre randomised controlled clinical trial. Lancet Neurol 2006;5:310–316.

10. Allais G, De Lorenzo C, Quirico PE, Lupi G, Airola G, Mana O, Benedetto C. Non-pharmacological approaches to chronic headaches: transcutaneous electrical nerve stimulation, lasertherapy and acupuncture in transformed migraine treatment. Neurol Sci 2003;24:S138–S142

11. Vickers AJ, Rees RW, Zollman CE, McCarney R, Smith CM, Ellis N, Fisher P, Van Haselen R. Acupuncture for chronic headache in primary care: large, pragmatic, randomised trial. BMJ 2004; 328:744

12. Linde M, Fjell A, Carlsson J, Dahlof C. Role of the needling per se in acupuncture as prophylaxis for menstrually related migraine: a randomized placebo-controlled study. Cephalalgia 2005;25: 41–47

13. Holroyd KA, Penzien DB. Pharmacological versus non-pharmacological prophylaxis of recurrent migraine headache: a meta-analytic review of clinical trials. Pain 1990;42:1–13

14. Lemstra M, Stewart B, Olszynski WP. Effectiveness of multidisciplinary intervention in the treatment of migraine: a randomized controlled trial. Headache 2002;42:845–854

15. Scharff L, Marcus DA, Masek BJ. A controlled study of minimal-contact thermal biofeedback treatment in children with migraine. J Pediatr Psychol 2002;27:109–119

16. Fichtel A, Larsson B. Relaxation treatment administered by school nurses to adolescents with recurrent headaches. Headache 2004;44:545–554

17. Kaushik R, Kaushik RM, Mahajan SK, Rajesh V. Biofeedback assisted diaphragmatic breathing and systematic relaxation versus propranolol in long term prophylaxis of migraine. Complement Ther Med 2005;13:165–174

18. NIH Technology Assessment Statement. Integration of behavioral and relaxation approaches into the treatment of chronic pain and insomnia. NIH Technol Assess Statement 1995;16–18:1–34

19. Larsson B, Carlsson J, Fichtel A, Melin L. Relaxation treatment of adolescent headache sufferers: results from a school-based replication series. Headache 2005;45:692–704

20. Hermann C, Kim M, Blanchard EB. Behavioral and prophylactic pharmacological intervention studies of pediatric migraine: an exploratory meta-analysis. Pain 1995;60:239–256

21. Egger J, Carter CM, Wilson J, Turner MW, Soothill JF. Is migraine food allergy? A double-blind controlled trial of oligoantigenic diet treatment. Lancet 1983;2:865–869

22. Mansfield LE, Vaughan TR, Waller SF, Haverly RW, Ting S. Food allergy and adult migraine: double-blind and mediator confirmation of an allergic etiology. Ann Allergy 1985;55:126–129

23. Grossman M, Schmidramsl H. An extract of *Petasites hybridus* is effective in the prophylaxis of migraine. Int J Clin Pharmacol Ther 2000;38:430–435

24. Diener HC, Rahlfs VW, Danesch U. The first placebo-controlled trial of a special butterbur root extract for the prevention of migraine: reanalysis of efficacy criteria. Eur Neurol 2004;51:89–97

25. Pittler MH, Ernst E. Feverfew for preventing migraine. The Cochrane Database of Systematic Reviews 2004, Issue 1. Art No.: CD002286

26. Diener HC, Pfaffenrath V, Schnitker J, Friede M, Henneicke-von Zepelin HH. Efficacy and safety of 6.25 mg t.i.d. feverfew CO_2-extract (MIG-99) in migraine prevention – a randomized, double-blind, multicentre, placebo-controlled study. Cephalalgia 2005;25: 1031–1041

27. Hu ZQ, Song LG, Mei T. Clinical and experimental study on treatment of migraine with shutianing granule. [In Chinese.] Zhongguo Zhong Xi Yi Jie He Za Zhi 2002;22:581–583

28. Burke BE, Olson RD, Cusack BJ. Randomized, controlled trial of phytoestrogen in the prophylactic treatment of menstrual migraine. Biomed Pharmacother 2002;56:283–288

29. Ernst E. Homeopathic prophylaxis of headaches and migraine? A systematic review. J Pain Symptom Manage 1999;18:353–357

30. Straumsheim P, Borchgrevink C, Mowinckel P, Kierulf H, Hafslund O. Homeopathic treatment of migraine: a double-blind, placebo controlled trial of 68 patients. Br Homeopath J 2000;89:4–7

31. Bronfort G, Assendelft WJ, Evans R, Haas M, Bouter L. Efficacy of spinal manipulation for chronic headache: a systematic review. J Manipulative Physiol Ther 2001;24: 457–466

32. Astin JA, Ernst E. The effectiveness of spinal manipulation for the treatment of headache disorders: a systematic review of randomized clinical trials. Cephalalgia 2002;22:617–623

33. Sándor PS, Di Clemente L, Coppola G, Saenger U, Magis D, Seidel L, Agosti RM, Schoenen J. Efficacy of coenzyme Q10 in migraine prophylaxis: a randomized controlled trial. Neurol 2005; 64:713–715

34. Harel Z, Gascon G, Riggs S, Vaz R, Brown W, Exil G. Supplementation with omega-3 polyunsaturated fatty acids in the management of recurrent migraines in adolescents. J Adolesc Health 2002;31:154–161

35. Pradalier A, Bakouche P, Baudesson G, Delage A, Cornaille-Lafage G, Launay JM, Biason P. Failure of omega-3 polyunsaturated fatty acids in prevention of migraine: a double-blind study versus placebo. Cephalalgia 2001;21:818–822

36. Eftedal OS, Lydersen S, Helde G, White L, Brubakk AO, Stovner LJ. A randomized, double blind study of the prophylactic effect of hyperbaric oxygen therapy on migraine. Cephalalgia 2004;24:639–644

37. Pelka RB, Jaenicke C, Gruenwald J. Impulse magnetic-field therapy for migraine and other headaches: a double-blind, placebo-controlled study. Adv Ther 2001;18:101–109

38. Latha D, Kaliappan KV. Efficacy of yoga therapy in the management of headaches. J Indian Psychol 1992;10:41–47

39. Spigt MG, Kuijper EC, Schayck CP, Troost J, Knipschild PG, Linssen VM, Knottnerus JA. Increasing the daily water intake for the prophylactic treatment of headache: a pilot trial. Eur J Neurol 2005;12:715–718

MINOR TRAUMA

DEFINITION

For the purpose of this chapter, we define the following conditions as minor trauma: cuts, bruises, sprains and uncomplicated bone fractures.

RELATED CONDITIONS

Sport injuries, tendinopathies, repetitive strain injury (see Tennis elbow, p. 327), Whiplash injury, Burns (see p. 235).

CAM USAGE

No prevalence data are available; the use of 'folk remedies' seems to be widespread.

CLINICAL EVIDENCE

While there is a considerable amount of pre-clinical data,[1] clinical evidence remains scarce.

ACUPUNCTURE

A preliminary CCT suggested that electroacupuncture might accelerate the healing of wounds that were unresponsive to conventional therapy.[2]

HERBAL MEDICINE

A systematic review of CCTs of aloe (*Aloe vera*) found no conclusive evidence that it enhances wound healing.[3]

The results from an RCT involving 19 patients who were suffering from facial bruises after laser treatment for telangiectases who were treated with herbal arnica (*Arnica montana*) gel on one side and vehicle on the other side of the face[4] showed no differences in the prevention or resolution of bruises.

An ointment of comfrey (*Symphytum officinale*) root extract was tested against placebo in an RCT with 142 patients suffering from acute ankle sprain.[5] The active treatment was superior in terms of reduction of pain, oedema and immobility. The same group also showed in an equivalence RCT that comfrey ointment was as least as effective for this condition as diclofenac gel.[6]

A small ($n = 37$) RCT suggested that surgical wound healing can be accelerated by topically applying aqueous extracts of the bark of mangrove (*Rhizophora mangle*).[7]

HOMEOPATHY

A systematic review included seven CCTs of homeopathic *Arnica montana* for minor trauma. Collectively these data failed to convincingly show effectiveness.[8]

SECTION FIVE

HOMOTOXICOLOGY

A systematic review included three RCTs of Traumeel versus placebo for various forms of minor trauma.[9] All studies suggested effectiveness but there were several important caveats so the authors concluded that these trials failed to demonstrate efficacy.

HYPNOTHERAPY

An RCT ($n = 12$) tested whether bone fractures heal faster if, in addition to standard care, patients are hypnotised.[10] Even though there was a positive trend, the results failed to show that hypnotherapy accelerates the healing of bone tissue.

MANIPULATION

A single-blind CCT compared manual ankle adjustments with detuned ultrasound in 15 patients with ankle sprains.[11] The results suggested better pain control through manipulation. A similar trial confirmed these effects for osteopathic manipulative treatment.[12]

MUSIC THERAPY

An RCT with 77 patients suffering from minor musculoskeletal trauma showed no benefit of music therapy as an adjunct to standard care in terms of pain control.[13]

SPIRITUAL HEALING

Daniel Wirth has published at least five RCTs which uniformly show that spiritual healing enhances healing after various forms of minor trauma.[14] However, this body of research has recently been suspected to be fraudulent by his former supervisor among others.[15] We therefore believe that these results should not be regarded as reliable until the matter is clarified.

OVERALL RECOMMENDATION

Comfrey ointment or manual manipulation seem to be effective for reducing pain after ankle sprains but further studies would be necessary to be sure. Other CAM modalities offer few well-documented benefits for treating minor trauma.

Table 5.20 **Summary of clinical evidence for minor trauma**

Treatment	Weight of evidence	Direction of evidence	Serious safety concerns
Acupuncture	O	↗	Yes (see p. 96)
Herbal medicine			
Aloe vera	OO	↗	Yes (see p. 5)
Arnica	O	↘	Yes (see p. 176)
Comfrey	OO	↗	Yes (see p. 188)
Mangrove	O	↗	Yes (see p. 5)
Homeopathy	OO	→	No (see p. 124)
Homotoxicology	OO	↗	No (see p. 5)
Hypnotherapy	O	→	Yes (see p. 130)
Manipulation	OO	↗	Yes (see p. 112)
Music therapy	O	↘	No (see p. 142)
Spiritual healing	OO	→	No (see p. 162)

REFERENCES

1. Phan TT, Lee ST, Chan SY, Hughes MA, Cherry GW. Investigating plant-based medicines for wound healing with the use of cell culture technologies and *in vitro* models: a review. Ann Acad Med Singapore 2000;29:27–36

2. Sumano H, Mateos G. The use of acupuncture-like electrical stimulation for wound healing of lesions unresponsive to conventional treatment. Am J Acupunct 1999;27:5–14

3. Vogler BK, Ernst E. Aloe vera: a systematic review of its clinical effectiveness. Br J Gen Pract 1999;49:823–828

4. Alonso D, Lazarus MC, Baumann L. Effects of topical arnica gel on post-laser treatment bruises. Dermatol Surg 2002;8:686–688

5. Koll R, Buhr M, Dieter R, Pabst H, Predel HG, Petrowicz O, Giannetti B, Klingenburg S, Staiger C. Efficacy and tolerance of a comfrey root extract (Extr. Rad. Symphyti) in the treatment of ankle distorsions: results of a multicenter, randomized, placebo-controlled, double-blind study. Phytomedicine 2004;11:470–477

6. Predel HG, Giannetti B, Koll R, Bulitta M, Staiger C. Efficacy of a comfrey root extract ointment in comparison to a diclofenac gel in the treatment of ankle distortions: results of an observer-blind, randomized, multicenter study. Phytomedicine 2005;12:707–714

7. Fernandez O, Capdevila JZ, Dalla G, Melchor G. Efficacy of Rhizophora mangle aqueous bark extract in the healing of open surgical wounds. Fitoterapia 2002;73:564–568

8. Lüdtke R, Hacke D. Zur Wirksamkeit des homöopathischen Arzneimittels *Arnica montana*. Wien Med Wochenschr 2005;155:482–490

9. Ernst E, Schmidt K. Homotoxicology – a review of randomised clinical trials. Eur J Clin Pharmacol 2004;60:299–306

10. Ginandes CS, Rosenthal DI. Using hypnosis to accelerate the healing of bone fractures: a randomized controlled pilot study. Altern Ther Health Med 1999;5:67–75

11. Pellow JE, Brantingham JW. The efficacy of adjusting the ankle in the treatment of subacute and chronic grade I and grade II ankle inversion sprains. J Manipulative Physiol Ther 2001;24:17–24

12. Eisenhart AW, Gaeta TJ, Yens DP. Osteopathic manipulative treatment in the emergency department for patients with acute ankle injuries. J Am Osteopath Assoc 2003;103:417–421

13. Tanabe P, Thomas R, Paice J, Spiller M, Marcantonio R. The effect of standard care, ibuprofen, and music on pain relief and patient satisfaction in adults with musculoskeletal trauma. J Emerg Nurs 2001;27:124–131

14. Astin JA, Harkness EF, Ernst E. The efficacy of "Distant Healing": a systematic review of randomized trials. Ann Intern Med 2000;132:903–910

15. Solfvin J, Leskowitz E, Benor JD. Questions concerning the scientific credibility of wound healing studies authored by Daniel P. Wirth. Online. Available: http://www.wholistichealingresearch.com/WirthQ.asp Feb 18 2006

MYOFASCIAL PAIN

SYNONYMS

Muscle pain.

DEFINITION

A condition that affects the muscle and produces local and referred pain. It is characterised by motor and sensory abnormalities (tenderness and referred pain). It is classified as a musculoskeletal pain syndrome that can be acute or chronic, regional or generalised. It can be a primary disorder, causing local or regional pain, or a secondary disorder that occurs as a consequence of another condition. It tends to be associated with trauma, poor posture and may also develop from excessive strain on muscles or muscle groups.

RELATED CONDITIONS

Fibromyalgia.

SECTION FIVE

CAM USAGE
Massage, chiropractic, acupuncture.

CLINICAL EVIDENCE
ACUPUNCTURE
A Cochrane review aimed to determine the effects of dry needling on myofascial pain syndrome in the low-back region (see chapter on back pain, p. 230).[1] It concluded that dry needling appears to be a useful adjunct to other therapies for chronic low back pain. For treating myofascial trigger-point pain, a systematic review concluded that any effect is likely because of the needle or placebo.[2] Superficial needling followed by stretching was found to be more effective than stretching alone or no treatment in one RCT.[3] For temporomandibular joint dysfunction a systematic review included six RCTs, which overall suggest that acupuncture might be an effective option.[4] Subsequent studies reported mixed results in pain reduction compared with placebo/sham acupuncture[5,6] whereas another reported some beneficial effects compared with electrotherapy.[7] Overall, the data on acupuncture for myofascial pain suggest beneficial effects [see chapters on back (p. 230), neck (p. 286) and shoulder pain (p. 325)].[8–14]

BIOFEEDBACK
A systematic review (Box 5.32) of biofeedback-based treatments for temporomandibular disorders identified six RCTs;[15] two for each of surface EMG training of the masticatory muscles, surface EMG training combined with adjunctive cognitive–behavioural therapy techniques, and biofeedback-assisted relaxation training. It was suggested that these types of biofeedback training are probably effective for temporomandibular disorders.

COGNITIVE–BEHAVIOURAL THERAPY
Two RCTs were identified for treating patients with temporomandibular pain. One trial ($n = 61$) compared cognitive–behavioural therapy with hypnosis and reported similar decrements in pain.[16] The other compared cognitive–behavioural therapy with an education/attention control ($n = 158$).[17] Greater improvements at follow-up for each outcome, such as pain and function, were reported compared with controls.

OTHER THERAPIES
Two RCTs investigated the effects of repetitive magnetic stimulation for patients with myofascial pain syndrome.[18,19] In both trials beneficial effects on pain measures were reported.

Box 5.32 *Systematic review: biofeedback for temporomandibular disorders*[15]

- Fourteen controlled and uncontrolled studies of biofeedback-based treatments published since 1978 were identified
- Two RCTs of each of three types of biofeedback treatment were included: surface EMG training of the masticatory muscles, surface EMG training combined with adjunctive cognitive–behavioural therapy techniques, and biofeedback-assisted relaxation training
- Four RCTs reported biofeedback to be superior to sham/no treatment
- **Conclusion:** 'We conclude that surface EMG training with adjunctive cognitive behavioural therapy is an efficacious treatment for temporomandibular disorders and that both surface EMG training as the sole intervention and biofeedback-assisted relaxation training are probably efficacious treatments'

OVERALL RECOMMENDATION

The evidence suggesting that acupuncture has beneficial effects for patients with myofascial pain is convincing. Whether it is as effective as conventional treatments such as lidocaine injections is not clear. Given its favourable safety profile, however, it could be tried in patients who prefer acupuncture. For temporomandibular pain, biofeedback may have some beneficial effects, but as with other cognitive–behavioural treatments more trials are required for any firm recommendations to be made.

Table 5.21 **Summary of clinical evidence for myofascial pain**

Treatment	Weight of evidence	Direction of evidence	Serious safety concerns
Acupuncture	OOO	↑	Yes (see p. 96)
Biofeedback	OOO	↗	Yes (see p. 110)
Cognitive–behavioural therapy	OO	↗	Yes (see p. 5)

REFERENCES

1. Furlan AD, van Tulder MW, Cherkin DC, Tsukayama H, Lao L, Koes BW, Berman BM. Acupuncture and dry-needling for low back pain. The Cochrane Database of Systematic Reviews 2005, Issue1. Art. No.: CD001351
2. Cummings TM, White AR. Needling therapies in the management of myofascial trigger point pain: a systematic review. Arch Phys Med Rehabil 2001;82:986–992
3. Edwards J, Knowles N. Superficial dry needling and active stretching in the treatment of myofascial pain – a randomised controlled trial. Acupunct Med 2003;21:80–86
4. Ernst E, White AR. Acupuncture as a treatment for temporomandibular joint dysfunction: a systematic review of randomized trials. Arch Otolaryngol Head Neck Surg 1999;125:269–272
5. Schmid-Schwap M, Simma-Kletschka I, Stockner A, Sengstbratl M, Gleditsch J, Kundi M, Piehslinger E. Oral acupuncture in the therapy of craniomandibular dysfunction syndrome – a randomized controlled trial. Wien Klin Wochenschr 2006;118:36–42
6. Goddard G, Karibe H, McNeill C, Villafuerte E. Acupuncture and sham acupuncture reduce muscle pain in myofascial pain patients. J Orofac Pain 2002;16:71–76
7. Zhou FH, Zhao HY. Acupuncture and ultrasound therapy for temporomandibular disorders. Di Yi Jun Yi Da Xue Xue Bao 2004;24:720–721
8. Kamanli A, Kaya A, Ardicoglu O, Ozgocmen S, Zengin FO, Bayik Y. Comparison of lidocaine injection, botulinum toxin injection, and dry needling to trigger points in myofascial pain syndrome. Rheumatol Int 2005;25:604–611
9. Ilbuldu E, Cakmak A, Disci R, Aydin R. Comparison of laser, dry needling, and placebo laser treatments in myofascial pain syndrome. Photomed Laser Surg 2004;22:306–311
10. Chu J. Does EMG (dry needling) reduce myofascial pain symptoms due to cervical nerve root irritation? Electromyogr Clin Neurophysiol 1997;37:259–272
11. Irnich D, Behrens N, Gleditsch JM, Stor W, Schreiber MA, Schops P, Vickers AJ, Beyer A. Immediate effects of dry needling and acupuncture at distant points in chronic neck pain: results of a randomized, double-blind, sham-controlled crossover trial. Pain 2002;99:83–89
12. Birch S, Jamison RN. Controlled trial of Japanese acupuncture for chronic myofascial neck pain: assessment of specific and nonspecific effects of treatment. Clin J Pain 1998;14:248–255
13. Irnich D, Behrens N, Molzen H, Konig A, Gleditsch J, Krauss M, Natalis M, Senn E, Beyer A, Schops P. Randomised trial of acupuncture compared with conventional massage and 'sham' laser acupuncture for treatment of chronic neck pain. BMJ 2001;322:1574–1578
14. Ceccheerelli F, Bordin M, Gagliardi G, Caravello M. Comparison between superficial and deep acupuncture in the treatment of the shoulder's myofascial pain: a randomized and controlled study. Acupunct Electrother Res 2001;26:229–238

15. Crider A, Glaros AG, Gevirtz RN. Efficacy of biofeedback-based treatments for temporomandibular disorders. Appl Psychophysiol Biofeedback 2005;30:333–345

16. Stam HJ, McGrath PA, Brooke RI. The effects of a cognitive-behavioral treatment program on temporo-mandibular pain and dysfunction syndrome. Psychosom Med 1984; 46:534–545.

17. Turner JA, Mancl L, Aaron LA. Short- and long-term efficacy of brief cognitive-behavioral therapy for patients with chronic temporomandibular disorder pain: a randomized, controlled trial. Pain 2006;121:181–194

18. Smania N, Corato E, Fiaschi A, Pietropoli P, Aglioti SM, Tinazzi M. Repetitive magnetic stimulation: a novel therapeutic approach for myofascial pain syndrome. J Neurol 2005;252:307–314

19. Smania N, Corato E, Fiaschi A, Pietropoli P, Aglioti SM, Tinazzi M. Therapeutic effects of peripheral repetitive magnetic stimulation on myofascial pain syndrome. Clin Neurophysiol 2003; 114:350–358

NECK PAIN

SYNONYMS/SUBCATEGORIES

Mechanical neck disorder.

DEFINITION

Pain in the cervical region, with or without referral to the shoulder and arm. The symptom may arise from a broad range of conditions involving muscle, joint, disc, ligament or degenerative disorders. It may also occur with diffuse connective tissue diseases including rheumatoid arthritis, arthritis associated with spondylitis and a number of other systemic conditions. If symptoms persist for more than 3 months, the term chronic neck pain is used. Neck pain after whiplash injury is excluded from the following discussion.

CAM USAGE

According to survey data from the US,[1] 57% of people with neck pain used CAM in the previous 12 months, two-thirds visiting a practitioner. Manual therapies and acupuncture are commonly used.

CLINICAL EVIDENCE

ACUPUNCTURE

A systematic review of RCTs (Box 5.33) failed to provide evidence that acupuncture is superior to placebo.[2] Subsequent RCTs generated both positive[3–10] and negative results.[11] Other RCTs yielded ambiguous findings: acupuncture turned out to be less effective than spinal manipulation but superior to medication[12] or acupuncture 'produced a statistically, but not clinically, significant effect compared to placebo'.[13] An RCT suggested that intensive acupuncture/acupressure is better than sham treatment for a mixed group of patients suffering from chronic neck or shoulder pain.[14] A further systematic review that included some of these recent trials found 'modest' evidence in support of a specific effect of acupuncture.[15]

Box 5.33 *Systematic review: acupuncture for neck pain*[2]

- Fourteen RCTs involving 724 subjects with neck pain from various causes
- Seven studies were of good quality
- Acupuncture was superior to waiting list (one study), either no different from or superior to physiotherapy (three studies) and no different from placebo acupuncture (four out of five studies)
- **Conclusion**: no evidence that acupuncture is superior to placebo

EXERCISE

Both endurance and strength training exercises[16] but not dynamic muscle training[17] have been shown to alleviate chronic neck pain in large RCTs.

Positive findings were confirmed in an RCT ($n = 145$) that compared exercise with infrared radiation plus advice. The exercise group was superior in terms of pain and disability both in the short term as well as at 6-month follow-up.[18] When all systematic reviews on the subject were summarised, insufficient evidence was found that exercise therapy is effective for neck pain.[19]

MASSAGE

Regarding the effectiveness of massage for neck pain the trial data are somewhat contradictory. The above-mentioned RCT ($n = 177$) did not seem to indicate that massage (used as a control intervention) was effective.[4] On the other hand, an RCT with 29 patients suffering from neck, back or shoulder pain showed that massage generated more pain relief at the 3-month follow-up than standard medical care.[20]

SPINAL MANIPULATION

A Cochrane review (Box 5.34) found no strong evidence for the effectiveness of spinal manipulation in neck pain,[21] a finding that was confirmed also by other reviewers.[22] Systematic reviews authored by chiropractors[23,24] do, however, arrive at more optimistic conclusions. A subsequent large RCT ($n = 350$) showed that adding manipulative therapy to an exercise regimen was not followed by clinical improvements after the end of the 6-week intervention nor at a 6-month follow-up.[25] Further RCTs suggested that spinal manipulation may have immediate and long-term analgesic effects in patients with neck pain[26,27] and that osteopathic spinal manipulation generates results similar to those of a single dose of intramuscular ketorolac for acute neck pain.[28]

OTHER THERAPIES

Bitongxiao is a Chinese herbal decoction that was tested in a CCT ($n = 102$). The results suggest positive effects on pain.[29]

Low-level laser therapy is often used for neck pain. A systematic review of five RCTs found only limited evidence for the effectiveness of this approach compared to placebo.[30]

Magnetic-field therapy resulted in more pain reduction than placebo in a small ($n = 34$) RCT with patients suffering from neck pain as a result of cervical osteoarthritis.[31]

A small RCT ($n = 37$) suggested that a 7-week programme of applied relaxation generates better long-term pain control than a standard physiotherapeutic approach.[32]

An RCT ($n = 68$) of spiritual healing for improvement of restricted neck movement found no pain relief through this intervention.[33]

Box 5.34 *Systematic review: spinal manipulation and mobilisation for neck pain*[21]

- Thirty-three RCTs were included
- Forty-two per cent were of high methodological quality
- No benefit against placebo or other treatments for acute, subacute or chronic pain
- Combined with exercise there was evidence of benefit
- **Conclusion**: the evidence did not favour mobilisation or manipulation when carried out alone

OVERALL RECOMMENDATION

The evidence for CAM in the treatment of neck pain is either ambiguous or not convincing. Therefore it cannot be recommended as an option for treating neck pain. Active physiotherapy is a recognised effective conventional therapy.

Table 5.22 **Summary of clinical evidence for neck pain**

Treatment	Weight of evidence	Direction of evidence	Serious safety concerns
Acupuncture	OOO	↗	Yes (see p. 96)
Exercise	OO	↗	Yes (see p. 5)
Massage	OO	→	No (see p. 137)
Spinal manipulation	OOO	↗	Yes (see p. 112)

REFERENCES

1. Eisenberg DM, Davis R, Ettner SL, Appel S, Wilkey S, Rompay MV. Trends in alternative medicine use in the United States, 1990–1997. JAMA 1998;280:1569–1575
2. White AR, Ernst E. A systematic review of randomized controlled trials of acupuncture for neck pain. Rheumatol 1999;38:143–147
3. Heikkila H, Johansson M, Wenngren BI. Effects of acupuncture, cervical manipulation and NSAID therapy on dizziness and impaired head repositioning of suspected cervical origin: a pilot study. Man Ther 2000;5:151–157
4. Irnich D, Behrens N, Molzen H, Konig A, Gleditsch J, Krauss M, Natalis M, Senn E, Beyer A, Schops P. Randomised trial of acupuncture compared with conventional massage and 'sham' laser acupuncture for treatment of chronic neck pain. BMJ 2001;322:1574–1578
5. Seidel U, Uhlemann C. Behandlung der zervikalen Tendomyose. Dt Ztschr Akupunktur 2002;45:258–269
6. Irnich D, Behrens N, Gleditsch JM, Stor W, Schreiber MA, Schops P, Vickers AJ, Beyer A. Immediate effects of dry needling and acupuncture at distant points in chronic neck pain: results of a randomized, double-blind, sham-controlled crossover trial. Pain 2002; 99:83–89
7. Nabeta T, Kawakita K. Relief of chronic neck and shoulder pain by manual acupuncture to tender points – a sham-controlled randomized trial. Complement Ther Med 2002;10:217–222
8. Konig A, Radke S, Molzen H, Haase M, Muller C, Drezler D, Natalis M, Krauss M, Behrens N, Irnich D. Randomised trial of acupuncture compared with conventional massage and 'sham' laser acupuncture for treatment of chronic neck pain – range of motion analysis. Z Orthop Ihre Grenzgeb 2003;141:395–400
9. Sator-Katzenschlager SM, Szeles JC, Scharbert G, Michalek-Sauberer A, Kober A, Heinze G, Kozek-Langenecker SA. Electrical stimulation of auricular acupuncture points is more effective than conventional manual auricular acupuncture in chronic cervical pain: a pilot study. Anesth Analg 2003;97:1469–1473
10. He D, Veierstad KB, Hostmark AT, Medbo JI. Effect of acupuncture treatment on chronic neck and shoulder pain in sedentary female workers: a 6-month and 3-year follow-up study. Pain 2004;109: 299–307
11. Zhu XM, Polus B. A controlled trial on acupuncture for chronic neck pain. Am J Chin Med 2002;30:13–28
12. Giles LG, Muller R. Chronic spinal pain: a randomized clinical trial comparing medication, acupuncture, and spinal manipulation. Spine 2003;28:1490–1502
13. White P, Lewith G, Prescott P, Conway J. Acupuncture versus placebo for the treatment of chronic mechanical neck pain: a randomized, controlled trial. Ann Intern Med 2004;141:911–919
14. He D, Hostmark AT, Veiersted KB, Medbo JI. Effect of intensive acupuncture on pain-related social and psychological variables for women with chronic neck and shoulder pain – an RCT with six month and three year follow up. Acupunct Med 2005;23:52–61

15. Irnich D. Acupuncture for neck pain – review of recent randomised controlled trials. Dtsch Z Akupunkt 2005;48:40–43

16. Ylinen J, Takala EP, Nykanen M, Hakkinen A, Malkia E, Pohjolainen T, Karppi SL, Kautiainen H, Airaksinen O. Active neck muscle training in the treatment of chronic neck pain in women: a randomized controlled trial. JAMA 2003;289:2509–2516

17. Viljanen M, Malmivaara A, Utti J, Rinne M, Palmroos P, Laippala P. Effectiveness of dynamic muscle training, relaxation training, or ordinary activity for chronic neck pain: randomised controlled trial. BMJ 2003;327:475

18. Chiu TT, Lam TH, Hedley AJ. A randomized controlled trial on the efficacy of exercise for patients with chronic neck pain. Spine 2005;30:E1–E7

19. Smidt N, de Vet HCW, Bouter LM, Dekker J, Arendzen JH, de Bie RA, Bierma Zeinstra SMA, Helders PJM, Keus SHJ, Kwakkel G, Lenssen T, Oostendorp RAB, Ostelo RWJG, Reijman M, Terwee CB, Theunissen C, Thomas S, van Baar ME, van t Hul A, van Peppen RPS, Verhagen AP, van der Windt DAWM. Effectiveness of exercise therapy: a best evidence summary of systematic reviews. Aust J Physiother 2005;51:71–85

20. Walach H, Guthlin C, Konig M. Efficacy of massage therapy in chronic pain: a pragmatic randomized trial. J Altern Complement Med 2003;9:837–846

21. Gross AR, Hoving JL, Haines TA, Goldsmith CH, Kay T, Aker P, Bronfort G; Cervical Overview Group. A Cochrane review of manipulation and mobilization for mechanical neck disorders. Spine 2004;29:1541–1548

22. Sarigiovannis P, Hollins B. Effectiveness of manual therapy in the treatment of non-specific neck pain: a review. Phys Ther Rev 2005;10:35–50

23. Bronfort G, Haas M, Evans RL, Bouter LM. Efficacy of spinal manipulation and mobilization for low back pain and neck pain: a systematic review and best evidence synthesis. Spine J 2004;4:335–356

24. Haneline MT. Chiropractic manipulation and acute neck pain: a review of the evidence. J Manipulative Physiol Ther 2005;28:520–525

25. Dziedzic K, Hill J, Lewis M, Sim J, Daniels J, Hay EM. Effectiveness of manual therapy or pulsed shortwave diathermy in addition to advice and exercise for neck disorders: a pragmatic and randomized controlled trial in physical therapy clinics. Arthritis Rheum 2005;53:214–222

26. Cleland JA, Childs MJ, McRae M, Palmer JA, Stowell T. Immediate effects of thoracic manipulation in patients with neck pain: a randomized clinical trial. Manual Ther 2005;10:127–135

27. Palmgren PJ, Sandstrom PJ, Lundqvist FJ, Heikkila H. Improvement after chiropractic care in cervicocephalic kinesthetic sensibility and subjective pain intensity in patients with nontraumatic chronic neck pain. J Manipulative Physiol Ther 2006;29:100–106

28. McReynolds TM, Sheridan BJ. Intramuscular ketorolac versus osteopathic manipulative treatment in the management of acute neck pain in the emergency department: a randomized clinical trial. J Am Osteopath Assoc 2005;105:57–68

29. Li JX, Xiang CJ, Liu XQ. Clinical study on analgesic mechanism of bitongxiao in treating neck pain due to cervical spondylitis. [In Chinese.] Zhongguo Zhong Xi Yi Jie He Za Zhi 2001; 2197:516–518

30. Chow RT, Barnsley L. Systematic review of the literature of low-level laser therapy (LLLT) in the management of neck pain. Lasers Surg Med 2005;37:46–52

31. Sutbeyaz ST, Sezer N, Koseoglu BF. The effect of pulsed electromagnetic fields in the treatment of cervical osteoarthritis: a randomized, double-blind, sham-controlled trial. Rheumatol Int 2006;26:320–324

32. Gustavsson C, von Koch L. Applied relaxation in the treatment of long-lasting neck pain: a randomized controlled pilot study. J Rehabil Med 2006;38:100–107

33. Gerard S, Smith BH, Simpson JA. A randomized controlled trial of spiritual healing in restricted neck movement. J Altern Complement Med 2003;9:467–477

NEUROPATHIC/NEURALGIC PAIN

SYNONYMS

Nerve pain.

DEFINITION

Pain caused by a primary lesion or dysfunction in the nervous system. This can be peripheral or central neuropathic pain depending on whether the lesion or dysfunction affects the peripheral or central nervous system. Common causes are amputations, diabetes, multiple sclerosis, shingles and stroke. Neuropathic pain is often described by patients as burning, stabbing, tingling or numbing. Neuralgia is acute paroxysmal pain radiating along the course of one or more nerves usually without demonstrable changes in the nerve structure.

RELATED CONDITIONS

For lumbago see Back pain, p. 230.

CAM USAGE

Acupuncture, herbal medicine.

CLINICAL EVIDENCE

ACUPUNCTURE

A systematic review identified one RCT for post-herpetic neuropathy.[1] It reported that no analgesic benefit was associated with acupuncture compared with mock TENS. Another RCT found that neither acupuncture nor amitriptyline was more effective than placebo in relieving pain caused by human immunodeficiency virus-related peripheral neuropathy.[2] An RCT of 90 patients with primary trigeminal neuralgia compared two forms of acupuncture: deep needling and shallow routine needling both at local and distal acupoints.[3] The deep needling increased the therapeutic effect on trigeminal neuralgia.

ELECTROSTIMULATION

Three RCTs reported improvement of pain scores compared with baseline[4,5] and placebo[6] in patients with diabetic neuropathy using trans- or percutaneous electrical nerve stimulation. For patients suffering from hypersensitivity of the hand, differences were reported compared with placebo.[7]

HERBAL MEDICINE

A systematic review aimed to establish whether cannabis (*Cannabis sativa*) is an effective and safe treatment option in the management of all types of pain.[8] It found no RCTs that evaluated cannabis; all active substances tested were cannabinoids. The review concluded that, before cannabinoids can be considered for treating spasticity and neuropathic pain, further RCTs are needed. An RCT ($n = 66$) in patients with multiple sclerosis-related central neuropathic pain tested a whole-plant cannabis-based medicine delivered via an oromucosal spray.[9] Cannabis was superior to placebo in reducing mean pain intensity and was generally well tolerated, although more patients on cannabis reported dizziness, dry mouth and somnolence. For brachial plexus root avulsion a double-blind RCT reported no difference compared with placebo for mean pain severity.[10]

A double-blind RCT of geranium oil (*Pelargonium* spp.) for post-herpetic neuropathy reported a dose-dependent reduction in pain compared with placebo.[11]

A double-blind RCT ($n = 54$) of St John's wort (*Hypericum perforatum*) reported no effect on pain in polyneuropathy compared with placebo.[12]

MAGNETS

A systematic review of CAM treatments for diabetic neuropathy identified one RCT testing magnetised soles and reported reduction in numbness, tingling and burning compared with baseline.[13] Another systematic review aimed to assess the evidence of static magnets for pain relief.[14] It identified a further double-blind RCT for diabetic neuropathy, which reported reductions in pain, while beneficial effects were also reported in an RCT in patients with post-polio pain syndrome. An RCT testing electromagnetic neural stimulation reported a reduction in VAS pain scores compared with baseline.[15]

SUPPLEMENTS

Two RCTs of acetyl-L-carnitine for diabetic neuropathy suggested that it can give relief from pain.[16,17] Improvements were seen for chronic pain compared with placebo.

A systematic review identified six double-blind placebo-controlled trials ($n = 656$).[18] The relative benefit from topical capsaicin 0.075% compared with placebo was 1.4 (95% confidence interval 1.2–1.7) and the number needed to treat was 5.7 (4.0–10.0). It reported that for every six patients using topical capsaicin 0.075% for 8 weeks, one additional patient would benefit and concluded that it may be useful as an adjunct or sole therapy for some patients who are unresponsive to, or intolerant of, other treatments.

OTHER THERAPIES

Single trials showing positive results that require independent replication were reported for imagery,[19] whereas negative findings were reported for spiritual healing.[20]

OVERALL RECOMMENDATION

The evidence is not fully convincing for most CAM modalities in relieving neuropathic pain. However, for topically applied capsaicin, there is evidence of effectiveness. There is encouraging evidence for cannabis extract, magnetic insoles and electrostimulation.

Table 5.23 **Summary of clinical evidence for neuropathic/neuralgic pain**

Treatment	Weight of evidence	Direction of evidence	Serious safety concerns
Acupuncture	OO	→	Yes (see p. 96)
Electrostimulation	OO	↗	Yes (see p. 5)
Herbal medicine			
Cannabis	OO	↗	Yes (see p. 179)
Geranium	O	↗	Yes (see p. 5)
St John's wort	O	↘	Yes (see p. 5)
Magnets	OO	↗	Yes (see p. 164)
Supplements			
Acetyl-L-carnitine	OO	↗	Yes (see p. 5)
Capsaicin	OO	→	Yes (see p. 5)

SECTION FIVE

REFERENCES

1. Hempenstall K, Nurmikko TJ, Johnson RW, A'Hern RP, Rice AS. Analgesic therapy in postherpetic neuralgia: a quantitative systematic review. PLoS Med 2005;2:e164
2. Shlay JC, Chaloner K, Max MB, Flaws B, Reichelderfer P, Wentworth D, Hillman S, Brizz B, Cohn DL. Acupuncture and amitriptyline for pain due to HIV-related peripheral neuropathy: a randomized controlled trial. JAMA 1998;280:1590–1595
3. Zhang XY. Therapeutic effect of deep acupuncture at local acupoints on trigeminal neuralgia. Chin Acup Moxibustion 2005;25:549–550

4. Forst T, Nguyen M, Forst S, Disselhoff B, Pohlmann T, Pfutzner A. Impact of low frequency tran-scutaneous electrical nerve stimulation on symptomatic diabetic neuropathy using the new Salutaris device. Diabetes Nutr Metab 2004;17:163–168

5. Hamza MA, White PF, Craig WF, Ghoname ES, Ahmed HE, Proctor TJ, Noe CE, Vakharia AS, Gajraj N. Percutaneous electrical nerve stimulation: a novel analgesic therapy for diabetic neuropathic pain. Diabetes Care 2000;23:365–370

6. Kumar D, Marshall HJ. Diabetic peripheral neuropathy: amelioration of pain with transcutaneous electrostimulation. Diabetes Care 1997;20:1702–1705

7. Cheing GL, Luk ML. Transcutaneous electrical nerve stimulation for neuropathic pain. J Hand Surg 2005;30:50–55

8. Campbell FA, Tramer MR, Carroll D, Reynolds DJ, Moore RA, McQuay HJ. Are cannabinoids an effective and safe treatment option in the management of pain? A qualitative systematic review. BMJ 2001;323:13–16

9. Rog DJ, Nurmikko TJ, Friede T, Young CA. Randomized, controlled trial of cannabis-based medi-cine in central pain in multiple sclerosis. Neurology 2005;65:812–819

10. Berman JS, Symonds C, Birch R. Efficacy of two cannabis based medicinal extracts for relief of central neuropathic pain from brachial plexus avulsion: results of a randomised controlled trial. Pain 2004;112:299–306

11. Greenway FL, Frome BM, Engels TM 3rd, McLellan A. Temporary relief of postherpetic neuralgia pain with topical geranium oil. Am J Med 2003;115:586–587

12. Sindrup SH, Madsen C, Bach FW, Gram LF, Jensen TS. St John's wort has no effect on pain in polyneuropathy. Pain 2001;91:361–365

13. Huntley AL. CAM for the treatment of diabetic neuropathy. Focus Altern Complement Ther 2006;11:5–8

14. Eccles NK. A critical review of randomized controlled trials of static magnets for pain relief. J Altern Complement Med 2005;11:495–509

15. Bosi E, Conti M, Vermigli C, Cazzetta G, Peretti E, Cordoni MC, Galimberti G, Scionti L. Effectiveness of frequency-modulated electromagnetic neural stimulation in the treatment of painful diabetic neuropathy. Diabetologia 2005;48:817–823

16. Quatraro A, Roca P, Donzella C, Acampora R, Marfella R, Giugliano D. Acetyl-L-carnitine for symptomatic diabetic neuropathy. Diabetologia 1995;38:123

17. De Grandis D, Minardi C. Acetyl-L-carnitine (levacecarnine) in the treatment of diabetic neuropa-thy. A long-term, randomised, double-blind, placebo-controlled study. Drugs R D 2002;3:223–231

18. Liu JP, Manheimer E, Yang M. Herbal medicines for treating HIV infection and AIDS. The Cochrane Database of Systematic Reviews 2005, Issue 3. Art. No.: CD003937

19. Moseley GL. Graded motor imagery is effective for long-standing complex regional pain syn-drome: a randomised controlled trial. Pain 2004;108:192–198

20. Abbot NC, Harkness EF, Stevinson C, Marshall FP, Conn DA, Ernst E. Spiritual healing as a ther-apy for chronic pain: a randomized, clinical trial. Pain 2001;91:79–89

OSTEOARTHRITIS

SYNONYMS/SUBCATEGORIES

Degenerative arthritis, degenerative arthrosis, degenerative joint disease, hypertrophic arthritis, osteoarthrosis, gonarthrosis, coxarthrosis.

DEFINITION

Osteoarthritis is a condition for which the prevalence, risk factors, clinical manifestations and prognosis vary according to the joints affected. It most commonly affects hands, knees, hips and spinal apophyseal joints. It is usually defined by pathological or radiological crite-ria rather than clinical features, and is characterised by focal areas of damage to the cartilage surfaces of synovial joints, associated with remodeling of the underlying bone and mild syn-ovitis. When severe, there is characteristic joint-space narrowing and osteophyte formation, with visible subchondral bone changes on radiography.

Box 5.35 *Systematic review: acupuncture for peripheral joint osteoarthritis*[2]

- Eighteen RCTs were included
- Ten studies demonstrated greater pain reduction in acupuncture groups compared with controls
- Meta-analysis of three trials of manual acupuncture compared with sham acupuncture showed a significant effect (standardised mean difference 0.24, 95% CI 0.01 to 0.47, $P = 0.04$, $n = 329$)
- **Conclusion**: sham-controlled RCTs suggest that manual acupuncture has specific effects in reducing pain of osteoarthritis

CAM USAGE

In a US survey, 27% of people who described themselves as suffering from 'arthritis' had used CAM in the previous 12 months,[1] a third of them seeing a therapist. Acupuncture, massage, manipulation and homeopathy are the therapies most commonly used.

CLINICAL EVIDENCE

ACUPUNCTURE

Acupuncture is widely used for treating the pain of osteoarthritis. A systematic review identified evidence of efficacy of acupuncture for peripheral joint osteoarthritis (Box 5.35).[2] Ten trials tested manual acupuncture and eight trials tested electroacupuncture. The sham-controlled RCTs suggested that manual acupuncture has specific effects in reducing the pain of osteoarthritis. These findings are supported by systematic reviews assessing CAM therapies for osteoarthritis of the knee,[3] arthritis-related pain[4] and musculoskeletal pain.[5,6]

BALNEOTHERAPY

Balneotherapy or spa therapy is used to treat osteoarthritis, particularly in European countries. A Cochrane review[7] assessed the evidence and concluded that, although one cannot ignore the positive findings in most trials, firm statements about the efficacy of balneotherapy cannot be provided at present because of methodological flaws in the studies. For low back pain a meta-analysis concluded that, even though the data are scarce, there is some encouraging evidence suggesting that spa therapy and balneotherapy are effective.[8] Additional RCTs suggest beneficial effects of a balneotherapeutic regimen for the Lequesne index,[9] mud compresses for knee pain and the Lequesne index,[10] and a hydrotherapy-based strengthening programme for leg strength and distance walked.[11] The application of moist heat in the form of hot packs alone was found to be inferior to hot packs and chiropractic care.[12]

HERBAL MEDICINE

A Cochrane review assessed all placebo-controlled RCTs of herbal treatments for osteoarthritis.[13] Five trials of four different herbal interventions were identified. The data of the two studies testing avocado–soybean unsaponifiables were pooled and provided some positive evidence (Box 5.36). Another systematic review identified four double-blind, placebo-controlled RCTs of avocado–soybean unsaponifiables.[14] It concluded that the clinical evidence is, at present, not fully convincing.

A systematic review assessed the effects of devil's claw (*Harpagophytum procumbens*).[15] It included RCTs, quasi-RCTs and CCTs and concluded that there is limited evidence to support the use of an ethanolic extract containing <30 mg harpagoside per day in the treatment of knee and hip osteoarthritis. There is moderate evidence of effectiveness for the use

Box 5.36 *Systematic review: herbal therapy for osteoarthritis*[13]

- Five RCTs of four different herbal treatments were identified
- Two studies compared the effects of avocado/soybean unsaponifiables with placebo including 327 patients
- Both studies used 100-mm visual analogue scale for measuring pain. The weighted mean difference was -7.6, 95% CI -11.8 to -3.4)
- For the Lequesne's functional index the weighted mean difference was -1.7, 95% CI -2.4 to -1.0
- **Conclusion**: the current evidence for herbal treatment of osteoarthritis is generally sparse and therefore insufficient for a reliable assessment of efficacy

of a devil's claw powder containing 60 mg harpagoside in the treatment of osteoarthritis of the knee, hip and spine.

A systematic review assessed all RCTs of ginger (*Zingiber officinalis*).[16] It identified one double-blind RCT ($n = 56$), which reported no difference compared with placebo for pain and Lequesne index. A large ($n = 247$) double-blind RCT found a reduction in pain in the percentage of responders,[17] and another double-blind RCT reported no difference between a ginger extract and placebo after 3 months, but superiority over the placebo group at the end of 6 months.[18] A further double–blind RCT reported superiority of ginger extract and ibuprofen over placebo and no difference between ginger and ibuprofen.[19]

The efficacy of Phytodolor (a proprietary preparation which contains *Populus tremula*, *Fraxinus excelsior* and *Solidago virgaurea*) in painful arthritic conditions has been assessed in a number of studies. A systematic review identified at least six double-blind RCTs.[16] These trials suggest pain reduction, increase in mobility and a reduction in consumption of NSAIDs.

A systematic review of rose hip (*Rosa canina*) preparations identified four relevant RCTs and concluded that moderate evidence exists for the use of a powder of the seeds and husks of a rose hip subspecies in patients suffering from osteoarthritis.[20]

SKI 306X is a purified extract from a mixture of three herbs (*Clematis mandshurica*, *Trichosanthes kirilowii* and *Prunella vulgaris*). It was tested in patients with osteoarthritis of the knee and was found to be superior to placebo on both pain visual analogue scale and Lequesne index.[21] In a comparative trial against 300 mg diclofenac daily, the preparation showed similar effects on pain visual analogue scale.[22]

Single RCTs, which require independent replication, exist for willow bark (*Salix* spp),[23] Reumalex,[24] Tipi,[25] a herbomineral formulation[26] and Gitadyl.[27] Additional single RCTs are available for Eazmov,[28] stinging nettle (*Urtica dioica*),[29] boswellia (*Boswellia serrata*),[30] Duhuo Jisheng Wan[31] and Qianggu.[32]

HOMEOPATHY

A systematic review (Box 5.37) identified four trials of either oral or topically applied homeopathy, which were encouraging but insufficient to draw any conclusions for clinical practice.[33]

MAGNETS

Static magnets and electromagnetic fields are used to treat the symptoms of osteoarthritis. A Cochrane review assessed the evidence and found it limited (Box 5.38).[34] Further trials published since this review are available, which suggest some effects[35-38] but also include those which did not report a specific effect.[39-41]

Box 5.37 *Systematic review: homeopathy for osteoarthritis*[33]

- Four RCTs involving 406 patients with osteoarthritis were included
- All trials were of high quality
- Two positive and one negative comparisons with conventional oral drugs
- Topical homeopathic gel is no different in effect from conventional non-steroidal gel

Box 5.38 *Systematic review: magnetic fields for osteoarthritis*[34]

- Three RCTs including a total of 259 patients
- For pain relief the meta-analysis of two trials showed a standardised mean difference of -0.74, 95% CI -1.15 to -0.34
- Joint pain on motion improved (standardised mean difference -0.59, 95% CI -0.98 to -2.0)
- **Conclusion**: there is a need to confirm in larger trials whether the positive results point to clinically important benefits. The current limited evidence does not show a clinically important benefit for treating knee or cervical osteoarthritis

Box 5.39 *Meta-analysis: chondroitin sulphate for osteoarthritis*[43]

- Seven studies (372 patients) with duration of >3 months included
- Pain scores decreased progressively to 42% over the first 6 months of therapy (compared with 80% in placebo). Increased dosage did not result in better effectiveness
- Required daily dose of analgesic and NSAIDs was reduced
- **Conclusion**: evidence of clinically relevant efficacy of chondroitin sulphate on pain and function of knee and hip osteoarthritis, at least when given as an adjunct to standard analgesic and NSAIDs

PROLOTHERAPY

Prolotherapy uses injections of dextrose solutions, which causes a localised inflammation, increases the blood supply and is thought to stimulate tissue repair and pain relief. A systematic review concluded that there are limited high-quality data supporting the use of prolotherapy in the treatment of musculoskeletal pain or sport-related soft-tissue injuries.[42]

SUPPLEMENTS

A systematic review assessed all RCTs of capsaicin cream (0.025–0.075%).[16] It identified three double-blind RCTs ($n = 135$), which show beneficial effects on pain and articular tenderness. The meta-analysis of these data showed that it was better than placebo for treating osteoarthritis.

Chondroitin sulphate (Box 5.39)[43] and glucosamine (Box 5.40)[44] appear to be effective and have fewer adverse effects than NSAIDs. A meta-analysis[45] looked at data for both supplements and concluded that, although the effect sizes seen in the published studies are likely to be exaggerated by publication bias and quality issues, some degree of effectiveness appears probable for both preparations. A comprehensive meta-analysis suggested structural effectiveness for glucosamine and symptomatic effectiveness for glucosamine and chondroitin in knee osteoarthritis,[46] which is also supported for long-term treatment.[47] Further RCTs support this conclusion[48,49] although negative trials also exist, including one mega trial of 1583 patients.[50–52] Whether these supplements prevent further cartilage loss in patients is as yet not entirely clear.[53,54]

Green-lipped mussel (*Perna canaliculus*) was investigated in a double-blind controlled trial which included 28 rheumatoid and 38 osteoarthritis patients.[55] Full results are not given but 38% of those who received mussel improved compared with 14% of the placebo group. A further study by the same group[56] compared different preparations of mussel, again including patients with either rheumatoid or osteoarthritis. There were improvements in various outcomes in both groups. The evidence that green-lipped mussel has any effect in osteoarthritis is suggestive but not convincing.

The effectiveness of *S*-adenosylmethionine was assessed in a meta-analysis (Box 5.41).[57] There were beneficial effects when compared with placebo and it appears to be effective in reducing pain and in improving functional limitations.

Box 5.40 *Meta-analysis: glucosamine for osteoarthritis*[44]

- Twenty RCTs (*n* = 2570) included
- Analysis restricted to eight studies with adequate allocation concealment failed to show a benefit of glucosamine for pain and Western Ontario and McMaster Osteoarthritis Index (WOMAC) function
- Analysis of 10 RCTs testing the Rotta brand of glucosamine showed superiority for pain (standardised mean difference −1.31, 95% CI −1.99 to −0.64) and function using the Lequesne index (standardised mean difference −0.51, 95% CI −0.96 to −0.05) compared with placebo
- Comparing the Rotta brand of glucosamine with an NSAID, results were superior in two RCTs, and equivalent in two RCTs
- Glucosamine was as safe as placebo in terms of the number of subjects reporting adverse reactions
- **Conclusion**: results from studies using a non-Rotta preparation or adequate allocation concealment failed to show benefit in pain and WOMAC function while those studies evaluating the Rotta preparation show that glucosamine was superior to placebo in the treatment of pain and functional impairment resulting from symptomatic osteoarthritis

Box 5.41 *Meta-analysis: S-adenosylmethionine for osteoarthritis*[57]

- Eleven RCTs met the inclusion criteria
- When compared with placebo, *S*-adenosylmethionine is more effective in reducing functional limitation in patients with osteoarthritis (effect size 0.31, 95% CI 0.1 to 0.5)
- No effect for reducing pain (effect size 0.22, 95% CI −0.25 to 0.7) compared with placebo
- Compared with NSAIDs (pain: effect size 0.12, 95% CI −0.03 to 0.3; functional limitation: effect size 0.03, 95% CI −0.13 to 0.18)
- **Conclusion**: *S*-adenosylmethionine appears to be as effective as NSAIDs in reducing pain and improving functional limitation in patients with osteoarthritis without the adverse effects often associated with NSAID therapies

Further RCTs, which require independent replication, exist for vitamin E,[58] soy,[59] a milk-based micronutrient beverage[60] and Arthritis Relief Plus (also containing capsaicin 0.015%).[61]

TAI CHI

Similar to physical exercise, tai chi may be beneficial through maintaining balance and strength and through reducing the risk of falls. Two RCTs report less pain and stiffness in joints and improvements in physical functioning[62] as well as improved self-efficacy for arthritis symptoms.[63] Further trials are required for any recommendation to be made.

OTHER THERAPIES

Other RCTs, which require replication in independent trials, exist for hypnotherapy,[64] leech therapy,[65] music,[66] yoga,[67] imagery,[68] therapeutic touch[69] and biofeedback-assisted physical exercise.[70]

Table 5.24 **Summary of clinical evidence for osteoarthritis**

Treatment	Weight of evidence	Direction of evidence	Serious safety concerns
Acupuncture	OOO	↑	Yes (see p. 96)
Balneotherapy	OO	↗	Yes (see p. 126)
Herbal medicine			
Avocado–soybean unsaponifiables	OO	↗	Yes (see p. 178)
Boswellia serrata	O	↑	Yes (see p. 202)
Devil's claw	OO	↗	Yes (see p. 190)
Duhuo Jisheng Wan	O	↑	Yes (see p. 5)
Eazmov	O	↘	Yes (see p. 5)
Ginger	OO	↗	Yes (see p. 195)
Gitadyl	O	↑	Yes (see p. 5)
Herbomineral formulation	O	↗	Yes (see p. 5)
Phytodolor	OOO	↑	Yes (see p. 5)
Qianggu	O	↗	Yes (see p. 5)
Reumalex	O	↗	Yes (see p. 5)
Rose hip	OO	↗	Yes (see p. 5)
SKI 306X	OO	↑	Yes (see p. 5)
Stinging nettle	O	↑	Yes (see p. 207)
Tipi	O	↓	Yes (see p. 5)
Willow bark	O	↑	Yes (see p. 216)
Homeopathy	OO	↗	No (see p. 124)
Magnets	OO	↗	No (see p. 164)
Prolotherapy	OO	→	Yes (see p. 5)
Supplements			
Arthritis Relief Plus	O	↑	Yes (see p. 5)
Capsaicin	OO	↑	Yes (see p. 5)
Chondroitin	OOO	°	Yes (see p. 186)
Glucosamine	OOO	↗	Yes (see p. 197)
Green-lipped mussel	O	↗	Yes (see p. 199)
Micronutrient beverage	O	↑	Yes (see p. 5)
S-adenosylmethionine	OOO	↑	Yes (see p. 212)
Soy	O	↗	Yes (see p. 5)
Vitamin E	O	↓	Yes (see p. 5)
Tai chi	OO	↑	No (see p. 167)

OVERALL RECOMMENDATION

There is evidence to suggest that acupuncture is effective for pain control. Whether it is superior to conventional treatment is unclear. Other interventions with good evidence of effectiveness are the supplements chondroitin, glucosamine, *S*-adenosylmethionine and the herbal mixture phytodolor. Considering the favourable safety profile, balneotherapy and tai chi seem to be options worthy of consideration. For all other interventions more evidence is needed before firm recommendations can be made.

REFERENCES

1. Eisenberg DM, Davis R, Ettner SL, Appel S, Wilkey S, Rompay MV. Trends in alternative medicine use in the United States, 1990–1997. JAMA 1998;280:1569–1575
2. Kwon YD, Pittler MH, Ernst E. Acupuncture for peripheral joint osteoarthritis. A systematic review and meta-analysis. 2006;45:1331–1337
3. Ezzo J, Hadhazy V, Birch S, Lao L, Kaplan G, Hochberg M, Berman B. Acupuncture for osteoarthritis of the knee: a systematic review. Arthritis Rheum 2001;44:819–825
4. Soeken KL. Selected CAM therapies for arthritis-related pain: the evidence from systematic reviews. Clin J Pain 2004;20:13–18
5. Ernst E. Musculoskeletal conditions and complementary/alternative medicine. Best Pract Res Clin Rheumatol 2004;18:539–556
6. Weiner DK, Ernst E. Complementary and alternative approaches to the treatment of persistent musculoskeletal pain. Clin J Pain 2004;20:244–255
7. Verhagen AP, de Vet HC, de Bie RA, Kessels AG, Boers M, Knipschild PG. Balneotherapy for rheumatoid arthritis and osteoarthritis. The Cochrane Database of Systematic Reviews 2000, Issue 2. Art. No.: CD000518
8. Pittler MH, Karagulle MZ, Karagulle M, Ernst E. Spa therapy and balneotherapy for treating low back pain: meta-analysis of randomized trials. Rheumatology 2006;45:880–884
9. Sukenik S, Flusser D, Codish S, Abu-Shakra M. Balneotherapy at the Dead Sea area for knee osteoarthritis. Isr Med Assoc J 1999;1:83–85
10. Flusser D, Abu Shakra M, Friger M, Codish S, Sukenik S. Therapy with mud compresses for knee osteoarthritis. Comparison of natural mud preparations with mineral-depleted mud. J Clin Rheumatol 2002;8:197–203
11. Foley A, Halbert J, Hewitt T, Crotty M. Does hydrotherapy improve strength and physical function in patients with osteoarthritis – a randomised controlled trial comparing a gym based and a hydrotherapy based strengthening programme. Ann Rheum Dis 2003;62:1162–1167
12. Beyerman KL, Palmerino MB, Zohn LE, Kane GM, Foster KA. Efficacy of treating low back pain and dysfunction secondary to osteoarthritis: chiropractic care compared with moist heat alone. J Manipulative Physiol Ther 2006;29:107–114
13. Little CV, Parsons T, Logan S. Herbal therapy for treating osteoarthritis. The Cochrane Database of Systematic Reviews 2000, Issue 4. Art. No.: CD002947
14. Ernst E. Avocado-soybean unsaponifiables (ASU) for osteoarthritis – a systematic review. Clin Rheumatol 2003;22:285–288
15. Gagnier JJ, Chrubasik S, Manheimer E. *Harpagophytum procumbens* for osteoarthritis and low back pain: a systematic review. BMC Complement Altern Med 2004;4:13
16. Long L, Soeken K, Ernst E. Herbal medicines for the treatment of osteoarthritis: a systematic review. Rheumatology 2001;40:779–793
17. Altman RD, Marcussen KC. Effects of a ginger extract on knee pain in patients with osteoarthritis. Arthritis Rheum 2001;44:2531–2538
18. Wigler I, Grotto I, Caspi D, Yaron M. The effects of Zintona EC (a ginger extract) on symptomatic gonarthritis. Osteoarthritis Cartilage 2003;11:783–789
19. Haghighi M, Khalvat A, Toliat T, Jallaei S. Comparing the effects of ginger (*Zingiber officinale*) extract and ibuprofen on patients with osteoarthritis. Arch Iran Med 2005; 8:267–271
20. Chrubasik C, Duke RK, Chrubasik S. The evidence for clinical efficacy of rose hip and seed: a systematic review. Phytother Res 2006;20:1–3
21. Jung YB, Roh KJ, Jung JA, Jung K, Yoo H, Cho YB, Kwak WJ, Kim DK, Kim KH, Han CK. Effect of SKI 306X, a new herbal anti-arthritic agent, in patients with osteoarthritis of the knee: a double-blind placebo controlled study. Am J Chin Med 2001;29:485–491

22. Lung YB, Seong SC, Lee MC, Shin YU, Kim DH, Kim JM, Jung YK, Ahn JH, Seo JG, Park YS, Lee CS, Roh KJ, Han CK, Cho YB, Chang DY, Kwak WJ, Jung KO, Park BJ. A four-week, randomized, double-blind trial of the efficacy and safety of SKI306X: a herbal anti-arthritic agent versus diclofenac in osteoarthritis of the knee. Am J Chin Med 2004; 32:291–301

23. Biegert C, Wagner I, Ludtke R, Kotter I, Lohmuller C, Gunaydin I, Taxis K, Heide L. Efficacy and safety of willow bark extract in the treatment of osteoarthritis and rheumatoid arthritis: results of 2 randomized double-blind controlled trials. J Rheumatol 2004; 31:2121–2130

24. Mills SY, Jacoby RK, Chacksfield M, Willoughby M. Effect of a proprietary herbal medicine on the relief of chronic arthritic pain: a double-blind study. Br J Rheumatol 1996; 35:874–878

25. Bosi Ferraz M, Borges Pereira R, Iwata NM, Atra E. Tipi. A popular analgesic tea: a double-blind cross-over trial in arthritis. Clin Exper Rheumatol 1991;9:205–212

26. Kulkarni RR, Patki PS, Jog VP, Gandage SG, Patwardhan B. Treatment of osteoarthritis with a herbomineral formulation: a double-blind, placebo-controlled, cross-over study. J Ethnopharmacol 1991;33:91–95

27. Ryttig K, Schlamowitz PV, Warnoe O, Wilstrup F. Gitadyl versus ibuprofen in patients with osteoarthrosis. The result of a double-blind, randomized cross-over study. Ugeskrift for Laeger 1991;153:2298–2299

28. Biswas NR, Biswas K, Pandey M, Pandy RM. Treatment of osteoarthritis, rheumatoid arthritis and non-specific arthritis with a herbal drug: a double-blind, active drug controlled parallel study. JK Pract 1998;5:129–132

29. Randall C, Randall H, Dobbs F, Hutton C, Sanders H. Randomized controlled trial of nettle sting for treatment of base-of-thumb pain. J R Soc Med 2000;93:305–309

30. Kimmatkar N, Thawani V, Hingorani L, Khiyani R. Efficacy and tolerability of *Boswellia serrata* extract in treatment of osteoarthritis of knee – a randomized double blind placebo controlled trial. Phytomedicine 2003;10:3–7

31. Teekachunhatean S, Kunanusorn P, Rojanasthien N, Sananpanich K, Pojchamarnwiputh S, Lhieochaiphunt S, Pruksakorn S. Chinese herbal recipe versus diclofenac in symptomatic treatment of osteoarthritis of the knee: a randomized controlled trial. BMC Complement Altern Med 2004;4:19

32. Ruan XY, Liu YL, Peng ZL, Ji Y, Chen BY. Effect of qianggu capsule on the effective range of motion of knee joint in postmenopausal women with knee osteoarthritis. Chin J Clin Rehab 2005;9:170–171

33. Long L, Ernst E. Homeopathic remedies for the treatment of osteoarthritis: a systematic review. Br Homeopath J 2001;90:37–43

34. Hulme JM, Judd MG, Robinson VA, Tugwell P, Wells G, de Bie RA. Electromagnetic fields for the treatment of osteoarthritis. The Cochrane Database of Systematic Reviews 2002, Issue 1. Art. No.: CD003523

35. Battisti E, Piazza E, Rigato M, Nuti R, Bianciardi L, Scribano A, Giordano N. Efficacy and safety of a musically modulated electromagnetic field (TAMMEF) in patients affected by knee osteoarthritis. Clin Exp Rheumatol 2004;22:568–572

36. Nicolakis P, Kollmitzer J, Crevenna R, Bittner C, Erdogmus CB, Nicolakis J. Pulsed magnetic field therapy for osteoarthritis of the knee – a double-blind sham-controlled trial. Wien Klin Wochenschr 2002;114:678–684

37. Hinman MR, Ford J, Heyl H. Effects of static magnets on chronic knee pain and physical function: a double-blind study. Altern Ther Health Med 2002;8:50–55

38. Fischer G, Pelka RB, Barovic J. Adjuvant treatment of knee osteoarthritis with weak pulsing magnetic fields. Results of a placebo-controlled prospective clinical trial. Z Orthop Ihre Grenzgeb 2005;143:544–550

39. Harlow T, Greaves C, White A, Brown L, Hart A, Ernst E. Randomised controlled trial of magnetic bracelets for relieving pain in osteoarthritis of the hip and knee. BMJ 2004;329:1450–1454

40. Wolsko PM, Eisenberg DM, Simon LS, Davis RB, Walleczek J, Mayo-Smith M, Kaptchuk TJ, Phillips RS. Double-blind placebo-controlled trial of static magnets for the treatment of osteoarthritis of the knee: results of a pilot study. Altern Ther Health Med 2004; 10:36–43

41. Sutbeyaz ST, Sezer N, Koseoglu BF. The effect of pulsed electromagnetic fields in the treatment of cervical osteoarthritis: a randomized, double-blind, sham-controlled trial. Rheumatol Int 2006;26:320–324

42. Rabago D, Best TM, Beamsley M, Patterson J. A systematic review of prolotherapy for chronic musculoskeletal pain. Clin J Sport Med 2005;15:376–380

43. Leeb BF, Schweitzer H, Montag K, Smolen JS. A metaanalysis of chondroitin sulfate in the treatment of osteoarthritis. J Rheumatol 2000;27:205–211

44. Towheed TE, Anastassiades TP, Shea B, Houpt J, Welch V, Hochberg MC. Glucosamine therapy for treating osteoarthritis. The Cochrane Database of Systematic Reviews 2000, Issue 2. Art. No.: CD002946

45. McAlindon TE, LaValley MP, Gulin JP, Felson DT. Glucosamine and chondroitin for treatment of osteoarthritis. JAMA 2005;283:1469–1475

46. Richy F, Bruyere O, Ethgen O, Cucherat M, Henrotin Y, Reginster JY. Structural and symptomatic efficacy of glucosamine and chondroitin in knee osteoarthritis: a comprehensive meta-analysis. Arch Intern Med 2003;163:1514–1522

47. Poolsup N, Suthisisang C, Channark P, Kittikulsuth W. Glucosamine long-term treatment and the progression of knee osteoarthritis: systematic review of randomized controlled trials. Ann Pharmacother 2005;39:1080–1087

48. Uebelhart D, Malaise M, Marcolongo R, DeVathaire F, Piperno M, Mailleux E, Fioravanti A, Matoso L, Vignon E. Intermittent treatment of knee osteoarthritis with oral chondroitin sulfate: a one-year, randomized, double-blind, multicenter study versus placebo. Osteoarthritis Cartilage 2004;12:269–276

49. Cohen M, Wolfe R, Mai T, Lewis D. A randomized, double blind, placebo controlled trial of a topical cream containing glucosamine sulfate, chondroitin sulfate, and camphor for osteoarthritis of the knee. J Rheumatol 2003;30:523–528. Erratum in: J Rheumatol 2003;30:2512

50. Cibere J, Kopec JA, Thorne A, Singer J, Canvin J, Robinson DB, Pope J, Hong P, Grant E, Esdaile JM. Randomized, double-blind, placebo-controlled glucosamine discontinuation trial in knee osteoarthritis. Arthritis Rheum 2004;51:738–745

51. McAlindon T, Formica M, LaValley M, Lehmer M, Kabbara K. Effectiveness of glucosamine for symptoms of knee osteoarthritis: results from an internet-based randomized double-blind controlled trial. Am J Med 2004;117:643–649

52. Clegg DO, Reda DJ, Harris CL, Klein MA, O'Dell JR, Hooper MM, Bradley JD, Bingham CO 3rd, Weisman MH, Jackson CG, Lane NE, Cush JJ, Moreland LW, Schumacher HR Jr, Oddis CV, Wolfe F, Molitor JA, Yocum DE, Schnitzer TJ, Furst DE, Sawitzke AD, Shi H, Brandt KD, Moskowitz RW, Williams HJ. Glucosamine, chondroitin sulfate, and the two in combination for painful knee osteoarthritis. N Engl J Med 2006;354:795–808

53. Cibere J, Thorne A, Kopec JA, Singer J, Canvin J, Robinson DB, Pope J, Hong P, Grant E, Lobanok T, Ionescu M, Poole AR, Esdaile JM. Glucosamine sulfate and cartilage type II collagen degradation in patients with knee osteoarthritis: randomized discontinuation trial results employing biomarkers. J Rheumatol 2005;32:896–902

54. Michel BA, Stucki G, Frey D, De Vathaire F, Vignon E, Bruehlmann P, Uebelhart D. Chondroitins 4 and 6 sulfate in osteoarthritis of the knee: a randomized, controlled trial. Arthritis Rheum 2005;52:779–786

55. Gibson RG, Gibson SLM, Conway V, Chappell D. *Perna canaliculus* in the treatment of arthritis. Practitioner 1980;224:955–960

56. Gibson SLM, Gibson RG. The treatment of arthritis with a lipid extract of *Perna canaliculus*: a randomised trial. Complement Ther Med 1998;6:122–126

57. Soeken KL, Lee WL, Bausell RB, Agelli M, Berman BM. Safety and efficacy of S-adenosylmethionine (SAMe) for osteoarthritis. J Fam Pract 2002;51:425–430

58. Wluka AE, Stuckey S, Brand C, Cicuttini FM. Supplementary vitamin E does not affect the loss of cartilage volume in knee osteoarthritis: a 2 year double blind randomized placebo controlled study. J Rheumatol 2002;29:2585–2591

59. Arjmandi BH, Khalil DA, Lucas EA, Smith BJ, Sinichi N, Hodges SB, Juma S, Munson ME, Payton ME, Tivis RD, Svanborg A. Soy protein may alleviate osteoarthritis symptoms. Phytomedicine 2004;11:567–575

60. Colker CM, Swain M, Lynch L, Gingerich DA. Effects of a milk-based bioactive micronutrient beverage on pain symptoms and activity of adults with osteoarthritis: a double-blind, placebo-controlled clinical evaluation. Nutrition 2002;18:388–392

61. Gemmell HA, Jacobson BH, Hayes BM. Effect of a topical herbal cream on osteoarthritis of the hand and knee: a pilot study. J Manipulative Physiol Ther 2003;26:e15

62. Song R, Lee EO, Lam P, Bae SC. Effects of tai chi exercise on pain, balance, muscle strength, and perceived difficulties in physical functioning in older women with osteoarthritis: a randomized clinical trial. J Rheumatol 2003;30:2039–2044

63. Hartman CA, Manos TM, Winter C, Hartman DM, Li B, Smith JC. Effects of T'ai Chi training on function and quality of life indicators in older adults with osteoarthritis. J Am Geriatr Soc 2000;48:1553–1559

64. Gay MC, Philippot P, Luminet O. Differential effectiveness of psychological interventions for reducing osteoarthritis pain: a comparison of Erikson [correction of Erickson] hypnosis and Jacobson relaxation. Eur J Pain 2002;6:1–16

65. Michalsen A, Klotz S, Lüdtke R, Moebus S, Spahn G, Dobos GJ. Effectiveness of leech therapy in osteoarthritis of the knee: a randomized, controlled trial. Ann Intern Med 2003;139:724–730

66. McCaffrey R, Freeman E. Effect of music on chronic osteoarthritis pain in older people. J Adv Nurs 2003;44:517–524

67. Garfinkel MS, Schumacher HR, Husain A, Levy M, Reshetar RA. Evaluation of a yoga based regimen for treatment of osteoarthritis of the hands. J Rheumatol 1994;21:2341–2343

68. Baird CL, Sands L. A pilot study of the effectiveness of guided imagery with progressive muscle relaxation to reduce chronic pain and mobility difficulties of osteoarthritis. Pain Manag Nurs 2004;5:97–104

69. Eckes Peck SD. The effectiveness of therapeutic touch for decreasing pain in elders with degenerative arthritis. J Holistic Nurs 1997;15:176–198

70. Durmus D, Alayli G, Cantürk F. Effects of biofeedback assisted isometric exercise and electrical stimulation on pain, anxiety and depression scores in knee osteoarthritis. Turk Fiz Tip Rehab Derg 2005;51:142–145

OTITIS MEDIA

SYNONYMS/SUBCATEGORIES

Middle ear infection, purulent or suppurative otitis media.

DEFINITION

Infection of the middle ear, mostly of bacterial aetiology.

RELATED CONDITIONS

Infections of other parts of the ear, glue ear.

CAM USAGE

Otitis media is a common and painful, often recurring, condition affecting 65–95% of all children between birth and the age of 7. Many CAM interventions are promoted yet the prevalence of its use is unknown. Mothers using CAM for themselves are, however, known to try CAM for their children when they are ill.

CLINICAL EVIDENCE

Several reviews of the subject are available.[1,2]

ANTHROPOSOPHICAL MEDICINE

A non-randomised multicentre study compared 715 patients suffering from acute respiratory or ear infections consulting anthroposophical doctors with 301 patients who saw a conventional physician for the same condition.[3] Improvements were noted within 24 hours in 31% of the former and 17% of the latter group. These seemingly encouraging results could, however, be the result of selection bias and require confirmation in a randomised trial.

SECTION FIVE

HERBAL MEDICINE

Herbal ear drops containing four different plant extracts (Otikon Otic Solution) were compared to ear drops containing a local anaesthetic in an RCT of 103 children complaining of ear pain.[4] The results show beneficial effects on ear pain for both treatments. A slightly larger RCT ($n = 171$) employed a similar herbal mixture and compared it with anaesthetic ear drops with or without amoxicillin.[5] The results for ear pain were best in the groups receiving the herbal drops. An open non-randomised study suggested that a mixture of herbal extracts and homeopathic medicines has a similar effect to standard care but is better tolerated.[6] Encouraging findings also emerged from clinical trials testing the usefulness of Chinese herbal mixtures.[7–9]

HOMEOPATHY

Seventy-five children with acute otitis media were randomised to receive either individualised homeopathic remedies or placebo for 5 days.[10] The rates of treatment failures showed no differences but daily scores favoured the homeopathic approach. The findings of an earlier non-randomised study suggested that homeopathic treatment is superior to standard care.[11]

SPINAL MANIPULATION

A systematic review found no good RCT evidence that chiropractic spinal manipulation is an effective treatment for otitis media.[12] A small ($n = 57$) observational study suggested that osteopathic spinal manipulation may be a useful adjunct to prevent episodes of otitis media in children who suffer from this problem frequently.[13]

SUPPLEMENTS

A small observational study suggested that the intake of a multivitamin mineral supplement is associated with less antibiotic use during one otitis media session.[14] The birch-derived polyol sugar xylitol was tested in an RCT involving 306 children for the prevention of otitis media. The results suggest that, compared to placebo, regular xylitol consumption was associated with fewer episodes of otitis media.[15] This finding was confirmed in a subsequent RCT with 811 children.[16]

OVERALL RECOMMENDATION

There is no compelling trial evidence that any CAM approach is effective in alleviating the pain or other symptoms of otitis media. Xylitol may be effective in preventing otitis media but independent replication of these data seems necessary.

Table 5.25 **Summary of clinical evidence for otitis media**

Treatment	Weight of evidence	Direction of evidence	Serious safety concerns
Anthroposophical medicine	O	↗	No (see p. 5)
Herbal medicine	OO	↗	Yes (see p. 120)
Homeopathy	O	→	No (see p. 124)
Spinal manipulation	O	↘	Yes (see p. 112)
Supplements			
Multivitamin mineral	O	↗	Yes (see p. 5)
Xylitol	OO	↑	Yes (see p. 5)

REFERENCES

1. Yarnell E. Medicinal herbs for otitis media. Altern Complement Ther 1997;10:350–354
2. Cosford R. Otitis media. Complement Med 2004;16–22
3. Hamre HJ, Fischer M, Heger M, Riley D, Haidvogl M, Baars E, Bristol E, Evans M, Schwarz R, Kiene H. Anthroposophic vs. conventional therapy of acute respiratory and ear infections: a prospective outcomes study. Wien Klin Wochenschr 2005;117:256–268
4. Sarrell EM, Mandelberg A, Cohen HA. Efficacy of naturopathic extracts in the management of ear pain associated with acute otitis media. Arch Pediatr Adolesc Med 2001; 155:796–799
5. Sarrell EM, Cohen HA, Kahan E. Naturopathic treatment for ear pain in children. Pediatrics 2003;111:e574–579
6. Wustrow TP; Otovowen Study Group. Alternative versus conventional treatment strategy in uncomplicated acute otitis media in children: a prospective, open, controlled parallel-group comparison. Int J Clin Pharmacol Ther 2004;42:110–119
7. Li KY, Zhao NJ, Zhu JC. Clinical observation on treatment of chronic suppurative otitis media caused large tympanic membranes perforation by ear-dropping with combined Chinese and Western drugs. [In Chinese.] Zhongguo Zhong Xi Yi Jie He Za Zhi 2004;24: 989–991
8. Xu Y, Yu J, Song Q. Clinical and experimental study on treatment of chronic pyogenic tympanitis with shenlian ear-drops. [In Chinese.] Zhongguo Zhong Xi Yi Jie He Za Zhi 1999;19:477–480
9. Liao Y, Huang Y, Ou Y. Clinical and experimental study of Tongqiao tablet in treating catarrhal otitis media. [In Chinese.] Zhongguo Zhong Xi Yi Jie He Za Zhi 1998;18:668–670
10. Jacobs J, Springer DA, Crothers D. Homeopathic treatment of acute otitis media in children. Pediatr Infect Dis J 2001;20:177–183
11. Friese KH, Kruse S, Ludtke R, Moeller H. The homoeopathic treatment of otitis media in children – comparisons with conventional therapy. Int J Clin Pharmacol Ther 1997;35: 296–301
12. Ernst E. Chiropractic manipulation for non-spinal pain. NZ Med J 2003;116:U539
13. Mills MV, Henley CE, Barnes LL, Carreiro JE, Degenhardt BF. The use of osteopathic manipulative treatment as adjuvant therapy in children with recurrent acute otitis media. Arch Pediatr Adolesc Med 2003;157:861–866
14. Linday LA, Dolitsky JN, Shindledecker RD, Pippenger CE. Lemon-flavored cod liver oil and a multivitamin-mineral supplement for the secondary prevention of otitis media in young children: pilot research. Ann Otol Rhinol Laryngol 2002;111:642–652
15. Uhari M, Kontiokari T, Koskela M, Niemela M. Xylitol chewing gum in prevention of acute otitis media: double blind randomised trial. BMJ 1996;313:1180–1184
16. Uhari M, Kontiokari T, Niemela M. A novel use of xylitol sugar in preventing acute otitis media. Pediatrics 1998;102:879–884

PERI-OPERATIVE PAIN

SYNONYMS/SUBCATEGORIES

Surgical pain.

DEFINITION

Pain experienced before, during or after surgical interventions.

RELATED CONDITIONS

Procedural pain (see p. 312).

CAM USAGE

No prevalence figures seem to be available. Incidence of CAM use is likely to reflect that of the general population except for the CAM treatments that some people may take specifically for recovery after surgery, e.g. homeopathic arnica.

SECTION FIVE

CLINICAL EVIDENCE
ACUPUNCTURE

A systematic review[1] of all RCTs of acupuncture during the peri-operative period included 19 such studies. It failed to find conclusive evidence that acupuncture is effective for pain control during surgery (Box 5.42). RCTs of acupuncture for post-operative pain have generated both positive[2] and negative[3] results. Another systematic review[4] focused on acupuncture for dental pain. It found reasonably good evidence that acupuncture alleviates pain after dental operations.

HERBAL MEDICINE

Lubrication of endotracheal tubes with a chamomile (*Matricaria recutita*) extract was shown to be better than standard procedures in preventing post-operative sore throats in 161 surgical patients.[5]

An ointment with herbal arnica (*Arnica montana*) was compared to placebo in an RCT with 37 patients undergoing carpal tunnel release surgery;[6] 2 weeks after the operation patients receiving arnica complained of less pain than those in the placebo group.

HOMEOPATHY

The most recent systematic review included 20 CCTs of homeopathic arnica (*Arnica montana*) for peri-operative pain. Collectively their data failed to convincingly demonstrate effectiveness.[7] Individualised homeopathic prescriptions also did not generate better pain reduction than placebo in a placebo-controlled, crossover RCT with 24 patients after oral surgery.[8]

HYPNOTHERAPY

A systematic review and a meta-analysis (Box 5.43) of hypnotherapy used as an adjunct to standard care found good evidence to show that this technique is useful in post-operative pain management.[9,10] These beneficial effects also seem to extend to self-hypnosis.[11]

IMAGERY

An RCT compared peri-operative imagery plus standard care to standard care alone.[12] Its results demonstrated that the median increase in the worst pain following surgery was lower

Box 5.42 *Systematic review: acupuncture for pain during surgery*[1]

- Nineteen RCTs were included
- Methodological quality was mixed
- Seven RCTs suggested that acupuncture is effective as an adjunctive intervention during surgery
- Of nine high-quality RCTs only two suggested efficacy
- **Conclusion**: the evidence is inconclusive

Box 5.43 *Systematic review: hypnotherapy for post-operative pain*[10]

- Twenty controlled clinical trials were included
- Methodological quality was variable and often poor
- Hypnotherapy was associated with better outcomes, including less pain
- **Conclusion**: data strongly support the use of hypnosis with surgical patients

with imagery. Similarly encouraging findings were reported in an RCT with 73 children undergoing tonsillectomy,[13] an RCT with 208 patients having surgery for primary inguinal hernia or goiter[14] and an RCT with 86 patients after colorectal surgery.[15] More recently a three-armed RCT failed to show that either imagery or progressive muscle relaxation were effective in reducing pain after colorectal resections.[16]

MASSAGE

An RCT compared foot massage and standard care with standard care alone in 59 patients undergoing laparoscopic sterilisation.[17] The results failed to show relevant effects on pain. Mechanical abdominal wall massage was compared to no such adjunctive treatment in an RCT with 25 patients undergoing colectomy.[18] Massage was associated with less post-operative pain and less analgesic consumption. Swedish massage was compared to no such adjunctive treatment in an RCT of 105 women undergoing abdominal surgery.[19] Massage was more effective in alleviating post-operative pain than standard care alone. A similar RCT ($n = 202$) showed that patients receiving massage perceived a decline of the unpleasantness of post-operative pain.[20] An RCT ($n = 59$) showed that women who were taught a simple arm massage have less pain after lymph node resection than patients who did not use this technique.[21]

MUSIC THERAPY

An RCT with 60 post-operative patients failed to show an effect of listening to music on pain perception.[22] Similar results were obtained from an RCT with 84 patients who used either music therapy, relaxation, a combination of these or none of the adjunctive treatments after their operation.[23] Another RCT suggested that music reduces the distress of post-operative pain and showed that the choice of music is culturally determined.[24] A double-blind RCT with 90 patients undergoing hysterectomy found that intra-operative music under general anaesthesia was associated with less pain after surgery and earlier mobilisation.[25] This result was later confirmed in a follow-up RCT with 151 patients undergoing inguinal hernia repair.[26] An RCT with 61 patients undergoing open heart surgery suggested that listening to calming music was more effective in reducing post-operative pain than simple resting or having no such adjunctive intervention.[27] A further RCT suggested that music therapy plus standard care is more effective than standard care alone in reducing pain after laparoscopic gynaecological operations.[28]

RELAXATION

A systematic review of relaxation techniques included seven RCTs involving a total of 362 patients.[29] Three of these studies showed positive effects on sensation or distress of pain while four studies failed to demonstrate such benefits. Most studies suffered from methodological inadequacies. More recent RCTs have generated positive results[30-33] in terms of pain management in post-operative patients. One RCT, however, failed to show a reduction of analgesic use with relaxation as an adjunctive therapy after elective cholecystectomy.[34]

TRANSCUTANEOUS ELECTRICAL NERVE STIMULATION (TENS)

A meta-analysis including 21 placebo-controlled RCTs generated positive evidence for the efficacy of peri-operative TENS.[35] On average, analgesic consumption was reduced by 36%.

OTHER THERAPIES

EMG biofeedback was tested in an RCT with 12 patients after abdominal surgery.[36] Its results suggest that biofeedback can reduce post-operative pain in this situation. Oral proteolytic enzymes (Wobenzym) have generated encouraging results on post-operative pain in an RCT ($n = 80$).[37] An RCT of a purified flavonoid supplement with 60 patients after haemorrhoidopexy demonstrated no reduction of post-operative pain.[38] An RCT with 130 patients undergoing abdominal surgery suggested that reflexology alleviated post-operative pain.[39] An RCT of spinal manipulation after knee or hip arthroplasty failed to show positive effects on analgesic use compared to sham treatment.[40] A sham-controlled RCT of therapeutic touch found no effect of this intervention on post-operative pain.[41]

OVERALL RECOMMENDATION

A wide range of CAM treatments have been shown to be potentially useful adjuncts to standard peri-operative pain management. The most promising approaches included acupuncture, imagery, hypnotherapy, massage, music therapy, relaxation and TENS. None of these approaches should be used as an alternative to conventional peri-operative care.

Table 5.26 **Summary of clinical evidence for peri-operative pain**

Treatment	Weight of evidence	Direction of evidence	Serious safety concerns
Acupuncture	OOO	↗	Yes (see p. 96)
Herbal medicine			
Chamomile	O	↗	Yes (see p. 5)
Arnica ointment	O	↗	Yes (see p. 176)
Homeopathy	OO	↓	No (see p. 124)
Hypnotherapy	OOO	↑	No (see p. 130)
Imagery	OO	↗	No (see p. 132)
Massage	OOO	↗	No (see p. 137)
Music therapy	OOO	↗	No (see p. 142)
Relaxation	OOO	↗	No (see p. 158)
TENS	OOO	↑	No (see p. 5)

REFERENCES

1. Lee H, Ernst E. Acupuncture analgesia during surgery: a systematic review. Pain 2005;114: 511–517
2. Felhendler D, Lisander B. Pressure on acupoints decreases postoperative pain. Clin J Pain 1996; 12:326–329
3. Sakurai M, Suleman MI, Morioka N, Akca O, Sessler DI. Minute sphere acupressure does not reduce postoperative pain or morphine consumption. Anesth Analg 2003;96:493–497
4. Ernst E, Pittler MH. The effectiveness of acupuncture in treating acute dental pain: a systematic review. Br Dent J 1998;184:443–447
5. Charuluxananan S, Sumethawattana P, Kosawiboonpol R, Somboonviboon W, Werawataganon T. Effectiveness of lubrication of endotracheal tube cuff with chamomile-extract for prevention of postoperative sore throat and hoarseness. J Med Assoc Thai 2004;87(Suppl. 2):S185–S189
6. Jeffrey SL, Belcher HJ. Use of Arnica to relieve pain after carpal-tunnel release surgery. Altern Ther Health Med 2002;8:66–68
7. Lüdtke R, Hacke D. On the effectiveness of the homeopathic remedy *Arnica montana*. [In German.] Wien Med Wochenschr 2005;155:482–490
8. Lokken P, Straumsheim PA, Tveiten D, Skjelbred P, Borchgrevink CF. Effect of homeopathy on pain and other events after acute trauma: placebo controlled trial with bilateral oral surgery. BMJ 1995;310:1439–1442
9. Hauser W. The effectiveness of adjunctive hypnosis with surgical patients. A meta-analysis. [In German.] Schmerz 2003;17:374–376

10. Montgomery GH, David D, Winkel G, Silverstein JH, Bovbjerg DH. The effectiveness of adjunctive hypnosis with surgical patients: a meta-analysis. Anesth Analg 2002;94: 1639–1645

11. Ashton C Jr, Whitworth GC, Seldomridge JA, Shapiro PA, Weinberg AD, Michler RE, Smith CR, Rose EA, Fisher S, Oz MC. Self-hypnosis reduces anxiety following coronary artery bypass surgery. A prospective, randomized trial. J Cardiovasc Surg 1997;38: 69–75

12. Tusek DL, Church JM, Strong SA, Grass JA, Fazio VW. Guided imagery: a significant advance in the care of patients undergoing elective colorectal surgery. Dis Colon Rectum 1997;40: 172–178

13. Huth MM, Broome ME, Good M. Imagery reduces children's post-operative pain. Pain 2004;110: 439–448

14. Omlor G, Kiewitz S, Pietschmann S, Roesler S. Effect of preoperative visualisation therapy on postoperative outcome after inguinal hernia surgery and thyroid resection. [In German.] Zentralbl Chir 2000;125:380–385

15. Renzi C, Peticca L, Pescatori M. The use of relaxation techniques in the perioperative management of proctological patients: preliminary results. Int J Colorectal Dis 2000;15:313–316

16. Haase O, Schwenk W, Hermann C, Muller JM. Guided imagery and relaxation in conventional colorectal resections: a randomized, controlled, partially blinded trial. Dis Colon Rectum 2005;48:1955–1963

17. Hulme J, Waterman H, Hillier VF. The effect of foot massage on patients' perception of care following laparoscopic sterilisation as day case patients. J Adv Nurs 1999;30:460–468

18. Le Blanc-Louvry I, Costaglioli B, Boulon C, Leroi AM, Ducrotte P. Does mechanical massage of the abdominal wall after colectomy reduce postoperative pain and shorten the duration of ileus? Results of a randomized study. J Gastrointest Surg 2002;6:43–49

19. Taylor AG, Galper DI, Taylor P, Rice LW, Andersen W, Irvin W, Wang XQ, Harrell FE Jr. Effects of adjunctive Swedish massage and vibration therapy on short-term postoperative outcomes: a randomized, controlled trial. J Altern Complement Med 2003;9:77–89

20. Piotrowski MM, Paterson C, Mitchinson A, Kim HM, Kirsh M, Hinshaw DB. Massage as adjuvant therapy in the management of acute postoperative pain: a preliminary study in men. J Am Coll Surg 2003;197:1037–1046

21. Forchuk C, Baruth P, Prendergast M, Holliday R, Bareham R, Brimner S, Schulz V, Chan YC, Yammine N. Postoperative arm massage: a support for women with lymph node dissection. Cancer Nurs 2004;27:25–33

22. Heitz L, Symreng T, Scamman FL. Effect of music therapy in the postanesthesia care unit: a nursing intervention. J Post Anesth Nurs 1992;7:22–31

23. Good M, Stanton-Hicks M, Grass JA, Cranston Anderson G, Choi C, Schoolmeesters LJ, Salman A. Relief of postoperative pain with jaw relaxation, music and their combination. Pain 1999; 81:163–172

24. Good M, Chin CC. The effects of Western music on postoperative pain in Taiwan. Kaohsiung J Med Sci 1998;14:94–103

25. Nilsson U, Rawal N, Unestahl LE, Zetterberg C, Unosson M. Improved recovery after music and therapeutic suggestions during general anaesthesia: a double-blind randomised controlled trial. Acta Anaesthesiol Scand 2001;45:812–817

26. Nilsson U, Rawal N, Unosson M. A comparison of intra-operative or postoperative exposure to music – a controlled trial of the effects on postoperative pain. Anaesthesia 2003;58:699–703

27. Voss JA, Good M, Yates B, Baun MM, Thompson A, Hertzog M. Sedative music reduces anxiety and pain during chair rest after open-heart surgery. Pain 2004;112:197–203

28. Laurion S, Fetzer SJ. The effect of two nursing interventions on the postoperative outcomes of gynecologic laparoscopic patients. J Perianesth Nurs 2003;18:254–261

29. Seers K, Carroll D. Relaxation techniques for acute pain management: a systematic review. J Adv Nurs 1998;27:466–475

30. Miro J, Raich RM. Effects of a brief and economical intervention in preparing patients for surgery: does coping style matter? Pain 1999;83:471–475

31. Good M, Anderson GC, Stanton-Hicks M, Grass JA, Makii M. Relaxation and music reduce pain after gynecologic surgery. Pain Manag Nurs 2002;3:61–70

32. Roykulcharoen V, Good M. Systematic relaxation to relieve postoperative pain. J Adv Nurs 2004;48:140–148

33. Good M, Anderson GC, Ahn S, Cong X, Stanton-Hicks M. Relaxation and music reduce pain following intestinal surgery. Res Nurs Health 2005;28:240–251

34. Levin RF, Malloy GB, Hyman RB. Nursing management of postoperative pain: use of relaxation techniques with female cholecystectomy patients. J Adv Nurs 1987;12:463–472

35. Bjordal JM, Johnson MI, Ljunggreen AE. Transcutaneous electrical nerve stimulation (TENS) can reduce postoperative analgesic consumption. A meta-analysis with assessment of optimal treatment parameters for postoperative pain. Eur J Pain 2003;7:181–188

36. Madden C, Singer G, Peck C, Nayman J. The effect of EMG biofeedback on postoperative pain following abdominal surgery. Anaesth Intensive Care 1978;6:333–336

37. Hoernecke R, Doenicke A. Perioperative enzyme therapy. A significant supplement to postoperative pain therapy? [In German.] Anaesthesist 1993;42:856–861

38. Mlakar B, Kosorok P. Flavonoids to reduce bleeding and pain after stapled hemorrhoidopexy: a randomized controlled trial. Wien Klin Wochenschr 2005;117:558–560

39. Kesselring A, Spichiger E, Muller M. Foot reflexology: an intervention study. Pflege 1998; 11:213–218

40. Licciardone JC, Stoll ST, Cardarelli KM, Gamber RG, Swift JN Jr, Winn WB. A randomized controlled trial of osteopathic manipulative treatment following knee or hip arthroplasty. J Am Osteopath Assoc 2004;104:193–202

41. Meehan TC. Therapeutic touch and postoperative pain: a Rogerian research study. Nurs Sci Q 1993;6:69–78

PERIPHERAL ARTERIAL OCCLUSIVE DISEASE

SYNONYMS
Charcot's syndrome, myasthenia angiosclerotica, peripheral vascular disease.

DEFINITION
Peripheral arterial occlusive disease causing ischaemic pain arises as the result of significant narrowing of arteries distal to the arch of the aorta. Narrowing can be caused by arteritis, local thrombus formation, embolisation from the heart or more central arteries, or (most frequently) from arteriosclerotic changes in the arterial wall. Peripheral arterial occlusive disease stage I is when the narrowing does not yet cause symptoms. Stage II is called intermittent claudication and describes the situation where the narrowing is such that at increased oxygen demand (i.e. walking) the oxygen supply can no longer meet this demand – the result is ischaemic pain that subsides when the patient stops walking. Stage III is even more advanced narrowing such that pain is felt all the time. Stage IV is when ischaemia is so pronounced that it causes tissue necrosis or gangrene.

CAM USAGE
Hydrotherapy, chelation therapy, herbal medicine and lifestyle changes are interventions frequently used for the treatment of this condition.

CLINICAL EVIDENCE
BIOFEEDBACK

A systematic review[1] identified one RCT ($n = 12$), which tested biofeedback as an adjunctive treatment for patients with intermittent claudication. The treatment consisted of EMG feedback and skin temperature feedback from fingers and toes. Compared with baseline, the onset of ischaemic pain during walking was delayed, but there was no mention of intergroup differences.

Box 5.44 *Systematic review: chelation therapy for atherosclerotic cardiovascular disease*[2]

- Five double-blind, placebo-controlled RCTs
- Four of the studies (*n* = 250 patients) showed no difference in the following outcomes: direct or indirect measurement of disease severity and subjective measures of improvement
- For pain-free walking distance after 20 infusions, there was an effect in favour of placebo (weighted mean difference −16.4 m, CI −32.0 to −0.8, *n* = 167)
- Adverse events included faintness, hypocalcaemia, proteinuria and gastrointestinal symptoms
- **Conclusion**: there is not enough evidence to determine the effectiveness or otherwise of chelation therapy

Box 5.45 *Systematic review: garlic for peripheral arterial occlusive disease*[5]

- One double-blind, placebo-controlled RCT including 78 patients
- Men and women were included (age range 40–75 years)
- Treatment period was 12 weeks
- Pain-free walking distance increased from 161 to 207 m (garlic) and from 172 to 203 m (placebo)
- **Conclusion**: one small trial of short duration found no effect on walking distance

CHELATION THERAPY

A Cochrane review identified five RCTs (Box 5.44).[2] All studies compared chelation using ethylenediaminetetraacetic acid (EDTA) with isotonic NaCl solution or distilled water. There were no differences in favour of chelation therapy. For pain-free walking distance after 20 infusions the results of two trials (*n* = 167) were pooled and they suggest an effect in favour of placebo.

CO_2 APPLICATIONS

Subcutaneous CO_2 insufflations are being used as a treatment modality in continental Europe. A systematic review[3] identified three relevant RCTs. The data from one trial suggested differences for pain-free walking distance compared with patients on a waiting list, while two others reported mixed results compared with waiting list controls and patients receiving CO_2 baths. Another RCT (*n* = 24) assessed the effects of immersion in CO_2-containing water.[4] It reported an increase in pain-free walking distance after immersion of the lower extremities for 30 min five times weekly for 4 weeks compared with baseline.

HERBAL MEDICINE

A Cochrane review identified one double-blind RCT for garlic (*Allium sativum*) extract (Box 5.45).[5] Its results suggest that garlic powder given in a daily dose of 800 mg for 12 weeks increases pain-free walking distance more than placebo.[6]

The evidence for ginkgo (*Ginkgo biloba*) has been assessed in a meta-analysis.[7] According to these data and other evidence from comparative trials,[8] ginkgo extract increases pain-free and maximal walking distances to a similar degree compared with other conventional oral treatments. The overall effect, however, is modest. Another systematic review confirms the effectiveness of the special ginkgo extract EGb 761 (Box 5.46).[9]

Box 5.46 *Meta-analysis: ginkgo extract EGb 761 for peripheral arterial occlusive disease*[9]

- Nine double-blind, placebo-controlled RCTs
- All RCTs tested ginkgo extract EGb 761 in patients with peripheral arterial occlusive disease in Fontaine stage II
- Methodological quality and design of the trials were heterogeneous
- The data for pain-free walking distance show a beneficial effect over placebo (theta 1.23, 95% CI 1.16 to 1.31)
- **Conclusion**: this review confirms the efficacy of *Ginkgo biloba* special extract EGb 761

Box 5.47 *Systematic review: Padma 28 for peripheral arterial occlusive disease*[1]

- Five double-blind RCTs assessing 333 patients in Fontaine stage IIb
- Patients were treated with 1.5–2.3 g Padma 28 daily for 4 months
- The mean difference was 81.3 m (95% CI 65.5 to 97.1) in favour of Padma 28 compared with placebo
- Adverse events were exanthema, dermatosis and worsening of symptoms; there were four serious adverse events of which none were drug related
- **Conclusion**: the available evidence suggests that this herbal mixture is an option for patients with peripheral arterial occlusive disease

Padma 28 is a herbal mixture comprising 22 different ingredients. Data from five double-blind RCTs measuring maximal walking distance are available.[1] Based on these data, meta-analytical pooling suggests an increase in the walking distance with Padma 28 of about 81 m over placebo (Box 5.47).

SUPPLEMENTS

A Cochrane review of fish oil (omega-3 fatty acid) included four placebo-controlled RCTs.[10] Two trials that assessed walking distances suggested no changes for pain-free and maximal walking distances. It concluded that, although omega-3 fatty acids may positively affect the underlying arteriosclerotic process, there is no evidence of improved clinical outcomes in patients with peripheral arterial occlusive disease. More recently, an RCT with 60 patients with claudication showed that the supplementation of omega-3 fatty acids over 12 months prolongs pain-free walking distance more than placebo.[11]

One double-blind RCT investigated the effects of an L-arginine-enriched food bar.[12] After 2 weeks of administering the food bar, the pain-free walking distance had increased by 66% while the maximal walking distance had increased by 23%. These effects were not observed in the placebo group. An RCT with 80 claudicants demonstrated no effect of L-arginine supplementation (0, 3, 6 or 9 g/day) for 12 weeks on walking distance.[13]

Another Cochrane review assessed the evidence for vitamin E and identified three double-blind RCTs.[14] The authors concluded that there is insufficient evidence to determine whether vitamin E is effective for treating patients with peripheral arterial occlusive disease. The meta-analysis of two trials, which included one non-randomised trial, suggested a relative risk of 0.6 (95% CI 0.3 to 1.2) for patients' subjective evaluation of the treatment.

OVERALL RECOMMENDATIONS

For intermittent claudication, no therapy is as effective as conventional regular physical exercise. It can be recommended as a beneficial lifestyle change in addition to smoking cessation. Convincing evidence exists for the effectiveness of ginkgo extract, which seems to be as effective as other conventional oral interventions. Although the overall effect seems modest, given the relative lack of serious adverse events, it can be recommended. Padma 28 also seems to be of benefit. For other interventions, such as CO_2 applications and vitamin E, the evidence is encouraging but insufficient for firm recommendations to be made.

Table 5.27 **Summary of clinical evidence for peripheral arterial occlusive disease**

Treatment	Weight of evidence	Direction of evidence	Serious safety concerns
Biofeedback	O	↗	Yes (see p. 110)
Chelation therapy	OOO	↓	Yes (see p. 5)
CO_2 applications	OO	↗	Yes (see p. 5)
Herbal medicine			
Garlic	O	↗	Yes (see p. 5)
Ginkgo	OOO	↑	Yes (see p. 5)
Padma 28	OOO	↑	Yes (see p. 5)
Supplements			
Fish oil	OO	↘	Yes (see p. 5)
L-arginine-enriched bar	O	↗	Yes (see p. 5)
Vitamin E	OO	↗	Yes (see p. 5)

REFERENCES

1. Pittler MH, Ernst E. Complementary therapies for peripheral arterial disease: systematic review. Atherosclerosis 2005;181:1–7
2. Villarruz MV, Dans A, Tan F. Chelation therapy for atherosclerotic cardiovascular disease. The Cochrane Database of Systematic Reviews 2002, Issue 4. Art. No.: CD002785
3. Brockow T, Hausner T, Dillner A, Resch KL. Clinical evidence of subcutaneous CO_2 insufflations: a systematic review. J Altern Comp Med 2000;6:391–403
4. Hartmann BR, Bassenge E, Hartmann M. Effects of serial percutaneous application of carbon dioxide in intermittent claudication: results of a controlled trial. Angiology 1997;48:957–963
5. Jepson RG, Kleijnen J, Leng GC. Garlic for peripheral arterial occlusive disease. The Cochrane Database of Systematic Reviews 1997, Issue 2. Art. No.: CD000095
6. Kiesewetter H, Jung F, Jung EM, Blume J, Mrowietz C, Birk A, Koscielny J, Wenzel E. Effects of garlic coated tablets in peripheral arterial occlusive disease. Clin Invest 1993;71:383–386
7. Pittler MH, Ernst E. *Ginkgo biloba* extract for the treatment of intermittent claudication: a meta-analysis of randomized trials. Am J Med 2000;108:276–281
8. Böhmer D, Kalinski S, Michaelis P, Szögy A. Behandlung der PAVK mit *Ginkgo-biloba*-extrakt (GBE) oder Pentoxifyllin. Herz Kreislauf 1988;20:5–8
9. Horsch S, Walther C. *Ginkgo biloba* special extract EGb 761 in the treatment of peripheral arterial occlusive disease (PAOD) – a review based on randomized, controlled studies. Int J Clin Pharmacol Ther 2004;42:63–72
10. Sommerfield T, Hiatt WR. Omega-3 fatty acids for intermittent claudication. The Cochrane Database of Systematic Reviews 2004, Issue 1. Art. No.: CD003833
11. Carrero JJ, Lopez-Huertas E, Salmeron LM, Baro L, Ros E. Daily supplementation with (n-3) PUFAs, oleic acid, folic acid, and vitamins B6 and E increases pain-free walking distance and improves risk factors in men with peripheral vascular disease. J Nutr 2005;135:1393–1399
12. Maxwell AJ, Anderson BE, Cooke JP. Nutritional therapy for peripheral arterial disease: a double-blind, placebo-controlled, randomized trial of HeartBar. Vasc Med 2000;5: 11–19
13. Oka RK, Szuba A, Giacomini JC, Cooke JP. A pilot study of L-arginine supplementation on functional capacity in peripheral arterial disease. Vasc Med 2005;10:265–274
14. Kleijnen J, Mackerras D. Vitamin E for intermittent claudication. The Cochrane Database of Systematic Reviews 1998, Issue 1. Art. No.: CD000987

PROCEDURAL PAIN

DEFINITION

Pain related to diagnostic or non-surgical treatment procedures including dressing change, injections and physiotherapy. For Peri-operative pain see p. 303.

RELATED CONDITIONS

Peri-operative pain.

CAM USAGE

Acupuncture, hypnotherapy, mind–body therapies, relaxation and distraction therapies.

CLINICAL EVIDENCE

ACUPUNCTURE

A double-blind RCT ($n = 60$) testing whether acupressure could be an effective pre-hospital analgesic in patients with minor trauma reported less pain and anxiety, lower heart rates and a greater satisfaction in the group receiving acupressure compared to the sham acupressure point and no acupressure groups.[1] A systematic review ($n = 6$) of acupuncture for gastrointestinal endoscopy concluded that it was more effective than sham acupuncture and similar to conventional premedication in effect.[2]

A systematic review of acupuncture and other conscious sedation methods during oocyte retrieval included three trials of electroacupuncture in combination with paracervical block (Box 5.48).[3] It concluded that there was no superiority of any method; this finding was confirmed in a subsequent RCT.[4] In an RCT of 35 patients undergoing extracorporeal shockwave lithotripsy, reduced pain visual analogue scale scores were found with electroacupuncture for sedation and analgesia when compared with the combination of tramadol and midazolam.[5]

DISTRACTION THERAPY

A systematic review of the effects of distraction therapy on children's pain (10 clinical trials, $n = 535$) and distress (16 clinical trials, $n = 491$) during medical procedures concluded that the effect is influenced by moderator variables and has a positive influence on children's distress behaviour.[6] In an RCT of 80 adult patients undergoing flexible bronchoscopy, distraction therapy was reported to reduce pain compared to no distraction therapy.[7] An RCT ($n = 80$) compared the effects on pain and anxiety control during cataract surgery of different types and combinations of distraction interventions, involving massage, verbal coaching and slow breathing, with usual care.[8] It reported a reduction of discomfort or pain and anxiety when the distraction interventions were implemented during the ocular anaesthetic injection. Visual distraction alone did not decrease the dose of sedative medication required

Box 5.48 *Systematic review: electroacupuncture for procedure-related pain in oocyte retrieval*[3]

- Three trials were included which compared electroacupuncture with fentanyl, both administered in paracervical block
- Two trials found no differences in pain between groups
- One trial in which premedication was given to the fentanyl group but not the electroacupuncture group reported higher pain scores in the electroacupuncture group
- Combining pain assessment of these three trials favoured conventional analgesia with intravenous fentanyl plus paracervical block

for colonoscopy in an RCT ($n = 165$) but, when audio distraction was added, both the dose of sedative medication required and the pain scores decreased compared to patient-controlled sedation alone.[9]

HYPNOTHERAPY

A systematic review ($n = 8$) concluded that hypnosis has potential as a clinically valuable intervention for procedure-related pain and distress in paediatric cancer patients (Box 5.49).[10] An RCT of 44 children undergoing voiding cystourethrography compared hypnotherapy with routine care and indicated that the procedure was perceived as less traumatic and less distressing than previous procedures, that it was easier to conduct the procedure and that the procedure time was reduced when hypnotherapy was used.[11]

A small RCT ($n = 20$) found that hypnotherapy reduced post-procedural pain and distress in excisional breast biopsy compared to standard care.[12] Self-hypnotic relaxation and structured attention proved beneficial during percutaneous vascular and renal procedures compared to placebo, with hypnosis having more pronounced effects on pain and anxiety reduction.[13]

An RCT ($n = 44$) reported decreased degrees of pain and anxiety caused by physiotherapy in burns patients receiving hypnotherapy compared with controls not receiving hypnotherapy.[14] In an RCT of 30 severely burned patients, both hypnosis and a stress-reducing strategy reduced pain and increased patient satisfaction during dressing changes compared to baseline.[15]

In an RCT of 236 patients undergoing interventional radiological procedures, hypnotherapy as well as empathic attention reduced procedure time and medication use for all patients and provided better pain control than standard care for patients with low anxiety levels.[16]

MUSIC THERAPY

A systematic review of the effectiveness of music therapy for hospital patients included six RCTs of procedure-related pain.[17] Five RCTs found that music therapy was not superior to no music while only one RCT reported less narcotic analgesia administered during the procedure via a patient-controlled device in the music group. Single RCTs of music therapy report reduced pain during colposcopy,[18] colonoscopy,[19,20] tissue biopsy, port placement or removal[21] and debridement of burn wounds,[22] and reduced intravenous insertion pain.[23]

OTHER THERAPIES

In an RCT ($n = 78$) patients scheduled for an elective, diagnostic catheterisation based on routine clinical practices received either a 10-minute massage before the procedure or spent 10 minutes of quiet time with a massage therapist. No differences between groups regarding pain or discomfort were found.[24]

Box 5.49 *Systematic review: hypnotherapy for procedure-related pain in paediatric cancer patients*[10]

- Seven RCTs and one CCT were included
- Positive results were reported including reductions in pain and anxiety/distress
- A number of methodological limitations were identified
- **Conclusion**: hypnosis has potential as a clinically valuable intervention for procedure-related pain and distress in paediatric cancer patients but further research is recommended

SECTION FIVE

OVERALL RECOMMENDATION

Positive results exist for hypnotherapy (including in children), distraction therapy and music therapy. Given their relative safety they might be useful adjuncts in the management of pain during procedures.

Table 5.28 **Summary of clinical evidence for procedure-related pain**

Treatment	Weight of evidence	Direction of evidence	Serious safety concerns
Acupuncture			Yes (see p. 96)
Acupressure	O	↗	Yes (see p. 96)
Electroacupuncture	OO	→	Yes (see p. 96)
Distraction therapy	OOO	↑	No (see p. 5)
Hypnotherapy	OOO	↑	Yes (see p. 130)
Music therapy	OOO	↗	No (see p. 142)

REFERENCES

1. Kober A, Scheck T, Greher M, Lieba F, Fleischhackl R, Fleischhackl S, Randunsky F, Hoerauf K. Prehospital analgesia with acupressure in victims of minor trauma: a prospective, randomized, double-blinded trial. Anesth Analg 2002;95:723–727

2. Lee H, Ernst E. Acupuncture for GI endoscopy: a systematic review. Gastrointest Endosc 2004; 60:784–789

3. Kwan I, Bhattacharya S, Knox F, McNeil A. Conscious sedation and analgesia for oocyte retrieval during *in vitro* fertilisation procedures. The Cochrane Database of Systematic Reviews 2005, Issue 3. Art. No.: CD004829

4. Gejervall AL, Stener-Victorin E, Moller A, Janson PO, Werner C, Bergh C. Electro-acupuncture versus conventional analgesia: a comparison of pain levels during oocyte aspiration and patients' experiences of well-being after surgery. Hum Reprod 2005;20:728–735

5. Resim S, Gumusalan Y, Ekerbicer HC, Sahin MA, Sahinkanat T. Effectiveness of electro-acupuncture compared to sedo-analgesics in relieving pain during shockwave lithotripsy. Urol Res 2005;33:285–290

6. Kleiber C, Harper DC. Effects of distraction on children's pain and distress during medical procedures: a meta-analysis. Nurs Res 1999;48:44–49

7. Diette GB, Lechtzin N, Haponik E, Devrotes A, Rubin HR. Distraction therapy with nature sights and sounds reduces pain during flexible bronchoscopy: a complementary approach to routine analgesia. Chest 2003;123:941–948

8. Simmons D, Chabal C, Griffith J, Rausch M, Steele B. A clinical trial of distraction techniques for pain and anxiety control during cataract surgery. Insight 2004;29:13–16

9. Lee DW, Chan AC, Wong SK, Fung TM, Li AC, Chan SK, Mui LM, Ng EK, Chung SC. Can visual distraction decrease the dose of patient-controlled sedation required during colonoscopy? A prospective randomized controlled trial. Endoscopy 2004;36: 197–201

10. Richardson J, Smith JE, McCall G, Pilkington K. Hypnosis for procedure-related pain and distress in pediatric cancer patients: a systematic review of effectiveness and methodology related to hypnosis interventions. J Pain Symptom Manage 2006;31:70–84

11. Butler LD, Symons BK, Henderson SL, Shortliffe LD, Spiegel D. Hypnosis reduces distress and duration of an invasive medical procedure for children. Pediatrics 2005;115:e77–85

12. Montgomery GH, Weltz CR, Seltz M, Bovbjerg DH. Brief presurgery hypnosis reduces distress and pain in excisional breast biopsy patients. Int J Clin Exp Hypn 2002;50:17–32

13. Lang EV, Benotsch EG, Fick LJ, Lutgendorf S, Berbaum ML, Berbaum KS, Logan H, Spiegel D. Adjunctive non-pharmacological analgesia for invasive medical procedures: a randomised trial. Lancet 2000;355:1486–1490

14. Harandi AA, Esfandani A, Shakibaei F. The effect of hypnotherapy on procedural pain and state anxiety related to physiotherapy in women hospitalized in a burn unit. Contemp Hypn 2004; 21:28–34
15. Frenay MC, Faymonville ME, Devlieger S, Albert A, Vanderkelen A. Psychological approaches during dressing changes of burned patients: a prospective randomised study comparing hypnosis against stress reducing strategy. Burns 2001;27:793–799
16. Schupp CJ, Berbaum K, Berbaum M, Lang EV. Pain and anxiety during interventional radiologic procedures: effect of patients' state anxiety at baseline and modulation by nonpharmacologic anal-gesia adjuncts. J Vasc Interv Radiol 2005;16:1585–1592
17. Evans D. The effectiveness of music as an intervention for hospital patients: a systematic review. J Adv Nurs 2002;37:8–18
18. Chan YM, Lee PW, Ng TY, Ngan HY, Wong LC. The use of music to reduce anxiety for patients undergoing colposcopy: a randomized trial. Gynecol Oncol 2003;91:213–217
19. Lee DW, Chan KW, Poon CM, Ko CW, Chan KH, Sin KS, Sze TS, Chan AC. Relaxation music decreases the dose of patient-controlled sedation during colonoscopy: a prospective randomized controlled trial. Gastrointest Endosc 2002;55:33–36
20. Uedo N, Ishikawa H, Morimoto K, Ishihara R, Narahara H, Akedo I, Ioka T, Kaji I, Fukuda S. Reduction in salivary cortisol level by music therapy during colonoscopic examination. Hepatogastroenterology 2004;51:451–453
21. Kwekkeboom KL. Music versus distraction for procedural pain and anxiety in patients with can-cer. Oncol Nurs Forum 2003;30:433–440
22. Fratianne RB, Prensner JD, Huston MJ, Super DM, Yowler CJ, Standley JM. The effect of music-based imagery and musical alternate engagement on the burn debridement process. J Burn Care Rehabil 2001;22:47–53
23. Jacobson AF. Intradermal normal saline solution, self-selected music, and insertion difficulty effects on intravenous insertion pain. Heart Lung 1999;28:114–122
24. Okvat HA, Oz MC, Ting W, Namerow PB. Massage therapy for patients undergoing cardiac catheterization. Altern Ther Health Med 2002;8:68–75

RAYNAUD'S PHENOMENON

SYNONYMS/SUBCATEGORIES
Raynaud's disease, Raynaud's syndrome.

DEFINITION
Raynaud's phenomenon is episodic vasospasm of the peripheral arteries, causing pallor followed by cyanosis and redness with pain and sometimes paraesthesia, and, rarely, ulceration of the fingers and toes (and in some cases of the ears or nose). Primary or idiopathic Raynaud's phenomenon (Raynaud's disease) occurs without an underlying dis-ease and its cause is unknown. Secondary Raynaud's phenomenon (Raynaud's syndrome) occurs in association with an underlying disease – usually connective tissue disorders such as scleroderma, systemic lupus erythematosus, rheumatoid arthritis or polymyositis. It was named after Maurice Raynaud (1834–1881), a French physician who first described the condition.

RELATED CONDITIONS
Frostbite.

CAM USAGE
Biofeedback is used for this condition.

CLINICAL EVIDENCE
ACUPUNCTURE

Two small RCTs ($n = 33$, $n = 19$) tested the effects of acupuncture in outpatients with primary Raynaud's phenomenon.[1,2] Reductions in attack frequency compared with baseline were reported but no changes in duration and severity of attacks. Another RCT assessed patients with secondary Raynaud's phenomenon and reported no beneficial effects on symptoms.[3]

AUTOGENIC TRAINING

A meta-analysis was performed to evaluate the clinical effectiveness of autogenic training (Box 5.50).[4] The demonstrated effects are encouraging but not convincing.

BIOFEEDBACK

Two RCTs were identified that assessed the effects of temperature biofeedback. Patients with secondary Raynaud's phenomenon as a result of scleroderma were included in one trial which compared finger temperature biofeedback, frontalis EMG biofeedback and autogenic training.[5] No group showed symptomatic improvement. A large ($n = 313$) RCT compared the effectiveness of temperature biofeedback and sustained-release nifedipine in patients with primary Raynaud's phenomenon.[6] Whereas nifedipine-treated patients showed a reduction in attacks compared with placebo, temperature biofeedback training did not reduce attacks compared with control (EMG) biofeedback.

HERBAL MEDICINE

A small ($n = 21$) double-blind trial tested evening primrose oil (*Oenothera biennis*) and reported an improvement in the severity of attacks.[7] No changes in hand temperatures were seen in either group.

One double-blind RCT investigated the clinical effectiveness of a standardised *Ginkgo biloba* extract in the treatment of primary Raynaud's phenomenon.[8] A decrease in the number of daily attacks compared with placebo was reported.

OVERALL RECOMMENDATION

There are very few data from rigorous trials of complementary therapies for treating Raynaud's phenomenon. The same is, however, also true for conventional treatments with the exception of nifedipine. Given its good safety profile, autogenic training may be worth a try.

Box 5.50 *Systematic review: autogenic training for all conditions*[4]

- A total of 35 RCTs were included; six RCTs assessed 108 patients with Raynaud's phenomenon
- Patients with primary and secondary Raynaud's phenomenon ($n = 12$) were included
- Analysis of pre–post comparisons indicate an effect across different outcome measures (effects size 0.47, $P < 0.01$)
- Compared to no-treatment control groups the effects are not significant
- **Conclusion**: '... autogenic training proved its effectiveness in more than one study in [...] Raynaud's disease'

Table 5.29 **Summary of clinical evidence for Raynaud's phenomenon**

Treatment	Weight of evidence	Direction of evidence	Serious safety concerns
Acupuncture	OO	→	Yes (see p. 96)
Autogenic training	OO	↗	Yes (see p. 106)
Biofeedback	OO	↘	Yes (see p. 110)
Herbal medicine			
Evening primrose oil	O	↗	Yes (see p. 191)
Ginkgo biloba	O	↑	Yes (see p. 5)

REFERENCES

1. Appiah R, Hiller S, Caspary L, Alexander K, Creutzig A. Treatment of primary Raynaud's syndrome with traditional Chinese acupuncture. J Intern Med 1997;241:119–124

2. Steins A, Jünger M, Rösch G, Möhrle M, Blum A, Lorenz F et al. Wirkungen der Akupunktur bei akralen Durchblutungsstörungen gezeigt an Patienten mit primärem Raynaud-Phänomen. Phlebol 1996;25:139–143

3. Hahn M, Steins A, Mohrle M, Blum A, Junger M. Is there a vasospasmolytic effect of acupuncture in patients with secondary Raynaud phenomenon? J Dtsch Dermatol Ges 2004;2:758–762

4. Stetter F, Kupper S. Autogenic training: a meta-analysis of clinical outcome studies. Appl Psychophysiol Biofeedback 2002;27:45–98

5. Freedman RR, Ianni P, Wenig P. Behavioral treatment of Raynaud's phenomenon in scleroderma. J Behav Med 1984;7:343–353

6. Raynaud's Treatment Study Investigators. Comparison of sustained-release nifedipine and temperature biofeedback for treatment of primary Raynaud phenomenon. Results from a randomized clinical trial with 1-year follow-up. Arch Intern Med 2000;160:1101–1108

7. Belch JJ, Shaw B, O'Dowd A, Saniabadi A, Leiberman P, Sturrock RD, Forbes CD. Evening primrose oil (Efamol) in the treatment of Raynaud's phenomenon: a double blind study. Thromb Haemost 1985;54:490–494

8. Muir AH, Robb R, McLaren M, Daly F, Belch JJ. The use of *Ginkgo biloba* in Raynaud's disease: a double-blind placebo-controlled trial. Vasc Med 2002;7:265–267

RHEUMATOID ARTHRITIS

SYNONYMS

Arthritis deformans, arthritis nodosa, nodose rheumatism.

DEFINITION

Rheumatoid arthritis is a chronic inflammatory disorder. It is characterised by a chronic polyarthritis that primarily affects the peripheral joints and related periarticular tissues and causes pain. It usually starts as an insidious symmetric polyarthritis, often with non-specific systemic symptoms. Diagnostic criteria include arthritis lasting longer than 6 weeks, positive rheumatoid factor and radiological signs of damage.

RELATED CONDITIONS

Other inflammatory rheumatic diseases such as ankylosing spondylitis and psoriatic arthritis.

CAM USAGE

Rheumatoid arthritis is associated with a high level of CAM usage. In particular, patients often try herbal treatments and other nutritional supplements.[1] Modifications of the regular diet are also frequent (e.g. vegetarianism); most of the dietary approaches, however, are considered conventional. In a survey of CAM organisations the following treatments were recommended for arthritis: aromatherapy, homeopathy, hypnotherapy, magnet therapy, massage, nutrition, reflexology and yoga.

CLINICAL EVIDENCE

ACUPUNCTURE

A Cochrane review[2] evaluated the evidence for efficacy of acupuncture or electroacupuncture in patients with rheumatoid arthritis (Box 5.51). Two RCTs were identified; one for acupuncture reporting no differences for pain visual analogue scale and one for electroacupuncture reporting a decrease of knee pain compared with placebo. It was concluded that the available data are too scarce to allow recommendations of acupuncture or electroacupuncture for treating rheumatoid arthritis. A similar conclusion was reached for bee venom acupuncture.[3]

BALNEOTHERAPY

Balneotherapy is one of the oldest forms of therapy for people with arthritis. A Cochrane review (Box 5.52) concluded that, although one cannot ignore the positive findings reported in most studies, the evidence is insufficient with regard to pain, function and quality of life.[4] High-quality research is needed in this area.

DIET

Various (mostly conventional) dietary approaches have been tried for rheumatoid arthritis. Trials from Scandinavia show encouraging effects for fasting followed by a vegetarian diet. A

Box 5.51 *Systematic review: acupuncture for rheumatoid arthritis*[2]

- Two RCTs ($n = 84$) were included
- One assessed acupuncture, the other assessed electroacupuncture
- For acupuncture, there were no effects on C-reactive protein, pain and other outcome measures
- For electroacupuncture, a decrease in knee pain was reported compared to placebo
- **Conclusion**: although some positive results are reported, the effects are only short-term, not exceeding 24 hours of relief. The poor quality of the trials preclude the recommendation of acupuncture in patients with rheumatoid arthritis

Box 5.52 *Systematic review: balneotherapy for rheumatoid arthritis*[4]

- Six RCTs met the inclusion criteria ($n = 355$)
- Most studies were methodologically flawed to some extent
- Three studies compared balneotherapy with other forms of baths
- **Conclusion**: there is insufficient evidence that one type of bath is more effective than another or other treatments or no treatment

systematic review included four such studies.[5] The meta-analysis of these data suggests long-term improvements in pain and related outcomes. Both fasting and strict vegetarian diets are associated with the risk of malnutrition, thus adequate medical supervision is advisable. Further CCTs[6] and RCTs[7,8] support the observed benefits associated with the Mediterranean diet and gluten-free diets.

HERBAL MEDICINE

A systematic review assessed the evidence from all RCTs testing the effectiveness of Ayurvedic medicine (Box 5.53).[9] It is reported that there is a paucity of RCTs of Ayurvedic medicines for rheumatoid arthritis.

A double-blind RCT assessed a cannabis-based medicine (Sativex) in 58 patients.[10] In comparison with placebo, cannabis produced improvements in pain on movement, pain at rest and quality of sleep.

An extract of cat's claw (*Uncaria tomentosa*) was tested in 40 patients undergoing sulfasalazine or hydroxychloroquine treatment.[11] Twenty-four weeks of treatment with the extract resulted in a modest reduction of the number of painful joints compared to placebo. This small preliminary study requires independent replication.

A Cochrane review of herbal treatments for rheumatoid arthritis concluded that there appears to be beneficial effects on pain visual analogue scale from γ-linolenic acid although further studies are required to establish optimum dosage and duration of treatment.[12] A more recent assessment of the evidence largely corroborates these findings, suggesting moderate support for γ-linolenic acid found in some herbal medicines for reducing pain, tender joint count and stiffness (Box 5.54).[13]

Several herbal mixtures have been tested in clinical trials with positive results for rheumatoid arthritis patients. Of these preparations, only Phytodolor (a German proprietary

Box 5.53 *Systematic review: Ayurvedic medicine for rheumatoid arthritis*[9]

- Electronic databases, the abstract service of the Central Council for Research in Ayurveda and Siddha and one Sri Lankan and three Indian journals were searched
- Seven RCTs met the inclusion criteria
- Three trials tested Ayurvedic medicine against placebo and four tested against other Ayurvedic medicines.
- **Conclusion**: there is a paucity of RCTs of Ayurvedic medicines for rheumatoid arthritis. The existing RCTs fail to show convincingly that such treatments are effective therapeutic options for this condition

Box 5.54 *Systematic review: herbal medicines for rheumatoid arthritis*[13]

- Fourteen RCTs were included, all were double blind
- Meta-analyses of three trials of γ-linoleic acid ($n = 117$)
- Effect size for pain visual analogue scale was 0.76, 95% CI 0.37 to 1.15
- Effect size for tender joint count was 0.93, 95% CI 0.47 to 1.38
- Effect size for stiffness was 0.23, 95% CI 0.02 to 0.90
- **Conclusion**: given the number of herbal medicines promoted for rheumatoid arthritis, further research is needed to examine their efficacy, safety and potential drug interactions

Box 5.55 *Systematic review: Phytodolor for rheumatoid arthritis*[14]

- Ten RCTs met the inclusion criteria (*n* = 1035). Six were conducted against placebo, four against reference medication
- Most studies included patients with various rheumatic diseases
- The quality of these trials was, on average, good
- The results imply that Phytodolor is superior to placebo and equally effective as standard NSAIDs in alleviating arthritic pain and restoring function
- **Conclusion:** Phytodolor is a safe and effective treatment for musculoskeletal pain

medicine containing extracts of *Populus tremula, Fraxinus excelsior* and *Solidago virgaurea*) has been submitted to independently replicated clinical trials (Box 5.55).[14]

Thunder god vine (*Tripterygium wilfordii*) is recommended in traditional Chinese medicine for a large range of conditions. RCTs suggested anti-inflammatory properties and effects in reducing the objective signs and subjective symptoms of rheumatoid arthritis.[15,16] A systematic review assessed the totality of the available evidence and concluded that because of the limited number of available RCTs and the reported serious adverse effects it cannot be recommended for use.[17]

Further single RCTs reporting some positive results, which require replication in independent trials, exist for biqi,[18] garlic (*Allium sativum*)[19] and tong luo kai bi tablets.[20]

Single RCTs reporting negative results exist for Indian frankincense[12] (*Boswellia serrata*), feverfew[12] (*Tanacetum parthenium*) and willow (*Salix* spp) bark extract.[21]

HOMEOPATHY

A review summarised three RCTs (*n* = 266) of homeopathic treatments of rheumatoid arthritis, which report mixed results.[22] An RCT published since this review found no evidence that homeopathy improves the symptoms of rheumatoid arthritis over 3 months in patients attending a routine clinic who are stabilised on NSAIDs or anti-rheumatic drugs.[23] Another systematic review found little evidence and concluded that high-quality research is needed, especially for herbal treatments and homeopathy.[24]

HYPNOTHERAPY

Most clinical trials on hypnotherapy suggest that it can be useful in pain management. In particular, pain perception seems to be influenced positively.[25] However, no rigorous RCTs exist specifically for rheumatoid arthritis.

MAGNETS

Two RCTs tested the effects of magnets on patients with rheumatoid arthritis.[26,27] Both trials reported encouraging results for pain relief. Further independent replications are required before any firm recommendations can be made.

RELAXATION

Several relaxation techniques are being advocated for rheumatoid arthritis. Muscle relaxation training was demonstrated to be superior to no intervention in an RCT (*n* = 68).[28] Patients received 30 minutes of relaxation training twice weekly for 10 weeks and subsequently showed improvement in both function and well-being. A systematic review of all RCTs on relaxation for chronic pain reported beneficial effects for rheumatoid arthritis compared with routine treatment.[29]

SPIRITUAL HEALING

Several RCTs of various forms of spiritual healing have been published.[30] The question of whether spiritual healing alleviates arthritic pain more than placebo does not find a uniform answer in these studies. Firm recommendations are therefore not possible at present.

SUPPLEMENTS

Elk velvet antler as an adjunctive treatment to conventional arthritis medications was compared with placebo.[31] There were no differences in terms of effectiveness and adverse events.

Fish oil is rich in the omega-3 fatty acids eicosapentaenoic acid and docosahexaenoic acid, which have anti-inflammatory activity through interfering with prostaglandin metabolism. The results of a meta-analysis suggested a reduction in tender joint counts and in morning stiffness,[32] which is confirmed by additional double-blind RCTs.[33,34] Another RCT reported no clinical benefit over placebo for a supplement containing omega-3 fatty acids.[35] The overall size of the effect seems modest. Interestingly, α-linolenic acid (e.g. from flaxseed oil), which is the precursor of these omega-3 polyunsaturated fatty acids, does not seem to have the same clinical effects.[36]

Green-lipped mussel (*Perna canaliculus*) was tested in an RCT in which 30 rheumatoid arthritis patients took either 1150 mg/day green-lipped mussel powder or 210 mg/day lipid extract of the green-lipped mussel.[37] The patients in both groups reported improvements in joint tenderness, morning stiffness and function compared with baseline. Results of a pain visual analogue scale did not improve in either group. As the trial did not include a placebo control group it was not possible to determine whether the two treatments were equally ineffective or effective.

A small ($n = 21$) RCT tested the effects of probiotics using *Lactobacillus rhamnosus*.[38] The mean number of tender and swollen joints decreased in the group given *Lactobacillus* and in the placebo group with no differences between them. There were no differences in arthritis activity.

In an open pilot study 20 rheumatoid arthritis patients received 20 μg or 1000 μg selenium orally for 4 weeks.[39] At the end of this treatment phase both immunological and clinical outcome variables suggested a positive effect. An RCT tested the effects of selenium-enriched yeast and assessed pain, Ritchie index, number of swollen and painful joints and morning stiffness.[40] There were no differences compared with placebo.

TAI CHI

A Cochrane review assessed the evidence for efficacy of tai chi for patients with rheumatoid arthritis (Box 5.56).[41] In terms of swollen/tender joints, it seems that it has no detrimental effects on the disease activity of rheumatoid arthritis whereas it appears to have a clinically important benefit on the range of motion outcomes of ankle plantar flexion. This is largely

Box 5.56 *Systematic review: tai chi for treating rheumatoid arthritis*[41]

- Three CCTs and one RCT met the inclusion criteria ($n = 206$)
- No clinically important effect on most outcomes, including activities of daily living, tender and swollen joints and patient global overall rating
- For range of motion, participants had clinically important improvements in ankle plantar flexion
- No adverse events were found
- **Conclusion**: tai chi does not exacerbate symptoms of rheumatoid arthritis. In addition, it has benefits on lower extremity range of motion, in particular ankle range of motion

supported by another systematic review that assessed the effects of tai chi on various chronic conditions.[42]

OTHER THERAPIES

An observational study suggested that aromatherapy massage increases the well-being of patients with rheumatoid arthritis.[43] Biofeedback and cognitive–behavioural therapy have been reported to have positive effects in rheumatoid arthritis.[44,45] Children with juvenile rheumatoid arthritis received massage therapy from their parents for 15 minutes daily for 30 days.[46] Subsequently, a decrease in self-reported and physician-assessed pain was noted. RCTs of the traditional Chinese medical treatment of 'softening and lubricating the joints'[47] and vedic vibration technology[48] reported some positive results. Some encouraging but mostly anecdotal evidence exists to suggest that yoga might benefit patients with rheumatoid arthritis.[49] Unfortunately this hypothesis has so far not been tested in rigorous clinical trials.

Table 5.30 **Summary of clinical evidence for rheumatoid arthritis**

Treatment	Weight of evidence	Direction of evidence	Serious safety concerns
Acupuncture	OO	→	Yes (see p. 96)
Balneotherapy	OO	↗	Yes (see p. 126)
Diet	OOO	↑	Yes (see p. 5)
Fasting and vegetarianism	OO	↑	Yes (see p. 5)
Herbal medicine			
Ayurvedic mixtures	OOO	↘	Yes (see p. 108)
Biqi	O	↗	Yes (see p. 5)
Cannnabis	O	↗	Yes (see p. 179)
Cat's claw	O	↗	Yes (see p. 182)
Feverfew	O	↘	Yes (see p. 194)
Garlic	O	↗	Yes (see p. 5)
γ-linolenic acid (e.g. borage)	OO	↗	Yes (see p. 5)
Indian frankincense	O	↘	Yes (see p. 202)
Phytodolor	OOO	↑	Yes (see p. 5)
Thunder god vine	OO	↘	Yes (see p. 5)
Tong luo kai bi	O	↗	Yes (see p. 5)
Willow bark	O	↘	Yes (see p. 216)
Homeopathy	OO	→	No (see p. 124)
Hypnotherapy	O	→	Yes (see p. 130)
Magnets	OO	↗	No (see p. 164)
Relaxation	OO	↗	No (see p. 158)
Spiritual healing	OO	→	No (see p. 162)
Supplements			
Elk velvet antler	O	↘	Yes (see p. 5)
Fish oil	OOO	↗	Yes (see p. 5)
Flaxseed oil (α-linoleic acid)	O	↓	Yes (see p. 5)
Green-lipped mussel	O	→	Yes (see p. 199)
Probiotics	O	↘	Yes (see p. 5)
Selenium	OO	→	Yes (see p. 5)
Tai chi	OO	↑	No (see p. 167)

OVERALL RECOMMENDATION

No disease-modifying complementary treatment of rheumatoid arthritis exists. The evidence for CAM reducing the pain of rheumatoid arthritis is mixed. Given the high rates of adverse effects with the synthetic drugs that are used for rheumatoid arthritis, the following CAM modalities would seem to be reasonable therapeutic options: Phytodolor, fish oil and tai chi. With all of these therapies the effect size is usually moderate to small. Thus, such CAM treatments would normally be reasonable adjuvant treatments rather than true therapeutic alternatives.

REFERENCES

1. Resch KL, Hill S, Ernst E. Use of complementary therapies by individuals with 'arthritis'. Clin Rheumatol 1997;16:391–395
2. Casimiro L, Brosseau L, Milne S, Robinson V, Wells G, Tugwell P. Acupuncture and electroacupuncture for the treatment of RA. The Cochrane Database of Systematic Reviews 2005, Issue 4. Art. No.: CD003788
3. Lee JD, Park HJ, Chae Y, Lim S. An overview of bee venom acupuncture in the treatment of arthritis. Evid Based Complement Altern Med 2005;2:79–84
4. Verhagen AP, Bierma-Zeinstra SMA, Cardoso JR, de Bie RA, Boers M, de Vet HCW. Balneotherapy for rheumatoid arthritis. The Cochrane Database of Systematic Reviews 2003, Issue 4. Art. No.: CD000518
5. Müller H, de Toledo FW, Resch KL. Fasting followed by vegetarian diet in patients with rheumatoid arthritis: a systematic review. Scand J Rheumatol 2001;30:1–10.
6. Kjeldsen-Kragh J. Rheumatoid arthritis treated with vegetarian diets. Am J Clin Nutr 1999;70:594S–600S
7. Hafstrom I, Ringertz B, Spangberg A, von Zweigbergk L, Brannemark S, Nylander I, Ronnelid J, Laasonen L, Klareskog L. A vegan diet free of gluten improves the signs and symptoms of rheumatoid arthritis: the effects on arthritis correlate with a reduction in antibodies to food antigens. Rheumatology (Oxford) 2001;40:1175–1179
8. Skoldstam L, Hagfors L, Johansson G. An experimental study of a Mediterranean diet intervention for patients with rheumatoid arthritis. Ann Rheum Dis 2003;62:208–214
9. Park J, Ernst E. Ayurvedic medicine for rheumatoid arthritis: a systematic review. Semin Arthritis Rheum 2005;34:705–713
10. Blake DR, Robson P, Ho M, Jubb RW, McCabe CS. Preliminary assessment of the efficacy, tolerability and safety of a cannabis-based medicine (Sativex) in the treatment of pain caused by rheumatoid arthritis. Rheumatology (Oxford) 2006;45:50–52
11. Mur E, Hartig F, Eibl G, Schirmer M. Randomized double blind trial of an extract from the pentacyclic alkaloid-chemotype of *Uncaria tomentosa* for the treatment of rheumatoid arthritis. J Rheumatol 2002;29:678–681
12. Little CV, Parsons T. Herbal therapy for treating rheumatoid arthritis. The Cochrane Database of Systematic Reviews 2000, Issue 4. Art. No.: CD002948
13. Soeken KL, Miller SA, Ernst E. Herbal medicines for the treatment of rheumatoid arthritis: a systematic review. Rheumatology (Oxford) 2003;42:652–659
14. Ernst E. The efficacy of phytodolor for the treatment of musculoskeletal pain – a systematic review of randomized clinical trials. J Natural Med 1999;2:3–8
15. Cibere J, Deng Z, Lin Y, Ou R, He Y, Wang Z, Thorne A, Lehman AJ, Tsang IK, Esdaile JM. A randomized double blind, placebo controlled trial of topical *Tripterygium wilfordii* in rheumatoid arthritis: reanalysis using logistic regression analysis. J Rheumatol 2003;30:465–467
16. Tao X, Younger J, Fan FZ, Wang B, Lipsky PE. Benefit of an extract of *Tripterygium wilfordii* Hook F in patients with rheumatoid arthritis: a double-blind, placebo-controlled study. Arthritis Rheum 2002;46:1735–1743
17. Canter PH, Lee HS, Ernst E. A systematic review of randomised clinical trials of *Tripterygium wilfordii* for rheumatoid arthritis. Phytomedicine 2006;13:371–377
18. Liu W, Zhang L, Xu Z. Clinical observation on treatment of rheumatoid arthritis with biqi capsule. Zhongguo Zhong Xi Yi Jie He Za Zhi 2006;26:157–159.
19. Denisov LN, Andrianova IV, Timofeeva SS. Garlic effectiveness in rheumatoid arthritis. Tereapevticheskii Arkhiv 1999;71:55–58

SECTION FIVE

20. Shi Y, Zhang H, Du X, Zhang M, Yin Y, Zhou C, Song S, Fu X, Li S, Liu Y, Li H, Li X, Wu X, Zhu Y. A double blind observation for therapeutic effects of the tong luo kai bi tablets on rheumatoid arthritis. J Tradit Chin Med 1999;19:166–172

21. Biegert C, Wagner I, Lüdtke R, Kotter I, Lohmüller C, Gunaydin I, Taxis K, Heide L. Efficacy and safety of willow bark extract in the treatment of osteoarthritis and rheumatoid arthritis: results of 2 randomized double-blind controlled trials. J Rheumatol 2004;31:2121–2130

22. Jonas W, Linde L, Ramirez G. Homeopathy and rheumatic disease. Rheum Dis Clin North Am 2000;26:117–123

23. Fisher P, Scott DL. A randomized controlled trial of homeopathy in rheumatoid arthritis. Rheumatology (Oxford) 2001;40:1052–1055

24. Soeken KL. Selected CAM therapies for arthritis-related pain: the evidence from systematic reviews. Clin J Pain 2004;20:13–18

25. Weissenberg M. Cognitive aspects of pain and pain control. Int J Clin Exper Hypnosis 1998;46:44–61

26. Usichenko TI, Ivashkivsky OI, Gizhko VV. Treatment of rheumatoid arthritis with electromagnetic millimeter waves applied to acupuncture points – a randomized double blind clinical study. Acupunct Electrother Res 2003;28:11–18

27. Segal NA, Toda Y, Huston J, Saeki Y, Shimizu M, Fuchs H, Shimaoka Y, Holcomb R, McLean MJ. Two configurations of static magnetic fields for treating rheumatoid arthritis of the knee: a double-blind clinical trial. Arch Phys Med Rehabil 2001;82:1453–1460

28. Lundgren S, Stenstrom CH. Muscle relaxation training and quality of life in rheumatoid arthritis. A randomized controlled clinical trial. Scand J Rheumatol 1999;28:47–53

29. Carroll D, Seers K. Relaxation for the relief of chronic pain: a systematic review. J Adv Nurs 1998;27:476–487

30. Astin JA, Harkness E, Ernst E. The efficacy of 'distant healing': a systematic review of randomized trials. Ann Intern Med 2000;132:903–910

31. Allen M, Oberle K, Grace M, Russell A. Elk velvet antler in rheumatoid arthritis: phase II trial. Biol Res Nurs 2002;3:111–118

32. Fortin PR, Lew RA, Liang MH, Wright EA, Beckett LA, Chalmers TC, Sperling RI. Validation of a meta-analysis: the effects of fish oil in rheumatoid arthritis. J Clin Epidemiol 1995;48:1379–1390

33. Volker D, Fitzgerald P, Major G, Garg M. Efficacy of fish oil concentrate in the treatment of rheumatoid arthritis. J Rheumatol 2000;27:2343–2346

34. Berbert AA, Kondo CR, Almendra CL, Matsuo T, Dichi I. Supplementation of fish oil and olive oil in patients with rheumatoid arthritis. Nutrition 2005;21:131–136

35. Remans PH, Sont JK, Wagenaar LW, Wouters-Wesseling W, Zuijderduin WM, Jongma A, Breedveld FC, Van Laar JM. Nutrient supplementation with polyunsaturated fatty acids and micronutrients in rheumatoid arthritis: clinical and biochemical effects. Eur J Clin Nutr 2004;58:839–845

36. Nordstrom DCE, Honkanen VEA, Nasu Y, Antila E, Friman C, Konttinen YT. Alpha-linolenic acid in the treatment of rheumatoid arthritis: a double-blind, placebo-controlled and randomized study: flaxseed vs safflower seed. Rheumatol Int 1995;14:231–234

37. Gibson SLM, Gibson RG. The treatment of arthritis with a lipid extract of *Perna canaliculus*: a randomized trial. Complement Ther Med 1998;6:122–126

38. Hatakka K, Martio J, Korpela M, Herranen M, Poussa T, Laasanen T, Saxelin M, Vapaatalo H, Moilanen E, Korpela R. Effects of probiotic therapy on the activity and activation of mild rheumatoid arthritis – a pilot study. Scand J Rheumatol 2003;32: 211–215

39. Maleitzke R, Gottl KH. Treatment of rheumatoid arthritis with selenium. Therapiewoche 1996;46:1529–1532

40. Peretz A, Siderova V, Neve J. Selenium supplementation in rheumatoid arthritis investigated in a double blind, placebo-controlled trial. Scand J Rheumatol 2001;30:208–212

41. Han A, Judd MG, Robinson VA, Taixiang W, Tugwell P, Wells G. Tai chi for treating rheumatoid arthritis. The Cochrane Database of Systematic Reviews 2004, Issue 3. Art. No.: CD004849

42. Wang C, Collet JP, Lau J. The effect of Tai Chi on health outcomes in patients with chronic conditions: a systematic review. Arch Intern Med 2004;164:493–501

43. Brownfield A. Aromatherapy in arthritis: a study. Nurs Standard 1998;13:34–35

44. Evers AW. Cognitive-behavioral therapy in rheumatoid arthritis. Ned Tijdschr Fysioter 2005;115:143–146

45. Ernst E. Systematic reviews of biofeedback. Phys Med Rehab Kuror 2003;13:321–324

46. Field T, Hernandez-Reif M, Seligman S, Krasnegor J, Sunshine W, Rivas-Chacon R, Schanberg S, Kuhn C. Juvenile rheumatoid arthritis: benefits from massage therapy. J Paediatr Psychol 1997;22:607–617

47. Yang W, Ouyang J, Zhu K, Zhou S, Peng Z. TCM treatment for 40 cases of rheumatoid arthritis with channel blockage due to yin deficiency. J Tradit Chin Med 2003;23: 172–174

48. Nader TA, Smith DE, Dillbeck MC, Schanbacher V, Dillbeck SL, Gallois P, Beall-Rougerie S, Schneider RH, Nidich SI, Kaplan GP, Belok S. A double blind randomized controlled trial of Maharishi Vedic vibration technology in subjects with arthritis. Front Biosci 2001;6:H7–H17

49. Haslock I, Monro R, Nagarathna R, Nagendra HR, Raghuram NV. Measuring the effects of yoga in rheumatoid arthritis. Br J Rheumatol 1994;33:787–788

SHOULDER PAIN

SYNONYMS/SUBCATEGORIES

Rotator cuff disease, adhesive capulitis (frozen shoulder), myofascial pain, hemiparesis after stroke, arthritis and impingement syndrome are some of the underlying conditions causing shoulder pain.

DEFINITION

Pain in or around the shoulder, usually associated with restricted function. The symptoms can be caused by a multitude of pathologies.

CAM USAGE

No exact prevalence data are available specifically for shoulder pain. Chronic musculoskeletal problems (like shoulder pain) are the most common reason for consulting CAM practitioners.

CLINICAL EVIDENCE

Many CAM modalities are promoted for shoulder pain. Several reviews are available.[1–3]

ACUPUNCTURE

A Cochrane review of acupuncture for shoulder pain included nine RCTs (Box 5.57)[4] but all of this evidence failed to demonstrate that acupuncture is effective for this indication.

Box 5.57 *Systematic review: acupuncture for shoulder pain*[4]

- Nine RCTs met the inclusion criteria
- Methodology was highly variable
- All studies failed to include adequate descriptions of interventions
- For rotator cuff disease, acupuncture was not superior to placebo (two RCTs) in the short term
- Acupuncture was better than placebo at 4 weeks but at 4 months the effect was unlikely to be clinically relevant
- **Conclusion**: there is little evidence to support or refute the use of acupuncture for shoulder pain

ELECTRICAL STIMULATION

Various electrotherapeutic approaches are used (predominantly by physiotherapists). A Cochrane review included four RCTs and found no convincing evidence in favour of any form of electrical stimulation.[5]

EXERCISE

A systematic review found insufficient evidence for exercise as a treatment of shoulder pain.[6] One RCT ($n = 138$), however, demonstrated that physiotherapeutic exercise was equally effective in the short term to corticosteroid injections for shoulder pain of mechanical origin[7] and a further RCT ($n = 67$) found that construction workers with shoulder pain and impingement syndrome experience more benefit from exercise than patients not receiving exercise.[8]

MAGNETS

An RCT with 40 patients suffering from frozen shoulder pain suggested that treatment with a static magnet generated better pain relief than placebo.[9]

MASSAGE

An RCT with 102 patients suffering from shoulder pain following a stroke suggested that a series of slow-stroke back massages alleviated pain compared to no such therapy.[10] An RCT with 29 patients suffering from non-specific shoulder pain implied that six treatments of local soft-tissue massage improved pain and function more than no such treatment.[11]

SPINAL MANIPULATION

An RCT ($n = 150$) tested the relative value of spinal manipulation as an add-on therapy to normal care compared to normal care alone for patients with shoulder symptoms.[12] The results showed no immediate effects but suggested that manipulation accelerates recovery of shoulder symptoms in the long term. Similar results emerged from an RCT of a specific osteopathic 'Spencer' technique.[13] A further RCT failed to show that there are different long-term outcomes between treatment with corticosteroid injections, physiotherapy or manipulation.[14]

OTHER THERAPIES

One RCT suggested positive effects of internal qigong on shoulder/arm pain.[15]

OVERALL RECOMMENDATION

Shoulder pain has many causes and can be difficult to treat. The best evidence available to date is encouraging but not compelling for a number of approaches: exercise and spinal manipulation. On balance the treatment with the most favourable risk–benefit profile seems to be physiotherapeutic exercise.

Table 5.31 **Summary of clinical evidence for shoulder pain**

Treatment	Weight of evidence	Direction of evidence	Serious safety concerns
Acupuncture	OOO	→	Yes (see p. 96)
Electrical stimulation	OO	→	No (see p. 5)
Exercise	OO	↗	No (see p. 5)
Magnets	O	↗	No (see p. 164)
Massage	O	↗	No (see p. 137)
Spinal manipulation	OO	↗	Yes (see p. 112)

SECTION FIVE

REFERENCES

1. Speed C. Shoulder pain. In British Medical Journal. Clinical Evidence. British Medical Journal publishing group, 2006. Online. Available: http://www.clinicalevidence.com 6 Apr 2006
2. Johansson K, Oberg B, Adolfsson L, Foldevi M. A combination of systematic review and clinicians' beliefs in interventions for subacromial pain. Br J Gen Pract 2002;52:145–152
3. Green S, Buchbinder R, Glazier R, Forbes A. Interventions for shoulder pain. The Cochrane Database of Systematic Reviews 2000, Issue 2. Art. No.: CD001156
4. Green S, Buchbinder R, Hetrick S. Acupuncture for shoulder pain. The Cochrane Database of Systematic Reviews 2005, Issue 2. Art. No.: CD005319
5. Price CI, Pandyan AD. Electrical stimulation for preventing and treating post-stroke shoulder pain. The Cochrane Database of Systematic Reviews 2000, Issue 4. Art. No.: CD001698
6. Smidt N, de Vet HCW, Bouter LM, Dekker J, Arendzen JH, de Bie RA, Bierma Zeinstra SMA, Helders PJM, Keus SHJ, Kwakkel G, Lenssen T, Oostendorp RAB, Ostelo RWJG Reijman M, Terwee CB, Theunissen C, Thomas S, van Baar ME, van t Hul A, van Peppen RPS, Verhagen AP, van der Windt DAWM. Effectiveness of exercise therapy: a best-evidence summary of systematic reviews. Aust J Physiother 2005;51:71–85
7. Ginn K, Cohen M. Exercise therapy for shoulder pain aimed at restoring neuromuscular control: a randomized comparative clinical trial. J Rehabil Med 2005;37:115–122
8. Ludewig PM, Borstad JD. Effects of a home exercise programme on shoulder pain and functional status in construction workers. Occup Environ Med 2003;60:841–849
9. Kanai S, Taniguchi N, Kawamoto M, Endo H, Higashino H. Effect of static magnetic field on pain associated with frozen shoulder. Pain Clinic 2004;16:173–179
10. Mok E, Woo CP. The effects of slow-stroke back massage on anxiety and shoulder pain in elderly stroke patients. Complement Ther Nurs Midwifery 2004;10:209–216
11. van den Dolder PA, Roberts DL. A trial into the effectiveness of soft tissue massage in the treatment of shoulder pain. Aust J Physiother 2003;49:183–188
12. Bergman GJ, Winters JC, Groenier KH, Pool JJ, Meyboom-de Jong B, Postema K, van der Heijden GJ. Manipulative therapy in addition to usual medical care for patients with shoulder dysfunction and pain: a randomized, controlled trial. Ann Intern Med 2004;141:432–439
13. Knebl JA, Shores JH, Gamber RG, Gray WT, Herron KM. Improving functional ability in the elderly via the Spencer technique, an osteopathic manipulative treatment: a randomized, controlled trial. J Am Osteopath Assoc 2002;102:387–396
14. Winters JC, Jorritsma W, Groenier KH, Sobel JS, Meyboom-de Jong B, Arendzen HJ. Treatment of shoulder complaints in general practice: long term results of a randomised, single blind study comparing physiotherapy, manipulation, and corticosteroid injection. BMJ 1999;318:1395–1396
15. Youn HM, Kim MY, Kim YS, Lim JS. Effects of the doing gigong exercise on the shoulder-arm pain in women. J Korean Acu Moxibust Soc 2005;22:177–190

TENNIS ELBOW

SYNONYMS

Lateral elbow pain, lateral epicondylitis, rowing elbow, peritendinitis of the elbow.

DEFINITION

Tennis elbow is a condition characterised by pain and tenderness over the lateral epicondyle of the humerus and pain on resisted dorsiflexion of the wrist, middle finger, or both. The incidence of lateral elbow pain in general practice is 4–7 cases per 1000 people a year.[1,2] Tennis elbow is considered to be a repetitive strain injury, typically after minor and often unrecognised trauma of the extensor muscles of the forearm. Despite the title tennis elbow, tennis is a direct cause in only 5% of those with lateral epicondylitis.[3]

RELATED CONDITIONS

Other repetitive strain injuries.

CAM USAGE

Acupuncture is frequently used.

CLINICAL EVIDENCE

ACUPUNCTURE

A systematic review included four RCTs of which three compared acupuncture with placebo (Box 5.58).[4] It concluded that there appears to be some evidence to support the efficacy of acupuncture over a placebo for pain relief in short-term outcomes. This largely corroborates the conclusions of a Cochrane review[5] and another systematic review suggested strong evidence in favour of acupuncture in the short-term relief of lateral epicondyle pain.[6]

MANIPULATION

A systematic review reported three RCTs that assessed cervical or elbow manipulation and one that tested a wrist manipulation technique (Box 5.59).[4] It concluded that there appears to be some evidence of positive initial effects in favour of elbow manipulative therapy techniques. Two further RCTs report inferiority of chiropractic manipulation compared with ultrasound on pain-free function,[7] and greater improvement of pain measures with local manipulative treatment plus therapy aimed at the cervicothoracic spine compared with local treatment alone.[8] There was no difference between osteopathic treatment and chiropractic techniques for subjective pain sensation.[9]

MASSAGE

A Cochrane review assessed the efficacy of deep transverse friction massage for treating tendinitis pain.[10] It identified one RCT for tennis elbow, which showed no statistical difference

Box 5.58 *Systematic review: acupuncture for tennis elbow*[4]

- Four RCTs included
- Four studies used a blinded assessor and three also blinded the subjects
- One trial found that acupuncture resulted in relief of pain for a longer time than placebo (standardised mean difference 1.20, 95% CI 0.58 to 1.82) and was more likely to result in overall success (RR 3.17, 95% CI 1.54 to 6.52) after 10 treatments
- **Conclusion**: there appears to be some evidence to support the efficacy of acupuncture over a placebo as a treatment for tennis elbow in short-term outcomes

Box 5.59 *Systematic review: manipulation for tennis elbow*[4]

- Four RCTs included
- All four studies used a blinded assessor
- The pooled data from two studies showed a positive effect of manipulation on measures of pain-free grip strength (standardised mean difference 1.28, 95% CI 0.84 to 1.73) and pressure pain threshold (standardised mean difference 0.49, 95% CI 0.08 to 0.90)
- **Conclusion**: there appears to be some evidence of positive effects in favour of elbow manipulative therapy techniques

in pain relief, grip strength and function after nine consecutive sessions within 5 weeks compared with other physiotherapy.

OTHER THERAPIES

An RCT assessed the effects of an essential fatty acid supplement on pain. Compared with placebo there were no differences for pain visual analogue scale and maximal grip force.[11]

OVERALL RECOMMENDATION

There seems to be some indication that acupuncture and manipulative techniques are beneficial for short-term pain relief in tennis elbow. However, this is based on relatively few data. Given the limited options available in conventional medicine to treat this condition and a good safety profile of acupuncture and elbow manipulation these interventions seem worth a try in suitable cases.

Table 5.32 **Summary of clinical evidence for tennis elbow**

Treatment	Weight of evidence	Direction of evidence	Serious safety concerns
Acupuncture	OO	↗	Yes (see p. 96)
Manipulation	OO	↗	Yes (see p. 112)
Massage	O	→	Yes (see p. 137)

REFERENCES

1. Verhaar J. Tennis elbow: anatomical, epidemiological and therapeutic aspects. Int Orthop 1994;18:263–267
2. Hamilton P. The prevalence of humeral epicondylitis: a survey in general practice. J R Coll Gen Pract 1986;36:464–465
3. Murtagh J. Tennis elbow. Aust Fam Physician 1988;17:90–91,94–95
4. Bisset L, Paungmali A, Vicenzino B, Beller E. A systematic review and meta-analysis of clinical trials on physical interventions for lateral epicondylalgia. Br J Sports Med 2005;39:411–422
5. Green S, Buchbinder R, Barnsley L, Hall S, White M, Smidt N, Assendelft W. Acupuncture for lateral elbow pain. The Cochrane Database of Systematic Reviews 2002, Issue 1. Art. No.: CD003527
6. Trinh KV, Phillips SD, Ho E, Damsma K. Acupuncture for the alleviation of lateral epicondyle pain: a systematic review. Rheumatology 2004;43:1085–1090
7. Langen-Pieters P, Weston P, Brantingham JW. A randomized prospective pilot study comparing chiropractic care and ultrasound for the treatment of lateral epicondylitis. Eur J Chiropractic 2003;50:211–218
8. Cleland JA, Flynn TW, Palmer JA. Incorporation of manual therapy directed at the cervicothoracic spine in patients with lateral epicondylalgia: a pilot clinical trial. J Manual Manipul Ther 2005;13:143–151
9. Geldschlager S. Osteopathic versus orthopedic treatments for chronic epicondylopathia humeri radialis: a randomized controlled trial. Forsch Komplementarmed Klass Naturheilkd 2004;11:93–97
10. Brosseau L, Casimiro L, Milne S, Robinson V, Shea B, Tugwell P, Wells G. Deep transverse friction massage for treating tendinitis. The Cochrane Database of Systematic Reviews 2002, Issue 4. Art. No.: CD003528
11. Roe C, Odegaard TT, Hilde F, Maehlum S, Halvorsen T. No effect of supplement of essential fatty acids on lateral epicondylitis. Tidsskr Nor Laegeforen 2005;125:2615–2618

SECTION FIVE

Table 5.33 **Examples of other occasionally used treatments for specific conditions which lack sound evidence of effectiveness**

Abdominal pain
Abuta (*Cissampelos pareira*)
African wild potato (*Hypoxis hemerocallidea*)
Agrimony (*Agrimonia eupatoria, A. procera*)
Alfalfa (*Medicago sativa*)
Aloe (*Aloe vera*)
Alpinia (*Alpinia galanga*)
American pennyroyal (*Hedeana pulegioides*)
Applied kinesiology
Astragalus (*Astragalus membranaceus*)
Bacopa (*Bacopa monnieri*)
Barley (*Hordeum vulgare*), germinated barley foodstuff (GBF)
Belladonna (*Atropa belladonna*)
Bilberry (*Vaccinium myrtillus*)
Bitter melon (*Momordica charantia*)
Bitter orange (*Citrus aurantium*)
Black tea (*Camellia sinensis*)
Buchu (*Agathosma betulina*)
Calendula (*Calendula officinalis*)
Cascara sagrada (*Rhamnus purshiana*)
Cat's claw (*Uncaria tomentosa, U. guianensis*)
Chamomile (*Matricaria recutita, Chamaemelum nobile*)
Chicory (*Cichorium intybus*)
Clay
Clove (*Eugenia aromatica*) and clove oil (Eugenol)
Colon therapy/colonic irrigation
Cranberry (*Vaccinium macrocarpon*)
Dandelion (*Taraxacum officinale*)
Datura wrightii (California jimson weed)
Detoxification therapy (cleansing)
Devil's claw (*Harpagophytum procumbens*)
Dong quai (*Angelica sinensis*)
Echinacea (*Echinacea angustifolia, E. pallida, E. purpurea*)
Elder (*Sambucas nigra*)
Euphorbia spp.
Evening primrose oil (*Oenothera biennis*)
Eyebright (*Euphrasia officinalis*)
Feverfew (*Tanacetum parthenium*)
Flaxseed and flaxseed oil (*Linum usitatissimum*)
Fo-ti (*Polygonum multiflorum*)
Garcinia (*Garcinia cambogia*)
Garlic (*Allium sativum*)
Ginger (*Zingiber officinale*)
Ginseng
Globe artichoke (*Cynara scolymus*)
Green tea (*Camellia sinensis*)
Guided imagery
Gymnema (*Gymnema sylvestre*)
Hawthorn (*Crataegus laevigata, C. oxyacantha, C. monogyna, C. pentagyna*)
Holy basil (*Ocimum sanctum*)
Hops (*Humulus lupulus*)

table continues

Horsetail (*Equisetum arvense*)
Hydrotherapy
Juniper (*Juniperus communis*)
Kava (*Piper methysticum*)
Khella (*Ammi visnaga*)
Labrador tea (*Ledum groenlandicum*)
Relaxation therapy
Slippery elm (*Ulmus rubra, U. fulva*)
White horehound (*Marrubium vulgare*)
Yoga

Angina
Bilberry (*Vaccinium myrtillus*)
California jimson weed (*Datura wrightii*)
Coleus (*Coleus forskohlii*)
Detoxification therapy (cleansing)
Dong quai (*Angelica sinensis*)
Flaxseed and flaxseed oil (*Linum usitatissimum*)
Fo-ti (*Polygonum multiflorum*)
Germanium
Ginkgo (*Ginkgo biloba*)
Guided imagery
Hawthorn (*Crataegus laevigata, C. oxyacantha, C. monogyna, C. pentagyna*)
Khella (*Ammi visnaga*)
Kudzu (*Pueraria lobata*)
Ozone therapy
Prayer, distant healing
Tai chi
Yoga

Back pain
Alkanna (*Boraginaceae*)
Applied kinesiology
Arnica (*Arnica montana*)
Aromatherapy
Bacopa (*Bacopa monnieri*)
Belladonna (*Atropa belladonna*)
Black cohosh (*Actaea racemosa*)
Burdock (*Arctium lappa*)
Chamomile (*Matricaria recutita, Chamaemelum nobile*)
Chaparral (*Larea tridentata*)
Colon therapy/colonic irrigation
Detoxification therapy (cleansing)
Dong quai (*Angelica sinensis*)
Eucalyptus oil (*Eucalyptus* spp.)
Fo-ti (*Polygonum multiflorum*)
Goldenseal (*Hydrastis canadensis*)
Healing touch
Hellerwork
Holy basil (*Ocimum sanctum*)
Magnet therapy
Reflexology
Rehmannia (*Rehmannia glutinosa*)
Spiritual healing

SECTION FIVE

table continues

Stinging nettle (*Urtica dioica*)
Tai chi
Tamanu (*Calophyllum inophyllum*)

Burns
Acupuncture
Aloe (*Aloe vera*)
Aromatherapy
Astragalus (*Astragalus membranaceus*)
Burdock (*Arctium lappa*)
Calendula (*Calendula officinalis*)
California jimson weed (*Datura wrightii*)
Chamomile (*Matricaria recutita, Chamaemelum nobile*)
Chaparral
Danshen (*Salvia miltiorrhiza*)
Devil's club (*Oplopanax horridus*)
Echinacea (*E. angustifolia, E. pallida, E. purpurea*)
Elder (*Sambucas nigra*)
Eucalyptus oil (*Eucalyptus* spp.)
Fenugreek (*Trigonella foenum-graecum*)
Flaxseed and flaxseed oil (*Linum usitatissimum*)
Germanium
Ginger (*Zingiber officinale*)
Ginseng (*Panax ginseng*)
Gotu kola (*Centella asiatica*)
Hydrotherapy
Labrador tea (*Ledum groenlandicum*)
Marshmallow (*Althaea officinalis*)
Ozone therapy
Pantothenic acid (vitamin B5)
Passion flower (*Passiflora incarnata*)
Phosphates, phosphorus
Prayer, distant healing
Red clover (*Trifolium pratense*)
Reiki
Slippery elm (*Ulmus rubra, U. fulva*)
St. John's wort (*Hypericum perforatum*)
Stinging nettle (*Urtica dioica*)
Tamanu (*Calophyllum inophyllum*)
Tea tree oil (*Melaleuca alternifolia*)
Thyme (*Thymus vulgaris*)
Wheatgrass (*Triticum aestivum*)
White oak (*Quercus alba*)

Carpal tunnel syndrome
Alexander technique
Chamomile (*Matricaria recutita, Chamaemelum nobile*)
Healing touch
Hellerwork
Lavender (*Lavandula angustifolia*)
Reiki

Depression
Acerola (*Malpighia glabra, M. punicifolia*)
Aconite (*Aconitum napellus*)

table continues

Alexander technique
Art therapy
Ashwagandha (*Withania somnifera*)
Black cohosh (*Actaea racemosa*)
Cat's claw (*Uncaria tomentosa, U. guianensis*)
Detoxification therapy (cleansing)
Ephedra (*Ephedra sinica*)/Ma-huang
Evening primrose oil (*Oenothera biennis*)
Flaxseed and flaxseed oil (*Linum usitatissimum*)
Ginger (*Zingiber officinale*)
Ginseng (*Panax* spp.)
Gotu kola (*Centella asiatica*)
Healing touch
Hops (*Humulus lupulus*)
Hydrotherapy
Lavender (*Lavandula angustifolia*)
Liquorice (*Glycyrrhiza glabra*) and deglycyrrhizinated liquorice
Pet therapy
Prayer, distant healing
Qigong
Reflexology
Tai chi
Tribulus (*Tribulus terrestris*)
Valerian (*Valeriana officinalis*)

Dysmenorrhoea
Bee pollen
Bilberry (*Vaccinium myrtillus*)
Chamomile (*Matricaria recutita, Chamaemelum nobile*)
Chaparral (*Larrea tridentata*)
Devil's claw (*Harpagophytum procumbens*)
Dong quai (*Angelica sinensis*)
Fennel (*Foeniculum vulgare*)
Garlic (*Allium sativum*)
Ginger (*Zingiber officinale*)
Ginkgo (*Ginkgo biloba*)
Horse chestnut (*Aesculus hippocastanum*)
Horsetail (*Equisetum arvense*)
Hypnotherapy
Pycnogenol (*Pinus pinaster* ssp. *atlantica*)

Fibromyalgia
Alexander technique
Arnica (*Arnica montana*)
Cat's claw (*Uncaria tomentosa, U. guianensis*)
Devil's claw (*Harpagophytum procumbens*)
Ginseng (*Panax* spp.)
Hydrotherapy
Polarity
Qigong
Quercetin
Reflexology
Reiki
Spirulina
Tai chi

table continues

SECTION FIVE

Therapeutic touch
Yoga

Headache and migraine
Alexander technique
American pennyroyal (*Hedeoma pulegioides*), European pennyroyal (*Mentha pulegium*)
Applied kinesiology
Aromatherapy
Belladonna (*Atropa belladonna*)
Bitter orange (*Citrus aurantium*)
Black cohosh (*Actaea* syn. *Cimicifuga racemosa*)
Black tea (*Camellia sinensis*)
Burdock (*Arctium lappa*)
Calendula (*Calendula officinalis*), marigold
Chicory (*Cichorium intybus*)
Colon therapy/colonic irrigation
Dandelion (*Taraxacum officinale*)
Detoxification therapy (cleansing)
Devil's claw (*Harpagophytum procumbens*)
Dong quai (*Angelica sinensis*)
Echinacea (*E. angustifolia, E. pallida, E. purpurea*)
Elder (*Sambucas nigra*)
Eucalyptus oil (*Eucalyptus* spp.)
Garlic (*Allium sativum*)
Ginger (*Zingiber officinale*)
Ginkgo (*Ginkgo biloba*)
Ginseng (*Panax* spp.)
Green tea (*Camellia sinensis*)
Hellerwork
Holy basil (*Ocimum sanctum*)
Hydrotherapy
Kava (*Piper methysticum*)
Kudzu (*Pueraria lobata*)
Labrador tea (*Ledum groenlandicum*)
Lavender (*Lavandula angustifolia*)
Music therapy
Oregano (*Origanum vulgare*)
Qigong
Reiki
Rooibos (*Aspalathus linearis*)
Saw palmetto (*Serenoa repens*)
Spiritual healing
Tai chi
Tansy (*Tanacetum vulgare*)
Tribulus (*Tribulus terrestris*)
Valerian (*Valeriana officinalis*)

Neck pain
Alexander technique
Detoxification therapy (cleansing)
Hellerwork
Kudzu (*Pueraria lobata*)
Reflexology
Yoga

table continues

Neuralgia
Bitter orange (*Citrus aurantium*)
Black tea (*Camellia sinensis*)
Calendula (*Calendula officinalis*), marigold
Chamomile (*Matricaria recutita, Chamaemelum nobile*)
Devil's claw (*Harpagophytum procumbens*)
Ginseng (*Panax* spp.)
Guggul (*Commiphora mukul*)
Horse chestnut (*Aesculus hippocastanum*)
Hydrotherapy
Mastic (*Pistacia lentiscus*)
Peppermint (*Mentha* × *piperita*)

Osteoarthritis
Alexander technique
Ashwagandha (*Withania somnifera*)
Beta-carotene
Black tea (*Camellia sinensis*)
Boron
Boswellia (*Boswellia serrata*)
Cat's claw (*Uncaria tomentosa, U. guianensis*)
Chelation therapy
Chiropractic
Dandelion (*Taraxacum officinale*)
Guggul (*Commiphora mukul*)
Guided imagery
Hellerwork
Horse chestnut (*Aesculus hippocastanum*)
Kava (*Piper methysticum*)
Liquorice (*Glycyrrhiza glabra*) and deglycyrrhizinated liquorice
Massage
Relaxation therapy
Tai chi
Turmeric (*Curcuma longa*)

Rheumatoid arthritis
Abuta (*Cissampelos pareira*)
Alexander technique
Alfalfa (*Medicago sativa*)
Aloe (*Aloe vera*)
Alpinia (*Alpinia galanga*)
Arnica (*Arnica montana*)
Aromatherapy
Bacopa (*Bacopa monnieri*)
Bee pollen
Belladonna (*Atropa belladonna*)
Bilberry (*Vaccinium myrtillus*)
Bitter orange (*Citrus aurantium*)
Black cohosh (*Actaea* syn. *Cimicifuga racemosa*)
Boswellia (*Boswellia serrata*)
Buchu (*Agathosma betulina*)
Burdock (*Arctium lappa*)
Chamomile (*Matricaria recutita, Chamaemelum nobile*)
Chiropractic

table continues

Colon therapy/colonic irrigation
Couch grass (*Agropyron repens, Elymus repens*)
Cranberry (*Vaccinium macrocarpon*)
Dandelion (*Taraxacum officinale*)
Dong quai (*Angelica sinensis*)
Echinacea (*E. angustifolia, E. pallida, E. purpurea*)
Essiac
Eucalyptus oil (*Eucalyptus* spp.)
Feverfew (*Tanacetum parthenium*)
Garlic (*Allium sativum*)
Ginger (*Zingiber officinale*)
Guggul (*Commiphora mukul*)
Guided imagery
Horse chestnut (*Aesculus hippocastanum*)
Hydrotherapy
Juniper (*Juniperus communis*)
Kava (*Piper methysticum*)
Mistletoe (*Viscum album*)
Prayer, distant healing
Propolis
Relaxation therapy

Useful resources for pain manage-ment

USEFUL RESOURCES FOR PAIN MANAGEMENT

PAIN RESOURCES
PAIN RESOURCE WEBSITES

www.pain.com/ – Extensive information about pain and its treatment for professionals and patients

www.chronicpainsupport.org/ – Dedicated to supporting chronic pain patients

www.virtualpaincentre.com/ – Comprehensive information regarding pain

INTERNATIONAL PAIN SOCIETIES

International Association for the Study of Pain: www.iasp-pain.org/

NATIONAL PAIN SOCIETIES

American Pain Society: www.ampainsoc.org/

Australian Pain Society: www.apsoc.org.au/

British Pain Society: www.britishpainsociety.org/

Canadian Pain Society: www.medicine.dal.ca/cps/

UK PAIN SOCIETIES

Pain Research Institute: www.liv.ac.uk/pri/

Action on Pain: www.action-on-pain.co.uk

Pain Concern: www.painconcern.org.uk/

Pain Association of Scotland: www.painassociation.com/

The Pain Relief Foundation: www.painrelieffoundation.org.uk/

Patients' Association: www.patients-association.com

CONDITION-SPECIFIC UK SOCIETIES

National Association for Healthy Backs (UK): www.backpain.org

Vulval Pain Society (UK): www.vulvalpainsociety.org/

National Osteoporosis Society: www.nos.org.uk

MS Society of GB & NI: www.mssociety.org.uk

The National MS Society: www.nationalmssociety.org.uk

Migraine Trust: www.migrainetrust.org

Fibromyalgia Association UK: www.fibromyalgia-associationuk.org

The National Endometriosis Society: www.endo.org.uk

Arthritis & Musculoskeletal Alliance (ARMA): www.arma.uk.net

CancerBACUP: www.cancerbacup.org.uk

US PAIN SOCIETIES

The American Academy of Pain Medicine: www.painmed.org/

American Pain Society: www.ampainsoc.org/

American Pain Foundation: www.painfoundation.org/

Society for Pain Practice Management: www.sppm.org/

CONDITION-SPECIFIC US SOCIETIES

National Multiple Sclerosis Society: www.nmss.org/

National Migraine Association: www.migraines.org/

The National Fibromyalgia Association: www.fmaware.org/

National Vulvodynia Association: www.nva.org/

Arthritis Foundation: www.arthritis.org/

SECTION SIX

CAM RESOURCES

www.naturalstandard.com/ – Founded by clinicians and researchers to provide high quality, evidence-based information about CAM. This international multidisciplinary collaboration now includes contributors from more than 100 eminent academic institutions. A subscription is required.

http://nccam.nih.gov/about/aboutnccam/ – Dedicated to exploring CAM healing practices in the context of rigorous science, training researchers, and disseminating authoritative information to the public and professionals.

www.iscmr.org/index.html – The International Society for Complementary Medicine Research is an international scientific organisation of researchers, practitioners and policy makers that fosters complementary and integrative medicine research and provides a platform for knowledge and information exchange to enhance international communication and collaboration.

www.integrativeonc.org – Society of Integrated Oncology is a non-profit, multi-disciplinary organisation of professionals dedicated to studying and facilitating the cancer treatment and recovery process through the use of integrated complementary therapies. Their mission is to educate oncology professionals, patients, caregivers and relevant others about state-of-the-art integrative therapies, including their scientific validity, clinical benefits, toxicities, and limitations.

www.bcma.co.uk – The British Complementary Medicine Association supports and protects the integrity of its therapists and ensures the protection and well-being of their clients and the high-quality standards with which complementary medicine is delivered to the public.

www.quackwatch.org – A non-profit corporation whose purpose is to combat health-related frauds, myths, fads and fallacies. Its primary focus is on quackery-related information that is difficult or impossible to get elsewhere.

www.amfoundation.org/info.htm – The Alternative Medicine Foundation is a non-profit organisation, providing responsible and reliable information about alternative medicine to the public and health professionals.

www.fih.org.uk/ – The Prince's Foundation for Integrated Health aims to facilitate the development of safe, effective and efficient forms of health care to patients and their families by supporting the development and delivery of integrated health care.

POSTSCRIPT

Our main aim for this book was to summarise the evidence base for or against CAM in treating pain in an accessible fashion. As it turns out, this rigorous evidence-based approach generated highly variable results. Evaluating the 'weight' and the direction separately, we identified 21 pain syndromes or pain-related conditions for which the evidence for CAM is compelling, i.e. maximum weight and clearly positive direction of results (Table 6.1). For only one condition/treatment pair is the evidence compellingly negative (chelation therapy as a treatment of peripheral arterial occlusive disease).

In total, the evidence is at least encouraging ('positive' or 'tentatively positive' direction, any weight) for the majority ($n = 182$) of condition/treatment pairs. This indicates that CAM has a lot to offer for patients in pain.

We are sure that during the coming years we will be able to fill the many gaps in our current knowledge. As this happens we hope to be able to update this book. We are convinced that the evidence-based approach to CAM is the best way ahead for maximising patient benefits and minimising the risks.

Table 6.1 **Pain syndromes with compelling evidence for CAM**

Therapy	Condition
Acupuncture	Dental pain
Acupuncture	Myofascial pain
Acupuncture	Osteoarthritis (knee)
Biofeedback	Migraine
Diet	Rheumatoid arthritis
Distraction therapy	Procedure-related pain
Exercise	Fibromyalgia
Exercise	Depression
Ginkgo	Peripheral arterial occlusive disease
Hypnotherapy	Abdominal pain
Hypnotherapy	Labour pain
Hypnotherapy	Peri-operative pain
Hypnotherapy	Procedure-related pain
Padma 28	Peripheral arterial occlusive disease
Phytodolor	Osteoarthritis
Relaxation	Angina pectoris
Relaxation	Migraine
Relaxation	Depression
S-adenosylmethionine	Osteoarthritis
TENS	Peri-operative pain
Water immersion	Labour pain

TENS, transcutaneous electrical nerve stimulation.

Index